CONTEMPORARY GYNECOLOGIC PRACTICE

Edited by **Atef Darwish**

Contemporary Gynecologic Practice
http://dx.doi.org/10.5772/58510
Edited by Atef Darwish

Contributors

Wildemeersch, Fahimeh Ramezani Tehrani, Alan Sacerdote, Gul Bahtiyar, Ismail AbdulRahman Al-Badawi, Ahmed Abu-Zaid, Gautier Chene, Soundravally Rajendiran, Pooja Dhiman, Nyengidiki Tamunomie, Abam Dagogo, Julio Elito Jr., Eduardo Santana, Gustavo Nardini Cecchino, Atef M.M. Darwish

Published by InTech

Janeza Trdine 9, 51000 Rijeka, Croatia

Publishing Process Manager Danijela Duric
Technical Editor InTech DTP team
Cover InTech Design team

First published January, 2015
Printed in Croatia

Additional hard copies can be obtained from orders@intechopen.com

Contemporary Gynecologic Practice, Edited by Atef Darwish
p. cm.
ISBN 978-953-51-1736-0

For EU product safety concerns:
IN TECH d.o.o., Prolaz Marije Krucifikse Kozulić 3, 51000 Rijeka, Croatia,
info@intechopen.com or visit our website at intechopen.com.

Meet the editor

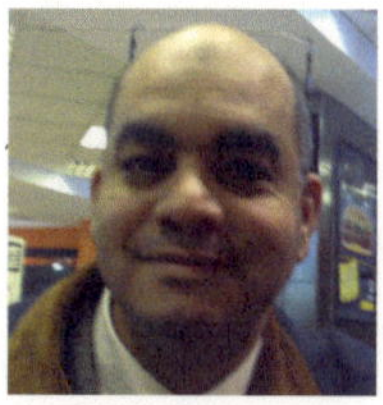

Dr Atef Darwish is a Professor of Obstetrics and Gynecology, Faculty of Medicine, Assiut University, Egypt since July 2005. Moreover, he is a consultant of Obstetrics and Gynecology in three hospitals and he is the moderator and lecturer of many endoscopic societies. He spent two years training in the endoscopic unit of Ulm university (Germany). He joined many centers in the US and Europe concentrating on the reproductive medicine He authored an internationally registered undergraduate book (Practical Obstetrics and Gynecology) and edited three InTech multi-author books. He presented more than 80 presentations in national and international meetings, delivered a lot of lectures in Egypt, some Arabian countries and the USA (Buffalo and Pennsylvania) and published more than 56 papers in international medical journals, and 7 papers in national journals. He received some congress prizes and awards due to his work in the field of reproductive medicine since 1995. He is a reviewer of many international journals and an associate editor of four of them. His special interest has been in the area of gynecologic laparoscopy, hysteroscopy, colposcopy, reproductive medicine, and assisted reproduction. He published some innovative procedures in the field of hysteroscopic, laparoscopic and minimal access surgeries in addition to drug therapy of hyperprolactinemia.
In 2009, he got a PhD degree in the reproductive medicine at the University of Utrichet, The Netherlands.

Contents

Preface IX

Section 1 Infertility 1

Chapter 1 **Endoscopic Explanation of Unexplained Infertility 3**
Atef M. Darwish

Section 2 Gynecologic Emergencies 31

Chapter 2 **Overview of Gynaecological Emergencies 33**
Dagogo Semenitari Abam

Chapter 3 **Biomarkers of Ectopic Pregnancy-Present and Future 51**
Soundravally Rajendiren and Pooja Dhiman

Section 3 Endocrinal Problems 77

Chapter 4 **Polycystic Ovary Syndrome 79**
Fahimeh Ramezani Tehrani and Samira Behboudi-Gandevani

Chapter 5 **Treatment of Congenital Adrenal Hyperplasia by Reducing Insulin Resistance and Cysticercosis Induced Polycystic Ovarian Syndrome 103**
Alan Sacerdote and Gül Bahtiyar

Section 4 Gynecologic Oncology 125

Chapter 6 **Screening Methods for Gynaecological Cancers 127**
T.K. Nyengidiki

Chapter 7 **From the Ovary to the Fallopian Tube: A History of Ovarian Carcinogenesis 143**
G. Chene, G. Lamblin, K. Le Bail-Carval, P. Chabert, J.D. Tigaud and G. Mellier

Chapter 8 **Past, Present and Future Perspectives on the Management of Endometrial Cancer— A Comprehensive Review 157**
Ahmed Abu-Zaid and Ismail A. Al-Badawi

Chapter 9 **Endometrial Cancer Prevention with Levonorgestrel-Releasing Intrauterine System 183**
Dirk Wildemeersch, Maciej Jóźwik and Marcin Jóźwik

Section 5 Twins Pregnancy 201

Chapter 10 **Monochorionic Twin Pregnancy— Potential Risks and Perinatal Outcomes 203**
Julio Elito Júnior, Eduardo Félix Martins Santana and Gustavo Nardini Cecchino

Preface

Gynecology is a dynamic medical specialty. Thanks to the implication of assisted reproduction and minimally access therapy, all gynecologic subspecialties showed marvelous development in recent years. The field of infertility is expanding due to the implication of sophisticated diagnostic aids. In modern practice, it seems illogic that we consider a case as unexplained infertility without endoscopic evaluation. In this book, you will read many fertility-related gynecologic abnormalities detected by laparoscopy or hysteroscopy.

Gynecologists are accused to be calmer and less energetic than obstetricians. In this book, your will find many gynecologic situations that necessities emergency diagnostic work up and crash intervention in the same way like crash cesarean section. Detection of early markers for diagnosis of ectopic pregnancy as well as step-by- step approach for all gynecologic emergencies are present in two chapters of this book.

Some gynecologic endocrinal problems continue to be a real challenge for gynecologists. The most famous syndrome is polycystic ovarian syndrome commonly encountered among infertile women and those with abnormal menstrual patterns. Congenital adrenal hyperplasia is an important issue in this context. Both abnormalities are discussed in two separate chapters in this book.

Prevention, screening as well as early management of gynecologic malignancies should be in the core of any gynecologist's job. Gynecologic examination is the best chance for detection of any pre-malignant lesion of the genital tract. The gynecologist has no excuse to miss any of them or to underestimate female genital tract screening for malignant or pre-malignant lesion. Four chapters of this book will tackle this topic in details.

Thanks to liberal use of drugs for induction of superovulation and the wide spread of IVF/ICSI, gynecologists commonly encounter a lot of cases of multiple pregnancy that require prompt early management starting from prevention, fetal reduction and subsequent antenatal management. More details are demonstrated on the last chapter on monchorionic twin pregnancy.

In short, I am sure that you will enjoy refreshing your knowledge and adding some new information on many gynecologic subspecialties if you go through this book.

Dr. Atef Darwish
Department of Obstetrics and Gynecology,
Woman's Health University Hospital
Assiut, Egypt

Section 1

Infertility

Chapter 1

Endoscopic Explanation of Unexplained Infertility

Atef M. Darwish

Additional information is available at the end of the chapter

http://dx.doi.org/10.5772/59948

1. Introduction

1.1. Dilemma of definition of Unexplained Infertility (UI)

Infertility is a continuous challenge for all gynecologists worldwide. Unexplained infertility (UI) is infertility in which the cause of the fertility impairment cannot be detected by use of standard diagnostic measures like semen analysis, tests for ovulation and tubal patency. It remains a clinical and scientific challenge [1]. Unexplained infertility is a source of anxiety for couples desiring pregnancy. It can be diagnosed after a complete evaluation [2]. The Practice Committee of the American Society for Reproductive Medicine (ASRM) has published guidelines for a standard infertility evaluation [3]. UI does not mean there is no physical explanation for the infertility, but that is just, medical tests have not identified any specific problems [4, 5]. A quarter of infertility range (25%) cannot be explained because of current tests are not perfect in finding all problems., the problem preventing pregnancy is not covered by the usual range of tests for assessing infertility, or causes which are not yet understood by scientists [4]. In the past decades, tremendous advancement in the field of infertility has been made. The development of better methods of diagnosis due to better understanding of physiology of ovulation, advent of ultrasound, endoscopy and other modern equipments have changed the whole approach to this problem. [6]. Possible Etiologies for UI may include hostile cervical mucus [7], subtle ovulatory dysfunction [8], luteal-Phase Defect [9], impaired fertilizing ability of oocytes specially when associated with raised LH levels, hyperprolactinemia [10], sperm dysfunction and antisperm Antibodies (151endometrial Steroid receptor defects [12], some genetic [13], psychological [14] or immunological Causes [15]. Prospective studies appear to have clearly demonstrated the substantial importance of even minimal endometriosis, which has been shown to be associated with impaired fertilization ability of oocyte and presumably impaired follicular function. Changes in the intraperitoneal environment leading to an inflammatory process in the absence of visible abnormalities have been suggested as being causal in some cases of unexplained infertility [11]. Scientific curiosity must take second place to a more pragmatic approach, which takes into account the clinical and financial costs of making a more accurate diagnosis [5]. Laparoscopy is generally accepted as a good standard for diagnosing tubal pathology or other pelvic reproductive diseases, such as adhesions and endometriosis. Once identified, appropriate surgical treatment can be given, enhancing the chance of spontaneous conception. Furthermore, in cases with poor prognosis, laparoscopy could accelerate the commencement of (IVF), bypassing unnecessary cycles of ovulatory stimulation with or without intrauterine insemination [16].

1.2. Is it logic to omit laparoscopy and hysteroscopy from the definition of UI?

There is a general consensus among gynecologists that tubal patency at HSG is quite assuring about tubal factor and they proceed to investigate other factors or advise patients to try assisted reproduction. On reviewing literature, Kahyaogla [17] found that laparoscopy can be omitted if there is no risk factor for pelvic pathology while it is recommended if suspected endometriosis or tubal pathology. Likewise, Bonneau et al. [16] examined 114 cases with UI by laparoscopy and detected abnormalities in 83.4% (n=95) of patients. More and more studies in addition to our day practice experience prefer to include laparoscopy and hysteroscopy in the evaluation of cases with UI. We believe that diagnostic laparoscopy is an integral step of the diagnostic work-up of any infertile couple before saying the term "unexplained". Laparoscopy can demonstrate previously undetected stage I or II endometriosis or periovarian or peritubal adhesions in a substantial proportion of women. Detection of these abnormalities may result in alternative treatment plans, such as surgery for endometriosis or direct referral to an IVF program if there are peritubal adhesions. The following factors would affect implication of laparoscopy as a routine test in all cases of UI including the availability of resources, the risk associated with laparoscopy, the knowledge that laparoscopy demonstrates abnormalities not otherwise detected by other infertility tests, and laparoscopic treatment of minimal and mild endometriosis enhances fecundity.

1.3. When to perform endoscopy?

Timing of performing combined laparoscopy and hysteroscopy for cases of UI is a controversial issue as well. In one study, they recommended that transvaginal hydrolaparoscopy and minihysteroscopy can be performed after a waiting period of 6-12 months in older women and particularly in women experienced infertility awareness methods [18]. In our practice, timing is a matter of individualization. If you have a patient with a persistent TVS abnormality that requires Endoscopic assessment, it is a waste of time to defer the decision. This decision is of high importance particularly if all other possible causes were excluded.

1.4. Current role of gynecologic endoscopy in UI

Including laparoscopy and hysteroscopy as a basic investigation for cases of UI would be expected to detect the following:

- Missed fallopian tubal causes.

- Hidden intrauterine infections.
- Missed ovarian causes.
- Missed intrauterine causes.
- Exploration of the fertilization site.
- Exploration of the implantation site.

2. Missed Fallopian tube abnormalities

Tubal factor infertility accounts for nearly one-quarter of all cases of infertility [19]. The fallopian tubes may be abnormal in structure or function. Structural disorders can block the fallopian tubes. They include tubal scarring or blockage most commonly from pelvic infections, prior abdominal surgeries and endometriosis. Practically, many gynecologists are reluctant when reporting on diagnostic laparoscopy. Some perform a single puncture intraumbilical procedure that neglects an auxillary portal for proper grasping of the adnexa and thorough evaluation of the ovarian fossa. Most of them comment on tubal patency only and neglect tubal morphology, size, length and proximity to the pouch of Douglas. Rarely, they comment on the mesosalpnix and Wolffian duct remnants.

2.1. What is the normal fallopian tube? It is a complex organ that should be

- Open with intact endosalpinx.: a patent tube per se is not a grantee that the tube is OK.
- Adequate length to reach the pelvic floor.
- Mobile to reach the site of released egg and to create a negative pressure in itself.
- Fimbria should be normal and freely mobile to direct the egg towards the tubal ostium.

3. Role of Hydatid of Morgagni in UI

The recommendations of all societies define UI after a free tubal patency test. They didn't define which test. One of the great advantages of diagnostic laparoscopy is proper visualization of the genital organs and the pelvis. Some Wollfian duct vestigial remnants could be easily seen by laparoscopy like Hydatif of Morgagni and paratubal cysts and of course are not visible by HSG.

Hydatid of Morgagni is commonly underestimated finding even by expert laparoscopists. Tubal heaviness, possible fimbrial occlusion and restricted tubal mobility hindering ovum pick-up from the pouch of Douglas are possible mechanisms of infertility. Whether they are definite cause of infertility or not was studied in a randomized study [20]. They recruited a total 455 patients. The 240 of them were pregnant to whom planned cesarean section (C/S) and the other 215 were infertile one who have undergone diagnostic laparoscopy. Fertile Group (Group 1) consisted of women whom have become spontaneously pregnant without any kind of infertility management. These are planned to undergo C/S with different indications. Infertile group (Group 2) consisted of women diagnosed as unexplained infertility and planned to undergo diagnostic laparoscopy according to ASRM 2006 guidelines. The frequency, number, and the bilaterality of the MH were evaluated during the C/S in fertile group and diagnostic laparoscopy in infertile group. SPSS was used for statistical analyses. The Morgagni hydatids (MH) frequency was higher in Group 2 than Group 1 ($P < 0.05$). The bilaterality of MHs was significantly higher in Group 2 than Group 1 ($P < 0.05$). The number of the MHs was significantly higher in Group 2 than Group 1 ($P < 0.05$). They concluded that these findings suggest a possible effect of MH on fertility. The theory of MH disturbing tubal motility with respect to the pick-up and transport of ovum appears logical in this aspect.

Another non-randomized study [21] was conducted on two hundred and thirteen patients with unexplained infertility and hydatid of Morgagni diagnosed at laparoscopy were included. The laterality (bilateral vs unilateral), location (fimbrial vs juxta-fimbrial), number (single vs multiple) and diameter of the hydatids of Morgagni were recorded. Patients were allocated to a study group (n=127) who underwent laparoscopic excision of hydatid of Morgagni and a control group (n=86) who underwent no intervention. Patients were followed for six months without any infertility or hormonal treatment to detect spontaneous pregnancy. Patients missed during the follow-up or who received infertility treatment was excluded. Statistical analysis was done using Chi-square test and Student's t-test. To find the most important character of hydatid of Morgagni which impedes pregnancy, logistic regression analysis of the dependent variable (no pregnancy) and independent variables (different characters ofhydatid of Morgagni) was carried out in the control group. Hydatid of Morgagni was detected in 52.1% of patients with unexplained infertility compared to 25.6% of those with explained infertility ($p<0.001$). The pregnancy rate was higher in the study group than the control group (58.7% vs 20.6%, $p<0.001$). The pregnancy rate was significantly higher in the study group than the control group if the hydatid cystwas bilateral (85.7% vs 5.3%, $p<0.001$), fimbrial (85.6% and 9.1%, $p<0.001$), single (57.6% and 30.3%, $p<0.001$) or 1-2 cm in diameter (58.1% and 25.5%, $p<0.001$). Logistic analysis showed that the bilaterality and fimbrial location of thehydatid of Morgagni were the most significant characteristics impeding pregnancy (odds ratio=7.27 and 3.67 respectively). They concluded that Hydatid of Morgagni is a possible underestimated cause of unexplained infertility. Laparoscopic removal of hydatid of Morgagni in patients with unexplained infertility was followed with a high spontaneous pregnancy rate. This is particularly obvious with bilateral and fimbrial hydatid of Morgagni.

4. Undescended tubes

Sometimes during laparoscopy you may notice that the tubes are congenitally nearer to the lateral pelvic wall or even adherent to it. By this way, the tubes are expected to be out of function due to the wide distance between the fimbria and the pouch of Douglas. It is commonly seen with some Mullerian duct anomalies.

4.1. Subtle tubal endometriosis

These lesions are only seen by laparoscopy which may include: tubal sacculations. Diverticulae [22], convolutions, phimosis, fimbrial agglutination or other subtle lesions (red, white or vesicular lesions).

4.2. Typical tubal endometriosis

Black or blue lesions could be seen on the surface of the fallopian tube. It may affect tubal motility, may cause tubal constriction or even occlusion. Generally, there is low fecundibility rate in such cases. Laparoscopic coagulation would lead to fibrosis and subsequent constriction. No clear publication on this point found in literature so far.

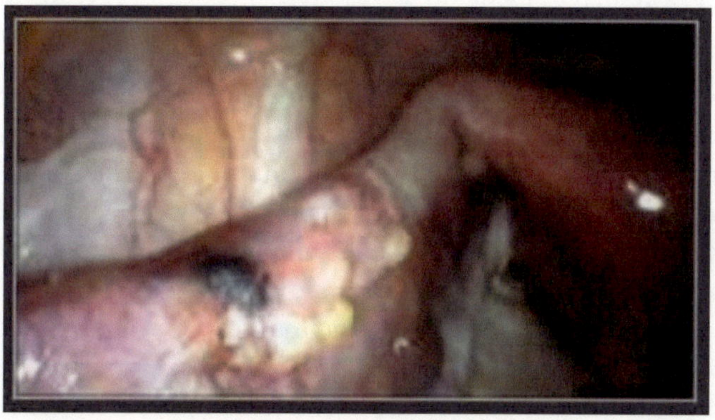

4.3. Role of tubal functions in UI

To achieve pregnancy, in addition to patency, two paradoxical types of peristaltic movements occur in the tubes. Muscular contractions of the distal part of tube and the cilia of its inner lining move the egg toward the interstitial segment of the tube which acts like a muscle sphincter and prevents the egg from being released into the uterus until it is ready for implantation. On the other hand, the proximal part of the tube expresses peristalsis to attract sperms to the site of implantation [23,24]. To date, tubal perstalsis and antiperstalsis are not well understood. Some invitro 3D studies were recently published but did not fully explain these complicated tubal phenomina [25]. Office hysteroscopy (OH) is a modern diagnostic tool with expanding popularity all over the world [26]. Adding vaginoscopic approach to office hysteroscopy is an extra simplification of the procedure with elimination of pain during examination [27].

4.4. New horizons for tubal patency detection

Since a long time, HSG is the classic tubal patency test. Lipiodol HSG has been shown to increase pregnancy rate which may be attributed to tubal patency or endometrial stimulation with possible enhanced receptivity of the endometrium to embryo implantation even in women with history of endometriosis [28,29]. Nevertheless, due to its well known drawbacks and complications (mainly pain), many women are afraid of doing HSG. Trials to improve its performance were described as elimination of traction on the cervix by tenaculum or usage of a pediatric Foley's catheter instead of the standard metal cannula [30] but still low patient acceptability of this invasive procedure is encountered. Saline infusion sonography (SIS) is an attractive alternative to HSG as it is a methodologically simple, cost effective, and time efficient comprehensive evaluation [31]. In 1999, we described a simplified technique of SIS utilizing a simple Nelaton catheter and 0.09% saline [32]. Despite its wide spread usage in many clinics, the main drawbacks of SIS are failure to localize the side of tubal patency and failure to properly visualize the tubes. Trials to improve results of SIS included the use of gel foam instead of saline [33], use of B-flow ultraspnography [34], 3D ultrasonography [35] or even sophisticated automated ultrasonography [36]. In the era of evidence-based medicine, Rubin pertubation tubal patency test is no longer implemented in modern practice [37] because it is very subjective and non-specific.

Definitely, hysteroscopy is the star of gynecologic endoscopy in recent years due to extended indications in modern practice. This position can be attributed to many factors including more technical refinement of instrumentation with better illumination and magnification, increased IVF/ICSI cycles practice and failures, increased interest in studying uterine factor of recurrent pregnancy loss (RPL), office usage with smaller caliber endoscopes omitting hospital admission, and increased product promotion. Most important, vaginoscopic approach with elimination of speculum insertion and traction on the cervix with a tenaculum had made hysteroscopy as simple as vaginal examination with high patient acceptability as shown in this study. OH saves money, omits stress for the patient, and improves health care services for the community at large. We believe that this attractive tool is not designed just to explore the endometrial cavity. The hysteroscopist should systematically examine the vagina, ectocervix, endocervical canal, endometrial cavity as well as the tubal ostea. Many tubal causes of infertility can be easily detected from the endoometrial cavity like polyps, fine adhesions or occlusion. These advantages are offered to the patient with minimal costs unlike other sophisticated and expensive approaches. For instance, MRI guided HSG was proved to be an effective patency test [38] but the costs and complicity of the technique are against the office principles.

Interest in hysteroscopic testing of tubal patency testing is not new. Hysteroscopic perturbation utilizing a fine catheter inserted into the tubal ostea followed by injection of methylene blue dye had been described [39]. If no reflux was seen, this means that the ostium was patent.

Unfortunately, they changed a simple office procedure into a complicated operation. They used a 5.5 mm operative bridge that would definitely increase pain. They used fine catheters and evaluated patency in a very subjective way without laparoscopic or even sonographic confirmation. Non-reflux of the dye doesn't necessarily mean patency. Intravasation or false passage due to unintentional perforation could be the cause. In short, their approach is similar to hysteroscopic tubal cannulation but in a blind manner without laparoscopic or sonographic monitoring.

On the other hand, hysteroscopic bubble suction test addressed in this study is a unique additional rapid costless step which could be done in every OH. What's new is to direct the attention of the hysteroscopist to its value. Not only did this study prove tubal patency, but it also clearly demonstrated an important tubal function which is tubal suction of sperms to the ampulla for fertilization which is mostly attributed to peristalsis of the proximal tube. This comes in accordance with recent interest in studying tubal function rather than just patency [40]. It should be mentioned that we didn't inject air into the tubal ostea but just observed tubal suction of the bubbles by the proximal part of the tube. Performing the procedure postmenstrual (with less vascular completely healed endometrium) together with the generation of minimal bubbles (that could pass through tubal ostia) and when needed slow injection of less than 2 ml of air (inside the bulb of the infusion device and not the tube) almost eliminate any risk of air embolism [41].

Two important issues that would compromise this test should be highlighted. The effect of increased intrauterine pressure was not responsible for positive bubble suction as we observed bubble suction after a while following uterine distension in a periodic manner despite keeping the same intrauterine pressure all the time and no suction occurred in some cases despite increased pressure up to 200 mmHg. The second issue is the possible effect of negative intrauterine pressure which is again excluded by observing bubble suction after a while of uterine cavity distension.

In this study, tubal block (even after increasing pressure into 200 mmHg) was suspected in 11.5% of women examined by OH (out of 76 women). Tubal block in the same set of women was found in 7.2% when examined through laparoscopy. There was some overestimation towards OH that may be attributed to subjective errors or tubal spasm. OH reports thick adhesions related to the proximal tubal end in 6 women (3.9%). Regarding other tubal abnormalities, normal laparoscopy was found to yield no abnormalities in HSG in 97% of cases while abnormal laparoscopy is found to meet with only 54.5% of abnormal HSG.

When OH is combined with HSG, diagnostic indices for tubal block were lowered rather than improved. This can be explained by that both OH and HSG diagnosed all the cases of tubal block with 100% sensitivity, adding both methods to each other didn't add to the strength of the detection. Contrarily, the false positive rates of the 2 methods add to each other and slightly decrease the diagnostic accuracy. The degree of agreement between OH and laparoscopy in evaluation of tubal patency was also quite interesting. Small sample size is a clear drawback of this study. From this study, it is concluded that hysteroscopic babble suction test is a costless, feasible and tolerable provisional test for tubal patency that should be attempted in every OH done for infertile women. Observation of movement of the peritubal bulge during bubble suction suggesting tubal peristalsis is interesting but requires more confirmatory studies.

5. Missed mesosalpingeal lesions

Mesosalpingeal lesions are perfectly seen by laparoscopy particularly if the lesion is small. They may include:

5.1. Paratubal cyst (Darwish et al., 2005) [42]

We constructed a study to define the proportion, methods of diagnosis and a simplified laparoscopic technique for treating paratubal and paraovarian cysts in a prospective cross-sectional study done at the Gynecologic Endoscopy Unit, Assiut University Hospital, Assiut, Egypt. It comprised a total of 1853 patients submitted to video-assisted laparoscopy. Transvaginal ultrasonography (TVS) was done in all cases to detect a paratubal or paraovarian cyst. Tubal shape and patency were evaluated using hysterosalpingography (HSG) in the infertile group. Diagnostic laparoscopy was done to confirm the diagnosis of paratubal or paraovarian cyst. Small cysts were punctured and coagulated, while larger cysts required cystectomty and extraction of the cysts using bipolar electrosurgery. Cystectomy was preceeded by endocystic visualization in all cases. Laparoscopically, only 118 patients (15.7%) were proved to have paratubal or paraovarian cysts. Preoperatively, TVS was able to diagnose paratubal or paraovarian cysts in 52 cases (44%) of them. Cysts less than 3 cm in size (34 cases) were treated with simple puncture and bipolar coagulation of the cyst wall whereas larger cysts (84 cases) were treated by cystectomy. Endocystic visualization using the 4-mm rigid hysteroscope was done in 84 cases (71%) with big cysts. There was statistically significant improvement of tubal patency after laparoscopic management. We concluded that sonographic diagnosis of the not uncommon paratubal and paraovarian cysts is not always feasible and requires more awareness and accuracy. The characteristic laparoscopic differentiation from ovarian cysts is the crossing of vessels over it. Endocystic endoscopic visualization is a valuable simple step prior to cystectomy. Bipolar coagulation or extraction of these cysts diagnosed at laparoscopy is easy and not time consuming and should be routinely done in all cases following the microsurgical laparoscopic principles. The significant effect of paratubal cystectomy on tubal patency and mobility supports the concept of routine removal of any paratubal or paraovarian cyst discovered at laparoscopy. Additional value of removal of these cysts detected at laparoscopy is exclusion of the rare possibility of malignancy (2-3%) and obtaining sufficient tissues for histopathologic evaluation. Lastly, its extraction is relatively easy and less time consuming unlike ovarian cystectomy.

5.2. Lipomesosalpnix

The classic tubal factors include post-inflammatory peritubal adhesions, prominal or diatal tubal occlusion [43] which can be easily diagnosed by most gynecologists based on HSG. Other rare tubal diseases are seldom investigated. For instance, salpingitis isthmica nodosa which is a nodular swelling of the isthmic segment of the fallopian tube are rarely reported [44]. Anatomically, mesosalpnix is defined as the part of the broad ligament enclosing a fallopian tube forming its mesentry. Histologically, it is formed of a thin layer of squamous epithelium and a small amount of loose areolar connective tissue [45,46]. It contains sympathetic ganglia and plexuses [47]. Laparoscopically, mesosalpnix is a thin vascular layer without evident fat in most cases.

With time interest to discover minute lesions that may affect fertility increased at our institution [42]. In practice, we observe some fatty tissue condensation in the mesosalpnix in some cases that deserved studying why it is present in some women. To make this study valuable,

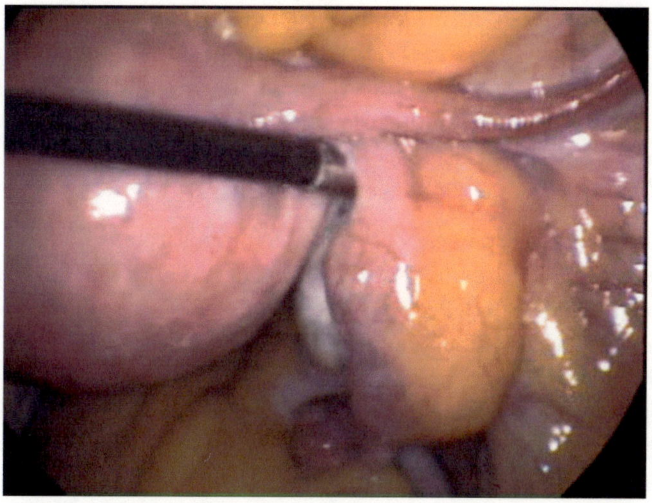

we considered mesosalpngeal adipose tissue significant if its caliber was at least similar or exceeds the caliber of the ampulla of the ipsilateral fallopian tube regardless the appearance of its borders.

We constructed a study to estimate the proportion of a significant mesosalpngeal adipose tissue condensation (lipomesosalpnix, at least of a caliber similar to the ampulla of the ipsilateral tube regardless with well-defined or poorly defined margins) among infertile women subjected to diagnostic laparoscopy. It was a cross sectional study done at a specialized endoscopic center. It comprised all infertile women scheduled for diagnoastic/therapeutic laparoscopy during the period between July 1994 and December 2012 were included in this study. Preoperative hysterosalpingography (HSG), transvaginal ultrasonography (TVS) as well as body mass index (BMI) for all cases. Laparoscopic documentation of a significant mesosalpingeal condensation of adipose tissue. Histopathologic assessment of the adipose tissues in some cases. Main outcome measures included number of cases with unilateral or bilateral lipomesosalpnix Significant lipomesosalpnix was diagnosed in 145 cases (5.7%) out of 2563 cases examined by laparoscopy. In all but 7 cases, lipomesosalpnix was seen bilaterally (99.7%). There was insignificant correlation between those cases and high BMI when compared to the rest of cases. Infertility was unexplained by laparoscopy in 621 cases (24.3%) while laparoscopy diagnosed etiologic factors in 1942 (75.7%) cases. Lipomesosalpnix was seen in 46 (7.4 %) and 79 (3.9%) of the unexplained cases and explained cases respectively without a statistically significant difference (P 0.48). We concluded that despite being a rare laparoscopic finding, significant lipomesosalpnix should be reported and documented as a possible missed tubal factor of infertility. Whether to treat lipomesosalpnix or not, bilaterally or unilaterally and by which means require further studies with proper second look laparoscopy.

This study directs attention towards more concentration on some factors that would affect tubal motility and commonly missed by gynecologists. Previously, some authors reported on Hydatid of Morgagni as a cause of UI [21]. Likewise, an old study [48] diagnosed fimbrial agglutinations (25%), accessory tubes (13%), accessory ostia (10%), phimoses (13%), and sacculations (7%) more in the infertile women. Tubal abnormalities would affect the prognosis of natural pregnancy as well as assisted reproduction [49, 50]. At our institution, we consider tubal sacculations, diverticulae, convolutions, phimosis or fimbrial agglutination as laparoscopic criteria of subtle tubal endometriosis specially if seen with other typical or atypical endometriotic tubal or peritoneal lesions. Proper endoscopic training would eliminate all these mistakes that would affect diagnosis as well as therapy.

Mesosalpingeal lesions include paratubal cyst [42], leiomyosarcoma of the broad ligament [51], Choristoma of Heterotopic Adrenal Tissue [52], primary Fallopian Tube Carcinoma [53] or lipoma of the Broad Ligament [54]. Preciously, among 1853 cases subjected to laparoscopy, we succeeded to diagnose a paratubal or paraovarian cyst in 118 patients (15.7%) [42]. Fat condensation in the mesosalpnix is not described in text books on histology, pathology or even endoscopic surgery as far as I know. Due to our interest in missed factors of infertility we tried to study the clinical significance of lipomesosalpnix. To be practical, we excluded cases with small amount of adipose tissue that wouldn't expect to affect tubal motility. In this study, preoperative TVS failed to diagnose lipomesosalpnix in all cases. Fallopian tubes are not usually visualized on a routine transvaginal sonographic examination unless outlined by fluid. However, the interstitial segment may be identified on TVS as an echogenic line arising from the endometrial canal and extending through the uterine wall. When surrounded by intraperitoneal fluid, the remaining segments of the fallopian tubes are commonly seen as tubular structures extending between the uterus and the ovaries. Fallopian tubes are best visualized on sonography when thickened or fluid-filled as a result of pelvic inflammatory disease, torsion, ectopic pregnancy, or tumors [55]. Nevertheless, we still recommend performing TVS routinely prior to laparoscopy to detect important findings like paraovarain cysts [42] and more importantly intrauterine lesions that would make concomitant hysteroscopy a mandatory step.

Despite similarity of the histopathologic appearance of lipomesosalpnix to any adipose tissue in the body, failure to prove any correlation between lipomesosalpnix and obesity would support screening for lipomesosalpnix in all infertile women.

To date, there is no uniform definition for unexplained infertility (UI) [56]. With the marvelous advancement in illumination and magnification, endoscopy would add a lot for the diagnostic work-up for cases with UI. The findings of this and our previous [42] studies would support the central role of dual endoscopy (combined laparoscopy and hysteroscopy) in all cases of infertility despite not being clearly stated by most of the infertility-interested societies when defining UI. One of the promising and attractive options for evaluation of subtle tubal and mesosalpingeal lesions is hydrolaparoscopy which offers a comparable accuracy to laparoscopy in 96.1% of cases [55].

Despite being described since a long time [57], the impact of fatty condensation of the mesosalpnix on fertility is not yet studied so far and this is the first study in English literature to address this point and to report it in 5.7% of infertile women. Lipomesosalpnix would theoretically affect tubal motility and more importantly leads to failure to reach the pouch of Douglas for ovum pick up despite being a patent tube. Nevertheless, the results of this study failed to prove a positive correlation between lipomesosalpnix and unexplained infertility.

http://dx.doi.org/10.5772/59948

This calls for a more large sample sized multicentric study. The main value of this study is to direct attention to mesosalpngeal lesions that would affect fertility.

6. Hidden Douglas pouch abnormalities

Douglas pouch is the site of ovum pick-up by the healthy fimbria. Sometimes, hidden factors contributing to infertility are seen in it. One of the best examples is subtle endometriosis which leads to changing environment and may hinder fimbrial pick up. One of the interesting laparoscopic findings is to see and cut fine adhesions that definitely affect ovum pick up. Such fine tiny lesions couldn't be seen by HSG. Practically, proper access to the pouch of Douglas can be aided by using a uterine manipulater with extreme anteversion of the uterus.

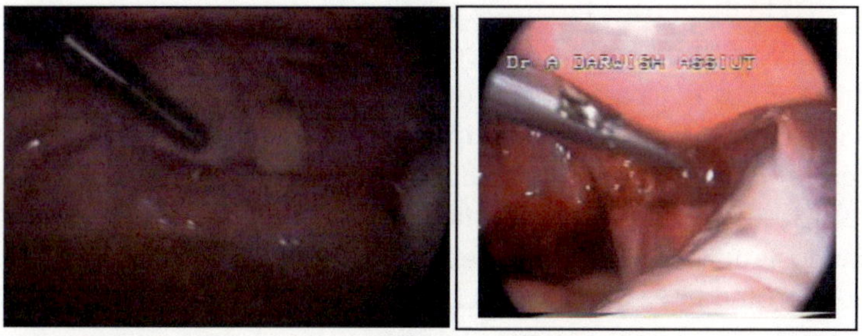

7. Uterovesical pouch abnormalities

Not uncommonly in post-cesarean section patients, we notice a thick central band between the uterus and the anterior abdominal wall attracting the uterus anteriorly causing severe anteversion. By this way infertility may occur due to relative shortening of the tubes as they will be far from the pouch of Douglas despite being completely healthy. The job of the laparoscopist in such cases is to cut this band to allow the tubes for proper function. One of the practical tricks, to know proper lysis is to test the level of the cervix by vaginal examination. Easy traction of the cervix is a good parameter of success. Moreover, the laparoscopist should look at the fimbrial relation to the pouch of Douglas. Care should be exerted to avoid bladder injury which can be easily induced particularly if a broad band with dense sealing is seen.

8. Role of Bacterial Vaginosis (BV) and the implementation of laparoscopy in these cases

We believe that occult infections are important explanation of UI particularly in patients who are unable to clearly give a history to explain a source for their tubal adhesions. BV infection was reported as a significant association with infertility and its proper treatment had lead to pregnancy, emphasizing the value and clinical implication of its screening and treatment [58]. It is hypothesized that immunity to infection might be correlated to sperm rejection in women with positive BV, leading to infertility [59]. On the other hand, low prevalence of BV (4.2%) was reported in a population of women undergoing in-vitro fertilization/embryo transfer (IVF-ET) where 331 infertile women were selected [60]. Variable results of many studies on the prevalence of BV among infertile women particularly UI were one of the main indications to construct a prospective study. Its aim was to estimate the prevalence of bacterial vaginosis (BV) among women with unexplained infertility (UI) and to describe laparoscopic appearances in positive cases. It was a prospective cross sectional comparative observational study done in a tertiary care referral facility and University hospital. It comprised one hundred and fifty women divided into UI study group (120 cases) and a control group (30 cases). Vaginal and cervical swabs form two subgroups of the UI group (60 cases each) and vaginal swabs from control group (30 cases). All swabs were tested using Amsel's criteria then cultured. Thereafter, UI group (60 cases) was subjected to diagnostic laparoscopy. Main outcome measures were the prevalence of BV among women with UI and laparoscopic findings among positive cases. In the study group, the number of positive cases of BV confirmed by culture was 51 cases (42.5 %) while it was diagnosed in only 3 cases (10%) in group B (p value 0.0001). BV was positive in 24 and 27 cases with periods of infertility less than and more than 3 years respectively and in 39 patients (32.5%) with recurrent vaginitis without statistical significance. There was an insignificant difference in diagnosis of BV whether the site of sample is vagina or cervix. Positive laparoscopic findings were reported in 77 patients (64.2 %). The most common laparoscopic abnormalities were hyperemic uterus and chronic salpingitis. In this study, we found that the prevalence of BV in women with UI is 42.5%, while the prevalence of BV in the fertile women (the control group) was 10% (P Value=0.0001). These results were similar to others who reported BV in 45.5% Vs 15.5% of the infertile and the control groups respectively [58]. On the other hand, BV was reported in only 18.9% of women with UI [61]. They reported rates of 12–15% in those with endometriosis and male factor infertility and 33–36% in those with anovulation and tubal infertility. Women with tubal factor were two to three times more likely to have BV than women with other types of infertility [62]. These findings highlight the importance of searching for BV in cases with tubal factor of infertility. This study reported no significant difference in the results of samples taken from the posterior fornix of vagina and those taken from the endometrial cavity (P Value=0.853). However, detection of clue cells in the endometrial cavity of women with UI demonstrates the possibility of ascending route of BV to the upper genital tract.

Regarding the role of culture for diagnosis of BV, we reported in 45.8% and 42.5% in culture and using Amsel`s criteria respectively without any significant difference. In this study, culture was a sensitive but not a specific method for diagnosing of BV compared to Amsel`s criteria which is demonstrated by ROC curve. Likewise, culture was unhelpful for the diagnosis of BV due to an imbalance of the normal organisms, without any pathogens necessarily being present [63].

The sensitivity and specificity of vaginal cultures for anaerobic bacteria (*Bacteroides* and *Peptostroptococcus*) and *Mycoplasma hominis* were reported in one study. They found that the presence of these organisms was a more specific indicator of BV than the presence of *G. vaginalis* but their detection had inadequate sensitivity [64]. Another group of anaerobic bacteria, Mobiluncus species, which is highly associated with BV, was very difficult to recover with culture methods [65].

In a previous study, 114 women with UI were examined laparoscopically Laparoscopy revealed pelvic pathology in 95 patients. Endometriosis, pelvic adhesions and tubal disease were observed and treated in 72, 46 and 24 patients, respectively. They could treat 72 patients of them, and 35 of them conceived using their own tubes. However they concluded that diagnostic laparoscopy should be strongly considered in UI work-up, and tubal efficacy should not be underestimated [66]. In this study, positive laparoscopic findings were reported in 77 patients (64.2 %). We found that laparoscopy can reveal upper genital tract pathology in 50% of positive cases with BV and it was negative in 35% of negative cases with BV (P Value=0.0001). There was a significant correlation between the positive cases of BV and the pathological lesions diagnosed by laparoscopy especially hyperemic uterus, chronic salpingitis and massive adhesions (P Value=0.0001) as shown in the following table.

9. Relation between positive cases of bacterieal vaginosis and laparoscopic findings

Subsequently, we recommend meticulous screening of women with these abnormal laparoscopic findings for possibility of hidden intrauterine infections. From this study, BV is strongly implicated in female infertility and it is probably an underestimated cause of UI. There is no extra benefit from using culture instead of Amsel's criteria for the diagnosis of BV. No difference in the site of sample taking in diagnosis of BV from posterior vaginal fornix or endometrial cavity. Laparoscopy is very beneficial in explaining the effect of BV on the upper genital tract. Further studies are required to test the impact of proper treating BV on subsequent fertility in case of UI.

diagnosis of bacterial vaginosis (Amsel`s criteria		chronic salpingitis	endometriosis	fine adhesions	hyperemic uterus	massive adhesions	normal	Total	P Value
+ve	Count	13	3	8	14	12	1	51	0.0001 (sig)
	% of Total	10.8%	2.5%	6.7%	11.7%	10.0%	0.8%	42.5%	
-ve	Count	7	5	5	8	2	42	69	
	% of Total	5.8%	4.2%	4.2%	6.7%	1.7%	35.0%	57.5%	
Total	Count	20	8	13	22	14	43	120	
	% of Total	16.7%	6.7%	10.8%	18.3%	11.7%	35.8%	100%	

10. Role of hidden intrauterine infections and the value of laparoscopy in these cases

Existing definitions of infertility lack uniformity, rendering comparisons in prevalence between countries or over time problematic. The absence of an agreed definition also compromises clinical management and undermines the impact of research findings [66]. Unexplained infertility is infertility that is idiopathic in the sense that its cause remains unknown even after basic infertility work-up, usually including semen analysis in the man and assessment of ovulation and fallopian tubes in the woman. The available diagnostic tools for intrauterine causes of infertility include transvaginal ultrasonograogy, hysterosalpingography (HSG) or sonohysterography [67]. Manifest uterine causes may include clinically symptomatizing uterine infections, intrauterine adhesions, polypi or uterine cavity malformations. Hidden uterine factors may include thin endometrium, poor endometrial receptivity, and immunological incompatibility which have received the most attention in recent years [68]. In literature, little attention was directed towards asymptomatic hidden intrauterine infections like Mycoplasma, Ureaplasma, Klebsiella and Chlamydia trachomatis particularly among infertile women [69].

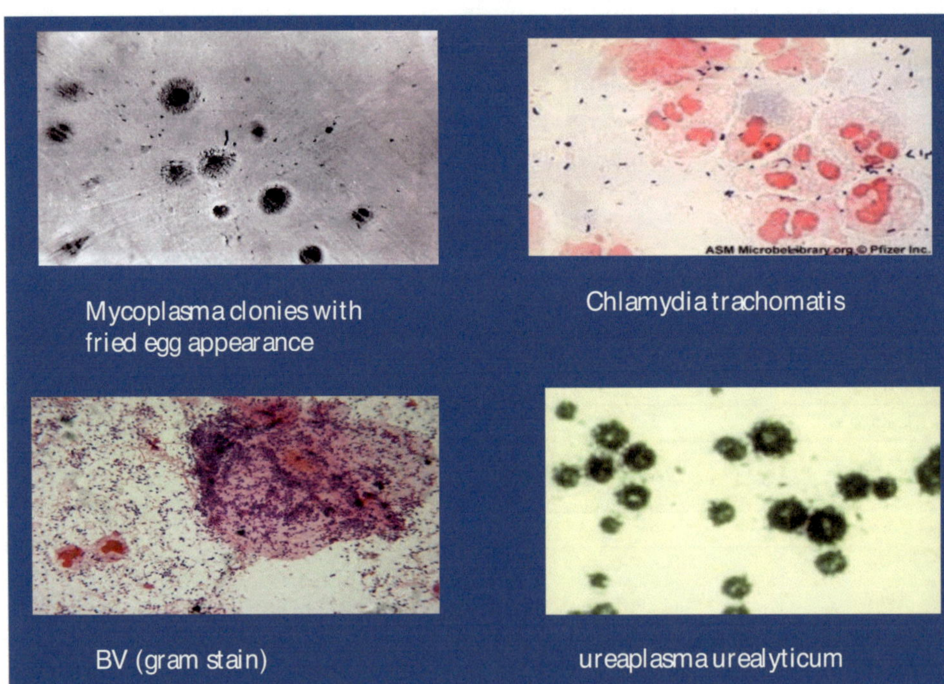

Subclinical infection can be a possible cause of unexplained infertility [70]. Changes in the intraperitoneal environment leading to an inflammatory process in the absence of visible abnormalities have been suggested as being causal in some cases of UI [71]. We believe that occult infections are important explanation of UI particularly in patients who are unable to clearly give a history to explain a source for their tubal adhesions.

We constructed a prospective study aimed to estimate the prevalence of hidden (asymptomatic) intrauterine infections among women with unexplained infertility in comparison to fertile women and to describe laparoscopic appearances in positive cases. It was a prospective cross sectional comparative observational study done at a tertiary care referral facility and University hospital. It comprised 50 women with unexplained infertility (study group A) and 50 fertile women (control group B) who came for contraceptive advice. Endouterine swab for bacteriologic study from all cases. Diagnostic laparoscopy for group A. Main outcome measures included prevalence of infections among both groups and to correlate laparoscopic findings to bacteriologic study in group A. There was statistically insignificant difference between both groups regarding the age and residence (p value >0.05) and it was highly significant regarding parity (p value <0.001). Hidden intrauterine infections were diagnosed by culture in 42 cases (84%) and 10 cases (20%) out of both groups respectively (P=0.001). The most common organisms detected in the study group were Mycoplasma (24%), klebsiella (20%), Chlamydia (18%) and Proteus (10%). In group A, positive laparoscopic findings were reported in 33 patients (66 %). There was a significant correlation between the positive cases of hidden intrauterine infections and abnormal laparoscopic findings (P Value=0.0001). The most common laparoscopic abnormalities were hyperemic uterus, peritubal adhesions and chronic salpingitis which were reported in 10 (20%), 6 (12%) and 4 (8%) cases respectively.

11. Hidden intrauterine microorganisms detected in both groups

Control group (B)		study group (A)		Organism
Percent	No (50)	Percent	No (50)	
2%	1	24%	12	*Mycoplasma*
8%	4	20%	10	*Klebsiella*
6%	3	18%	9	*Chlamydia*
0%	0	10%	5	*Proteus*
0%	0	6%	3	*Legionella*
2%	1	4%	2	*Ureaplasma*
0%	0	2%	1	*Staph.*
2%	1	0%	0	*Pseudomonous*
80%	40	16%	8	*Negative**

Control group (B)		study group (A)		Organism
Percent	No (50)	Percent	No (50)	
100%	50	100%	50	Total

12. Correlation between positive cases of hidden intrauterine infection and laparoscopic findings in UI group

Culture for intrauterine infection		Abnormal laparoscopic findings		Total	P Value
		+ve	-ve		
+ve	No.	30	12	42	0.0001
	% of Total	50%	16%	82%	
-ve	No.	3	5	8	
	% of Total	16%	18%	16%	
Total	No.	33	17	50	
	% of Total	66%	34%	100.0%	

13. Correlation between positive cases of hidden intrauterine infection and laparoscopic findings in UI group

We concluded that despite being an underestimated cause of female infertility, hidden intrauterine infections are frequent and strongly implicated in UI. Laparoscopy is very beneficial in explaining the effect of hidden intrauterine infections on the upper genital tract. We recommend postoperative screening for hidden intrauterine infections in UI cases with abnormal laparoscopic findings. Further studies are required to test pregnancy rate after proper treating of these infections in case of UI.

		chronic salpingitis	Endometriosis	fine peritubal adhesions	hyperemic uterus	Tubal block (uni/bi)	Fimbrial agglutination	Normal (17)	Total (50)
+ve (42)	No.	4	7	6	10	1	2	12	42
	% of Total	8%	14%	12%	20%	2%	4%	24%	84%
-ve (8)	No.	0	2	0	1	0	0	5	8

		chronic salpingitis	Endometriosis	fine peritubal adhesions	hyperemic uterus	Tubal block (uni/bi)	Fimbrial agglutination	Normal (17)	Total (50)
	% of Total	0	4%	0	2%	0	0	10%	16%
Total (50)	No.	4	9	6	11	1	2	17	50
	% of Total	8%	18%	12%	22%	2%	4%	34%	100%

In this study, we found that the prevalence of hidden intrauterine infections proved by culture of endouterine discharge in women with UI was 84% while the prevalence in the fertile women (the control group) was 20% (P Value=0.0001). Based on our results, we recommend that before starting a lengthy and costly list of sophisticated level II investigations of both partners, focusing attention to hidden uterine infections is very important basic step in UI. These results were similar to others who reported high prevalence of different types of infections [72]. It has been found that women with tubal factor were two to three times more likely to have genital tract infections than women with other types of infertility [73]. Likewise, our findings highlight the importance of searching for genital tract infections in cases with tubal factor of infertility. In this study we used culture of the intrauterine discharge as a diagnostic test for different infections. Biochemical confirmation was also performed. Others used more sophisticated tests like ELIZA and PCR [72,73]. We think that culture should be accepted as a basic screening tool due to availability and feasibility in many hospitals. Screening test should not be expensive or complicated to be extended to all hospitals particularly in low resource countries like ours.

This study demonstrated a high prevalence of Mycoplasma (24%), klebsiella (20%), Chlamydia (18%) and Proteus (10%) among women with UI. These results of high prevalence compared to fertile women would call for more attention to screening protocols in all infertility units dealing with UI ideally prior to laparoscopic intervention. Due to high prevalence of Chlamydia in infertile women in one previous study, screening for Chlamydia was recommended for cases with UI [72]. We reported Mycoplasma in about one quarter of positive cases. Likewise, mycoplasma was reported in 32% of infertile cases with a statistically significant difference from fertile group [77]. In this study, we cultured proteus infection in 10% of infected cases. This particular organism is commonly noticed in the urinary system. Reporting it in the genital tract would requires more studies to define its role in infertility. Unlike others, we reported low prevalence of Ureaplasma in only 4% of cases despite its previous reports of up to 32% infertile cases [72]. This wide difference may demonstrate the variability of frequency of hidden intrauterine infections in different populations and highlights detection of prevalence in each community.

The role of laparoscopy in the evaluation of infertility is crucial [78]. In this study we reported 33 case (66%) of abnormal laparoscopic findings in the infertile group. In a previous study [79], abnormal laparoscopic findings were reported in about 53 % of infertile women. Pelvic adhesions were the most frequent finding in their study. Others [80] reported a higher prevalence of abnormal laparoscopic findings in UI up to 87.2% who described endometriosis lesions, peritubal adhesions and tubal obstruction. In a previous study, 114 women with UI were examined laparoscopically. Laparoscopy revealed pelvic pathology in 95 patients. Endometriosis, ptielvic adhesions and tubal disease were observed and treated in 72, 46 and 24 patients, respectively. They could treat 72 patients of them, and 35 of them conceived using their own tubes. However they concluded that diagnostic laparoscopy should be strongly considered in UI work-up, and tubal efficacy should not be underestimated [65]. In this study, positive laparoscopic findings were reported in 33 patients (66 %). We found that laparoscopy can reveal upper genital tract pathology in 30 cases (71.4%) of positive cases with hidden infections (42 cases) and it was negative in 3 cases (37.5%) of negative cases with hidden intrauterine infections (P Value=0.0001). We reported a significant correlation between the positive cases of intrauterine infections and the pathological lesions diagnosed by laparoscopy especially hyperemic uterus, chronic salpingitis and peritubal adhesions (P Value=0.0001). Subsequently, we recommend meticulous screening of women with these abnormal laparoscopic findings for possibility of hidden intrauterine infections. Small sample size of individual types of hidden intrauterine infections and lake of precise description of a particular abnormal laparoscopic finding for each organism are clear limitations of this study. Diagnostic accuracy for Chlamydia detection would be better if we used Nucleic Acid Amplification (NAAT) instead of the only available direct immunofluorescence assay (IFA). From this study, we conclude that despite being an underestimated cause of female infertility, hidden intrauterine infections are frequent and strongly implicated in UI. Laparoscopy is very beneficial in explaining the effect of hidden intrauterine infections on the upper genital tract. We recommend postoperative screening for hidden intrauterine infections in UI cases with abnormal laparoscopic findings. Further studies are required to test the impact of proper treating these infections in cases of UI.

14. Hidden ovarian factors of infertility

The ovaries are easily and clearly seen by transvaginal ultrasonogtraphy. Intraovarian and capsular abnormalities can be detected in most of the cases. Despite properly confirmed ovulation in an otherwise normal couple, pregnancy could not be achieved. On doing diagnostic laparoscopy in those cases some tiny ovarian abnormalities could be diagnosed. Subtle surface ovarian endometriosis could be only diagnosed by laparoscopy. In such cases surface coagulation of red, white or vesicular lesions is easy. Moreover, typical black or blue lesions can be only seen and treated by laparoscopy. In some cases, we notice fine periovarian adhesions hindering rupture of the growing folloicles and preventing pick-up of the oocytes. In such cases, fine microsurgical adhesiolysis without capsular injuring using a delicate fine scissors is feasible by laparoscopy. We may see some dense ovarian adhesions to the lateral or anterior abdominal wall that clearly affect fertility In such cases, microsurgical adhesiolysis will regain the normal anatomy. Lastly, we may notice fine or dense adhesions between the ovary and the back of the uterus or the fallopian tubes. All these mechanical factors will not

http://dx.doi.org/10.5772/59948

be seen by HSG and highlight the importance of implication of dual laparoscopy and hysteroscopy in all cases of infertility particularly women with previous pelvic or uterine surgery.

15. Uterine causes of UI

Uterine factors account about 20% of all cases of infertility. Manifest uterine causes may include intrauterine adhesions, polypi or uterine cavity malformations. Hidden uterine factors may include thin endometrium, poor endometrial receptivity, and immunological incompatibility which have received the most attention in recent years. Some delicate endometrial lesions could be diagnosed by hysteroscopy as shown in this figure.

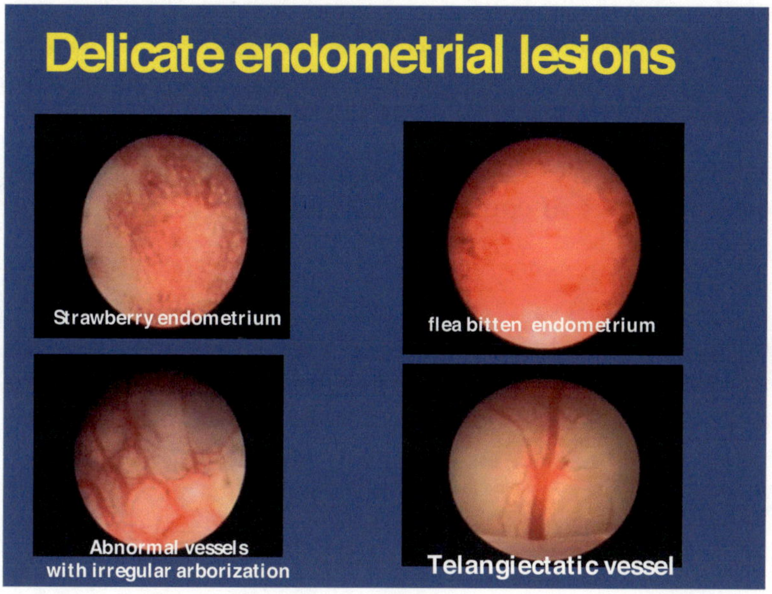

We constructed a study [81] aiming to estimate the safety, efficacy and patient acceptability of adding vaginoscopic office hysteroscopy (VOH) to the infertility diagnostic work-up prior to laparoscopy. It was a prospective comparative diagnostic trial done at a tertiary care referral facility and University hospital. A total of 156 infertile patients scheduled for laparoscopy. Seventy eight patients had VOH on one stop bases in addition to the usual infertility work-up were assigned as group B while a similar number was examined by the usual diagnostic work-up and assigned as group A. Main outcome measures included the diagnostic accuracy of VOH in diagnosing intrauterine abnormalities and tubal patency in comparison to hysterosalpingography (HSG) and diagnostic laparoscopy (DL). Combined VOH and HSG or DL assessment for diagnostic accuracy.

There was insignificant difference between both groups regarding sociodemographic and HSG data. Abnormal DL findings were more significant in group A. VOH detected 50% abnormal endometrial cavity in group B with a significant superiority over HSG. Blocked tubes were diagnosed in 9% and 11.5%, 5.1% and 6.4% and 3.8% and 5.1% using VOH, HSG and DL on right and left sides respectively. There was a high percentage of agreement in the diagnosis of uterine abnormalities between HSG and VOH (96%, k=0.394). n the other hand, the percentage of agreement between VOH and HSG is less (86%, k=0.214) and is much less between VOH and laparoscopy (82%, k=0.148) regarding tubal patency testing. Generally, VOH was an acceptable procedure with mild pain and feasible in most cases.

We concluded that VOH seems feasible, safe, simple, tolerable and quick out-patient procedure. It can diagnose intrauterine abnormalities in 23.7% of infertile women with normal HSG. VOH achieves marvelous agreement with HSG in diagnosing uterine abnormalities (96%), excellent agreement with HSG (86%) for tubal patency testing and very good agreement with DL (82%) regarding tubal patency. Diagnostic indices including accuracy of either HSG or DL would increase if combined with VOH. We recommend adding OH to the routine diagnostic work-up of infertile couples prior to laparoscopy. Nevertheless, whether its use would increase pregnancy rate among infertile women requires a further longitudinal comparative study.

16. Diagnostic accuracy of combined tests for assessment of uterine and tubal factors

	VOH + HSG (for assessment of uterine factor)	**VOH + HSG (for assessment of tubal patency)**	**VOH+ laparoscopy (for assessment of tubal patency)**
Sensitivity	97.4%	50%	94%
Specificity	56.2%	16.6%	33.3%
Positive predictive value	80.9%	76.2%	94%
Negative predictive value	90%	5.9%	33.3%
Accuracy	59.2%	44.7%	89.5%

17. Endoscopic exploration of the fertilization site

Sometimes the fallopian tubes appear normal at HSG and even laparoscopy but pregnancy doesnot occur due to some hidden intratubal fine lesions at the fertilization site (ampulla). Intratubal examination can only be done using falloposcopy (from the cervical side) or salpingoscopy (from the fimbrial side). Going inside the tube allows proper exploration of the endosalpnix. Lost or destroyed major or minor folds may explain infertility. Detection of fine adhesions or tiny polypi is feasible by salpingoscopy.

http://dx.doi.org/10.5772/59948

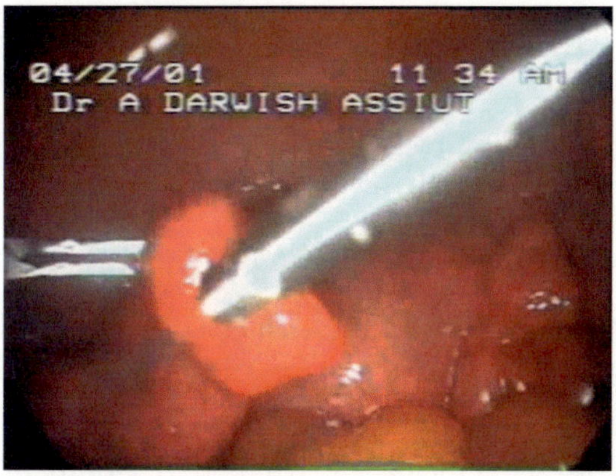

18. Exploration of the implantation site

Implantation site is located on the posterior endometrium at midline 10-15 mm from the fundus. Hysteroscopy can detect tiny lesions at the implantation site like fine adhesions, polypi or small septum. Implantation failure may be caused by abnormal cytokine expression by embryos and endometrium. As proved in many studies, endometrial injury would induce release of cytokines that may increase implantation. Practically, site-specific endometrial injury in the follicular phase with the edge of the office hysteroscopy lens would enhance implantation in cases with unexplained infertility. Nevertheless, the real implementation of this procedure requires more randomized studies.

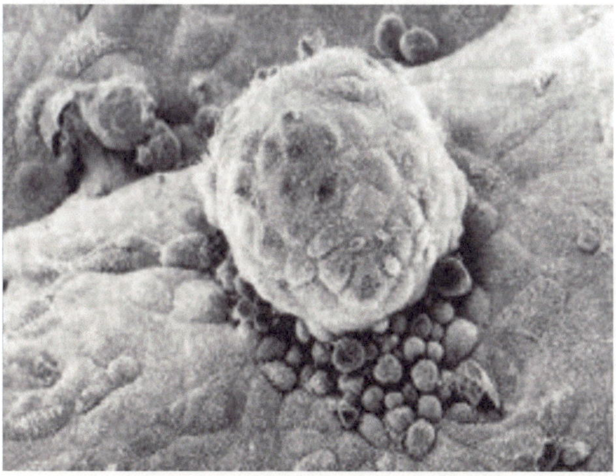

19. Keynote points

Unexplained infertility remains a clinical and scientific challenge.

Dual endoscopy (combined DL & DH) can explain a good percentage of cases with UI.

Nothing called UI without prior endoscopic assessment.

Office hysteroscopy (OH) is recommended even if HSG is normal.

Don't ignore hidden infections.

Try to explain UI but don't harm the patient. No need to perform unneeded procedure like overdoing of laparoscopic ovarian drilling that may invite adhesions and more importantly deleteriously affect ovarian reserve as shown in this figure.

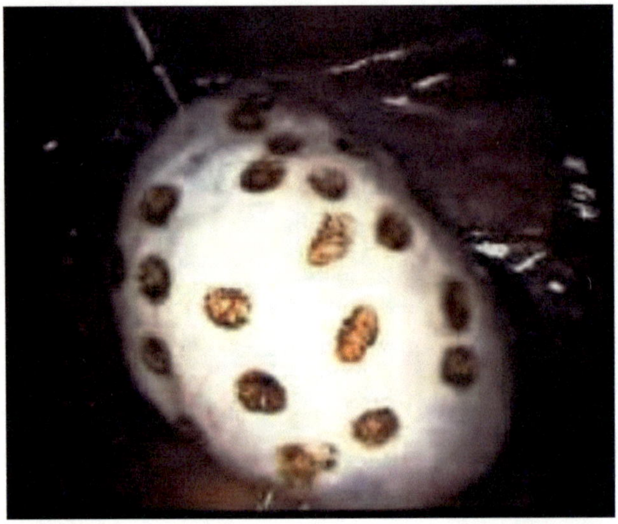

Author details

Atef M. Darwish*

Address all correspondence to: atef_darwish@yahoo.com

Department of Obstetrics and Gynecology, Woman's Health University Hospital, Faculty of Medicine, Assiut University, Egypt

References

[1] Siristatidis C, Bhattacharya S. Unexplained infertility: does it really exist? Does it matter? Hum Reprod. 2007;22(8):2084-7.

[2] Smith S, Pfiefer SM, Collins J. Diagnosis and management of female infertility. JAMA 2003; 290, 17.

[3] The Practice Committee of the American Society for Reproductive Medicine, authors. Optimal evaluation of the infertile female. Fertil Steril 2006; 86(5 suppl):S264–S267.

[4] Cahill DJ and Wardle PG. Management of infertility. British Medical Journal2002; 325:28-32.

[5] Randolph JF. Unexplained infertility. Clinical Obstetrics and Gynecology 2000; 43:897-901.

[6] Ray A, Shah A, Gudi A, Homburg R. Unexplained infertility: an update and review of practice. Reproductive Biomedicine Online 2012;24, 591-602.

[7] Querlen D. Fertility after conization. Rev Fr Gynecol and Obstet 1991;15;86(2):81-82.

[8] Paulson RJ. Unexplained infertility. MishelFs Textbook if infertility, Contraception and Reproductive Endocrine. 1997; Chapter (45): 743 – 753.

[9] Speroff L, Glass RH and Kase NG. Clinical gynecology Endocrine and infertility.5th ed. Williams &Wilkins Baltimore London. 2004;Vol. 11. p24.

[10] Balasch J, Fabregues F, Creus M, Casamitjana R, Peurto B and Vanrell JA. Recombinant human follicular stimulating hormone for ovulation induction in polycystic ovary syndrome: a prospective, randomized trial of two starting doses in a chronic low dose step up protocol. J Assist Reprod Genet 2000; 17(10):561-565.

[11] Cahill DJ, Wardle PG. Management of infertility. British Medical Journal 2002; 325:28-32.

[12] Schild RL, Knobloch C, Dorn C, Fimmers R, Van derv en H, Hansmann M. Endometrial receptivity in an in vitro fertilization program as assessed by spiral artery blood flow, Fertil Steril 2001;75:361-366.

[13] Li H, Chen S and Xing F. Expression of HOXA10 gene in human endometrium and its relationship with unexplained infertility. Chinese Journal of OB/GYN 2002; 37(1): 30-32.

[14] Collins JA Burrows EA, Willam AR. The prognosis for live birth among untreated infertile couples. Fertil Steril 1995; 64:22-28.

[15] Choudhury SR and Knapp LA. Human reproductive failure: Immunological factors. Hum Reprod Update 2001; 7(2):113-134.

[16] Bonneau C, Chanelles O, Sifer C, Poncelet C. Use of laparoscopy in unexplained infertility. European Journal of Obstetrics & Gynecology and Reproductive Biology 2012; 58-60.

[17] Kahyaoglu S. Does diagnostic laparoscopy have value in unexplained infertile couple? Review of the current literature. J Minimally Invasive Surgery Science. 2012 1;4: 124-128.

[18] De Wilde RL, Brosens I. Rationale of first-line endoscopy-based fertility exploration using transvaginal hydrolaparoscopy and minihysteroscopy. Hum Reprod. 2012 Aug;27(8):2247-53.

[19] Child T. Optimizing the management of patients with infertility. Practitioner. 2013;257(1759):19-22, 2-3.

[20] Cebesoy FB[1], Kutlar I, Dikensoy E, Yazicioglu C, Kalayci H. Morgagni hydatids: a new factor in infertility? Arch Gynecol Obstet. 2010 Jun;281(6):1015-7.

[21] Rasheed SM[1], Abdelmonem AM.Hydatid of Morgagni: a possible underestimated cause of unexplained infertility. Eur J Obstet Gynecol Reprod Biol. 2011 Sep;158(1): 62-6.

[22] Han H, Guan J, Wang Y, Zhang Q, Shen H. Diagnosis and treatment of tubal diverticula: report of 13 cases. J Minim Invasive Gynecol. 2014 Jan-Feb;21(1):142-6.

[23] Kunz G, Beil D, Deiniger H, Einspanier A, Mall G, Leyendecker G. The Uterine Peristaltic. The Fate of the Male Germ Cell. Advances in Experimental Medicine and Biology 1997; 424, 267-277.

[24] Maia H, Coutinho EM. Peristalsis and antiperstalsis of the human fallopian tube during the menstrual cycle. Biology of Reproduction. 1970;2,305-314.

[25] Aranda V, Cortez R, Fauci L. Stokesian peristaltic pumping in a three-dimensional tube with a phase-shifted asymmetry. Physics of Fluids 2011; 23, 081901.

[26] Darwish AM, Sayed EH, Mohammad SA, Mohammad II, Hassan HI. Reliability of out-patient hysteroscopy in one-stop clinic for abnormal uterine bleeding. Gynecologic Surgery 2012;9, 3, 289-295.

[27] Emanuel MH. New developments in hysteroscopy. Best Pract Res Clin Obstet Gynaecol. 2013 Feb 2. pii: S1521-6934(13)00005-9.

[28] Johnson NP Review of lipiodol treatment for infertility-an innovative treatment for endometriosis-related infertility?. Aust N Z J Obstet Gynaecol. 2014 Feb;54(1):9-12.

[29] Court KA, Dare AJ, Weston-Webb M, Hadden WE, Sim RG, Johnson NP. Establishment of lipiodol as a fertility treatment-Prospective study of the complete innovative treatment data set. Aust N Z J Obstet Gynaecol. 2014 Feb;54(1):13-19.

[30] Petri E, Berlit S, Sütterlin M, Hornemann A. Chromopertubation--presentation of a modification of the standard technique. Anticancer Res. 2013 Apr;33(4):1591-4.

[31] Saunders RD, Shwayder JM, Nakajima ST. Current methods of tubal patency assessment. Fertil Steril. 2011 Jun;95(7):2171-9.

[32] Darwish AM, Youssef AA. Screening sonohysterography in infertility. Gynecol Obstet Invest. 1999;48(1):43-7.

[33] Van Schoubroeck D, Van den Bosch T, Meuleman C, Tomassetti C, D'Hooghe T, Timmerman D. The use of a new gel foam for the evaluation of tubal patency. Gynecol Obstet Invest. 2013;75(3):152-6.

[34] Sladkevicius P, Zannoni L, Valentin L. Use of B-flow ultrasound facilitates visualization of contrast media during hysterosalpingo-contrast sonography (HyCoSy). Ultrasound Obstet Gynecol. 2013 Dec 20. doi: 10.1002/uog.

[35] Zhou L, Zhang X, Chen X, Liao L, Pan R, Zhou N, Di N. Value of three-dimensional hysterosalpingo-contrast sonography with SonoVue in the assessment of tubal patency. Ultrasound Obstet Gynecol. 2012 Jul;40(1):93-8.

[36] Exacoustos C, Di Giovanni A, Szabolcs B, Romeo V, Romanini ME, Luciano D, Zupi E, Arduini D. Automated three-dimensional coded contrast imaging hysterosalpingo-contrast sonography: feasibility in office tubal patency testing. Ultrasound Obstet Gynecol. 2013 Mar;41(3):328-35.

[37] Pavone ME, Hirshfeld-Cytron JE, Kazer RR. The progressive simplification of the infertility evaluation. Obstet Gynecol Surv. 2011 Jan;66(1):31-41.

[38] Ma L, Wu G, Wang Y, Zhang Y, Wang J, Li L, Zhou W. Fallopian tubal patency diagnosed by magnetic resonance hysterosalpingography. J Reprod Med. 2012 Sep-Oct; 57(9-10):435-40.

[39] Török P, Major T. Accuracy of assessment of tubal patency with selective pertubation at office hysteroscopy compared with laparoscopy in infertile women. J Minim Invasive Gynecol. 2012 Sep-Oct;19(5):627-30

[40] Kajanová M, L D, S P, Miko M, Urban L, Bokor T, Varga I. The structural basis for transport through the Fallopian tube. Ceska Gynekol. 2012 Dec;77(6):566-71.

[41] Groenman FA, Peters LW, Rademaker BM, Bakkum EA. Embolism of air and gas in hysteroscopic procedures: pathophysiology and implication for daily practice. J Minim Invasive Gynecol. 2008 Mar-Apr;15(2):241-7.

[42] Darwish AM, Amin AM, Mohammad SA. Laparoscopic management of paratubal and paraovarian cysts. Journal of the Society of Laparoendoscopic Surgeons 2003;7,2 :101-6.

[43] Gomel V, Taylor PJ, Yuzpe A, Roux J: Laparoscopy and Hysteroscopy in Gynecologic Practice. Chicago, Year Book, 1986.

[44] Chawla N, Kudesia S, Azad S, Singhal M, Rai SM.Salpingitis isthmica nodosa. Indian J Pathol Microbiol. 2009;52(3):434-5.

[45] Kessel R. Medical histology. Oxford University Press, London,P 486-1998

[46] Gartner LP, Hiatt JL. Color textbook of histology. Third Edition. Saunders, Elsevier, NewYork, P 477-78.

[47] Weiss L, Greep RO. Histology. Fourth Edition. McGraw-Hill Book Com, NewYork Page 920.

[48] Yablonski M, Sarge T, Wild RA. Subtle variations in tubal anatomy in infertile women. Fertil Steril. 1990 Sep;54(3):455-8.

[49] Hurst BS, Tucker KE, Awoniyi CA, Schlaff WD. Hydrosalpinx treated with extended doxycycline does not compromise the success of in vitro fertilization. Fertil Steril. 2001 May;75(5):1017-9.

[50] Fakih H, Marshall J. Subtle tubal abnormalities adversely affect gamete intrafallopian transfer outcome in women with endometriosis. Fertil Steril. 1994 Oct;62(4):799-801

[51] Kolusari A, Ugurluer G, Kosem M, Kurdoglu M, Yildizhan R, Adali E. Leiomyosarcoma of the broad ligament: a case report and review of the literature. Eur J Gynaecol Oncol. 2009;30(3):332-4.

[52] Janovski NA. Choristoma of heterotopic adrenal tissue in mesosalpinx. Obstet Gynecol. 1966 ;28(3):380-2.

[53] Huang WC, Yang SH, Yang JM. Ultrasonographic manifestations of fallopian tube carcinoma in the fimbriated end. J Ultrasound Med. 2005 ;24(8):1157-60; quiz 1161-2.

[54] Benjaminov O, Atri M. Sonography of the abnormal fallopian tube. AJR Am J Roentgenol. 2004 Sep;183(3):737-42.

[55] Ezedinma NA, Phelps JY. Transvaginal hydrolaparoscopy. JSLS. 2012;16(3):461-5.

[56] Ray A, Shah A, Gudi A, Homburg R. Unexplained infertility: an update and review of practice. Reprod Biomed Online. 2012;24(6):591-602.

[57] Lockyer C. Lipoma of the Broad Ligament. Proc R Soc Med. 1919;12(Obstet Gynaecol Sect):195-9.

[58] Rasheed M. Salah, Abdelmonem M. Allam, AminM. Magdy, Abeer Sh. Mohamed. Bacterial vaginosis and infertility: Cause or association ? European journal of obstetrics & gynecology and reproductive biology 2013; 167: 59-63.

[59] Mania-Pramanik J, Kerkar SC, Salvi VS. Bacterial vaginosis: a cause of infertility?. International Journal of STD & AIDS 2009; 20: 778–781.

[60] Spandorfer SD, Neuer A, Giraldo PC, Rosenwaks Z., Witkin SS. Relationship of abnormal vaginal flora, proinflammatory cytokines and idiopathic infertility in women undergoing IVF. J Reprod Med 2001; 46: 806-10.

[61] Janet D. Wilson, Susan G. Ralph, Anthony J. Rutherford. Rates of bacterial vaginosis in women undergoing in vitro fertilization for different types of infertility. BJOG: International journal of obstetrics and gynecology. 2002;109:714-717.

[62] Lamont RF. Bacterial vaginosis. Year book of obstetric and gynecology. 1998; 149:p154-158.

[63] Krohn MA, Hiller SL. Comparison of methods for diagnosiing bacterial vaginoss among pregnant women.J.Clin. Microbiol, 1989; 27:p1266-1271.

[64] Hiller SL, Krohn MA, Nugent RP. Characteristics of the vaginal flora patterns assessment by gram stain among pregnant women. Am. J. Obstet. Gynecol 1992;166:p938-949.

[65] Bonneau C, Chanelles O, Sifer C, Poncelet C. Use of laparoscopy in unexplained infertility. European Journal of Obstetrics & Gynecology and Reproductive Biology 2012; 58-60.

[66] Boivin J, Bunting L, Collins JA, Nygren KG. International estimates of infertility prevalence and treatment-seeking: potential need and demand for infertility medical care. Hum Reprod 2007;22:1506–1512.

[67] Darwish AM, Youssef AA. Screening sonohysterography in infertility. Gynecol Obstet Invest. 1999;48(1):43-7.

[68] Choudhury SR, Knapp LA. Human reproductive failure: Immunological factors. Hum Reprod Update 2001; 7(2):113-134.

[69] Cassell GH, Younger JB, Brown MB, Blackwell RE, Davis JK, Marriott P, Stagno S. Microbiologic study of infertile women at the time of diagnostic laparoscopy: Association of Ureaplasma urealyticum with a defined subpopulation. N Engl J Med 1983; 308: 502.

[70] The Practice Committee of the American Society for Reproductive Medicine, authors. Optimal evaluation of the infertile female. Fertil Steril 2006; 86(5 suppl):S264–S267.

[71] Siristatidis C, Bhattacharya S. Unexplained infertility: does it really exist? Does it matter? Hum Reprod. 2007;22(8):2084-7.

[72] Gupta A, Gupta A, Gupta S, Mittal A, Chandra P, Gill AK. Correlation of mycoplasma with unexplained infertility. Arch Gynecol Obstet 2009 Dec; 280(6):981-5.

[73] Cahill DJ, Wardle PG. Management of infertility. British Medical Journal 2002; 325:28-32.

[74] Hossein Rashidi B, Chamani Tabriz L, Haghollahi F, Jeddi-Tehrani M, Naghizadeh MM, Shariat M, et al. Effects of Chlamydia trachomatis Infection on Fertility; A Case-Control Study. J Reprod Infertil. 2013;14(2):67-72.

[75] Spandorfer SD, Neuer A, Giraldo PC, Rosenwaks Z., Witkin SS. Relationship of abnormal vaginal flora, proinflammatory cytokines and idiopathic infertility in women undergoing IVF. J Reprod Med 2001; 46: 806-10.

[76] Siam EM, Hefzy EM. The relationship between antisperm antibodies prevalence and genital chlamydia trachomatis infection in women with unexplained infertility. Afr J Reprod Health. 2011 Sep;15(3):93-101.

[77] Baczynska A, Friis Svenstrup H, Fedder J, Birkelund S, Christiansen G. The use of enzyme-linked immunosorbent assay for detection of Mycoplasma hominis antibodies in infertile women serum samples. Hum Reprod. 2005 May;20(5):1277-85.

[78] Tsuji I, Ami K, Miyazaki A, Hujinami N, Hoshiai H. Benefit of diagnostic laparoscopy for patients with unexplained infertility and normal hysterosalpingography findings. Tohoku J Exp Med. 2009;219(1):39-42.

[79] Gocmen, A. and T. Atak. "Diagnostic laparoscopy findings in unexplained infertility cases." Clin Exp Obstet Gynecol 2012;39(4): 452-453.

[80] Nakagawa, K., S. Ohgi, T. Horikawa, R. Kojima, M. Ito and H. Saito. "Laparoscopy should be strongly considered for women with unexplained infertility." J Obstet Gynaecol Res 2007;33(5): 665-670.

[81] Bonneau C, Chanelles O, Sifer C, Poncelet C. Use of laparoscopy in unexplained infertility. European Journal of Obstetrics & Gynecology and Reproductive Biology 2012; 58-60.

[82] Atef M. Darwish, Ahmad I. Hassanin, Mahmoud A. Abdel Aleem, Ibraheem I. Mohammad, Islam H. Aboushama. Routine vaginoscopic office hysteroscopy in modern infertility work-up: A randomized controlled trial. Gynecologic Surgery. April 2014 online.

Section 2

Gynecologic Emergencies

Chapter 2

Overview of Gynaecological Emergencies

Dagogo Sementari Abam

Additional information is available at the end of the chapter

http://dx.doi.org/10.5772/59107

1. Introduction

Gynaecological emergencies are disease conditions of the female reproductive system that threaten the life of the woman, her sexual function and the perpetuation of her fertility. Common gynaecological emergencies present as acute abdomen, abnormal vaginal bleeding, or a combination of both, and are often related to early pregnancy complications, pelvic inflammatory disease (PID) and contraceptive issues.

Some hospitals, mostly in the developed world, have specialist Emergency Gynaecology Units that provide fast intervention for acute gynaecological problems, such as pelvic pain, severe menorrhagia, vulvar problems, acute PID, hyperemesis gravidarum and post gynaecology surgical problems. These units are often manned by specialist nurses, sonologists and an on-call gynaecology medical team headed by a consultant gynaecologist. The aim of such a unit is to deliver adequate healthcare quickly, thus reducing the possible complications, and in so doing reducing the morbidity and mortality associated with such cases.

Advances in sonography, biochemical pregnancy testing, minimal access surgery and new antibiotics have led to early diagnosis of these conditions and adoption of more conservative approaches to treatment.

The basic objective of this chapter is to have an overview of these emergency gynaecological conditions on an individual basis, and their management. The management of these cases often requires history taking, clinical examination, investigations, both general and specific, and instituting the required treatment plan. Time is of the essence in these cases and so often there is an overlap in the management steps, with some requiring immediate resuscitation.

2. Ectopic pregnancy

Ectopic pregnancy is one in which the conceptus implants outside the normal endometrial lining of the uterus, with the vast majority, over 95%, occurring in the fallopian tube [1]. It is a life-threatening gynaecological emergency and a leading cause of maternal morbidity and mortality in the early half of pregnancy [2], [3].

The incidence of ectopic pregnancy is increasing worldwide [4], and reported incidence varies from 1:60 to 1:250 pregnancies, and is dependent on the incidence of genital tract pathology and contraceptive practices of the population studied [5].

Delay in the diagnosis of ectopic pregnancy can be catastrophic because of the associated haemorrhage. Ectopic pregnancy should always be ruled out when a woman in the reproductive age bracket presents with a missed period and abdominal pain.

There should be a high index of suspicion for early intervention and reduction of morbidity and mortality [6]. The presentation could be acute or chronic. Patients usually present with lower abdominal pain and minimal vaginal bleeding after 5-8 weeks period of amenorrhoea. There could also be shoulder tip pain and fainting spells if intraperitoneal bleeding is massive.

It is mandatory that patients with ectopic pregnancy be managed in a hospital. Sensitive pregnancy test and ultrasonography, preferably a transvaginal scan, aid in initial diagnosis. Laparoscopy may also be used to diagnose ectopic pregnancy, but fails to detect early ectopic pregnancies or those obscured by adhesion. Diagnostic mini-laparotomy comes into play here.

Expectant or medical management of ectopic pregnancy should be considered in selected cases, but they are not widely practiced [7]. Some ectopic pregnancies resolve spontaneously, and this is the basis for expectant management. Methotrexate is employed for medical management in patients with unruptured ectopic pregnancy who are haemodynamically stable [8].

Surgery remains the mainstay of treatment of ectopic pregnancy. Surgical management is carried out by laparoscopy (Fig. 1) or laparotomy. For tubal pregnancy surgery may be radical (salpingectomy) or conservative (usually salpingostomy). For patients with ruptured ectopic pregnancy, especially those who present late, resuscitation and emergency laparotomy and salpingectomy are often required [9].

Patients managed for ectopic pregnancy require counselling because of the risk of recurrence, which is up to 20.5%, and such cases often give rise to diagnostic dilemma, especially when it occurs in an ipsilateral location [10]. Misdiagnosis of ectopic pregnancy may lead to dire consequences and an increase in case fatality [11, 12].

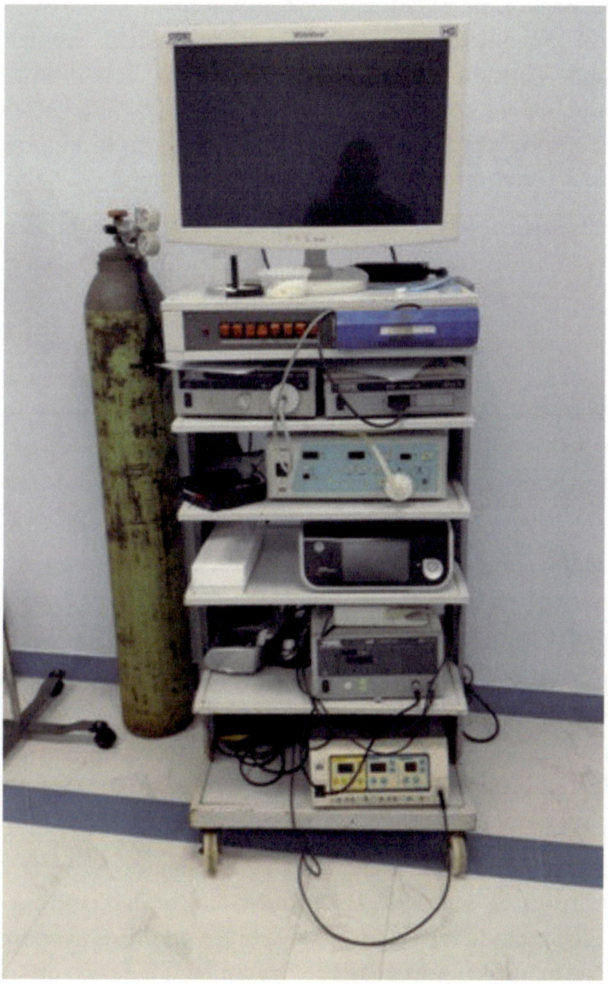

Figure 1. Laparoscopy equipment.

3. Miscarriage

The World Health Organization (WHO) defined abortion (preferably termed as miscarriage) as the termination of pregnancy prior to 20 weeks of gestation, or the birth of a fetus weighing less than 500g in case the period of gestation is not known. It is noteworthy to state here that a very early miscarriage can sometimes be assumed to be a delayed menstrual period.

There are several types of miscarriages – threatened, inevitable, incomplete, complete, missed, septic, spontaneous, habitual and induced. Miscarriages are a common problem. Approximately 75% of all miscarriages occur before 16 weeks of gestation and of these nearly three-quarters occur within the first 8 weeks of pregnancy [13].

Abortions, mostly the unsafe, are a leading cause of maternal mortality worldwide, accounting for a global average of 13% of fatalities related to pregnancy [14]. Estimates by the WHO give a global annual total of 42 million induced abortions, with 20 million being unsafe [15, 16]. About 98% of unsafe abortions occur in developing regions [16, 17]. Unsafe abortion generally refers to termination of unwanted pregnancy either by persons lacking the necessary skills or it being performed in an environment lacking the minimal medical standards, or both.

Vaginal bleeding with associated abdominal pain is a common complication in the first half of pregnancy, and most miscarriages present in this manner. There is a psychological impact of early pregnancy loss on women, their partners and families. For some there is need for psychological support.

For the management of miscarriages there is need for proper patient assessment with respect to the history and clinical evaluation, with the need to rule out ectopic gestation. If the vaginal bleeding is moderate to severe and the patient is in some distress or shock, an intravenous line should be set up with a wide bore cannula and crystalloids quickly infused, and blood samples collected for complete blood count and cross-matching of blood for possible transfusion.

Uterine evacuation is the management option for miscarriages, except for threatened miscarriage which requires a conservative approach. Retained products of conception may lead to infection and haemorrhage.

Surgical uterine evacuation is done either by vacuum aspiration or by sharp curettage. The use of the metal curette is not without complications, which invariably includes anaesthetic risk, risk of infection, bleeding, cervical trauma, uterine perforation, long term complications of decreased fertility and abnormal menstruation, including Asherman's syndrome. The suction curettage is safer and easier than the metal/sharp curettage.

Non-surgical management options for miscarriages include expectant management and medical treatment. Expectant management requires an understanding of the course of an abortive process, which includes resorption of early pregnancies to complete abortion. Here, there is a need for close monitoring and early intervention if the need arises. Medical treatment on the other hand involves the use of drugs to achieve uterine evacuation. The medications used here are the prostaglandins and their derivatives like misoprostol, and the antiprogestogens like mifepristone.

With expectant and medical treatment, the risks and side effects include unpredictability of the timing until the abortion is completed (with the possibility of significant pain and bleeding requiring an emergent curettage) and retained products of conception requiring surgical intervention. Expectant and medical treatments of abortion assume that prompt medical evaluation and possible intervention are immediately on ground if required, otherwise they should not be considered.

Septic abortion results from any type of miscarriage complicated by infection, especially unsafe abortion, resulting in foul smelling vaginal discharge and/or bleeding, with fever and lower abdominal pain/tenderness. Here, it is advised to cover with appropriate intravenous antibiotics for at least 6 hours prior to evacuation of retained products of conception. The antibiotics should be continued for a total of 14 days.

For missed abortion, there is a need to ripen the cervix before evacuation of retained products of conception after having confirmed the diagnosis by ultrasonography, which is often repeated in cases of very early gestations to ascertain non-viability, and making provisions for management of disseminated intravascular coagulopathy (DIC) if such should arise.

Habitual abortions, which entail at least three consecutive miscarriages, would require screening of patients before they embark on future pregnancy, but most turn out negative. Only a few, those positive for antiphospholipid antibodies (APA), can be treated with anticlotting agents, like aspirin, enoxaparin (clexane) and heparin, to improve outcome. For those with cervical incompetence resulting in second trimester miscarriages or early preterm births, cervical cerclage procedures may need to be performed between 14-16 weeks of gestation. Most of those with habitual abortion still have a successful pregnancy.

The complications of abortions, mostly haemorrhage and infection, and iatrogenic injuries like perforated uterus (Fig. 2) and gut injuries [18, 19, 20] cut across the different types of abortions, especially if the secondary care given for cases of spontaneous incomplete abortion is less than optimal. Laparoscopy, and/or laparotomy, is indicated to determine the extent of injury and to properly manage.

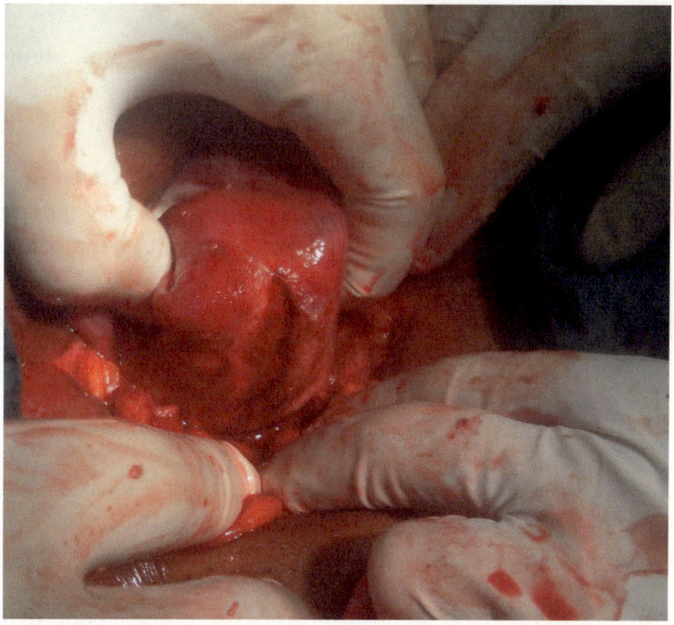

Figure 2. Perforation on the anterior uterine wall following instrumentation demonstrated at laparotomy.

Most healthcare systems expend far more resources treating complications of unsafe abortion than they would to provide safe abortion services [21, 22]. These costs are mostly on beds, antibiotics, blood transfusions services, surgeries and management of subsequent long term complications like ectopic pregnancy and infertility.

There is the need to send the specimen obtained from uterine evacuation for pathological analysis and for cervical/vaginal cultures to be obtained in cases of infection. Histopathological study may also exclude gestational trophoblastic diseases which can present in a similar manner to the miscarriages, may require suction evacuation of the uterus, but also do require a specific follow up plan, which may indicate the need for further treatment.

4. Severe pelvic pain

Based on the history pelvic pain could either be cyclical or non-cyclical. Cyclical pain is commonly as a result of pre-menstrual syndrome, pelvic endometriosis, primary dysmenorrhoea and ovulation pain (Mittelschmerz). For non-cyclical pain the common causes include pelvic inflammatory disease (PID), severe endometriosis, pelvic tumours, pelvic congestion syndrome and surgical causes like appendicitis and diverticulitis. A good history is required to make a possible diagnosis. The nature of the pain, whether cyclical or non-cyclical, acute or chronic (if present for 6 months or more), severity and exacerbating and relieving factors should be noted. Other associations to be noted include the parity, vaginal discharge, abnormal vaginal bleeding, dyspareunia, urinary symptoms, gastrointestinal symptoms, loss of appetite, weight loss and cervical smear.

Examination of the patient would involve general and systemic examinations, most especially the abdomen, pelvis and vagina. Pallor, wasting, abdominal distension, masses in the abdomen and pelvis, and abnormal growth in the lower genital tract should be sought for.

For the investigations, ultrasonography of the abdomen and the pelvis plays a key role. A growth in the lower genital tract may require a biopsy, and tumour marker screen for cancer antigen 125 (CA-125), carcino-embryonic antigen (CEA) and alpha feto-protein (AFP) may be required for pelvic tumours. A complete blood count, C-reactive protein and urine culture are often required. Diagnostic laparoscopy, when available, is a positive addition in the management of chronic pelvic pain when there is diagnostic difficulty, but not forgetting idiopathic pain.

5. Ovarian cysts

Tumours of the ovary are common in women, with about 80% being benign and occurring in the reproductive age group [23]. Ovarian tumours are multifaceted and their classification is based on the historical cell of origin [24, 25]. About 70-80% of primary ovarian tumours are epithelial in origin, 10% stromal and 5% germ cell, while the rest fall into other groups [26]. Dermoid cyst is one of the commonest ovarian tumours in child-bearing age [27], and 10% of cases are diagnosed during pregnancy [28].

Generally, ovarian cysts that are painful may be as a result of torsion (Fig. 3), haemorrhage, rupture, be endometriotic or cancerous. Torsion of ovarian cyst commonly presents as severe acute lower abdominal pain that is often associated with nausea and vomiting. The abdomen is usually tender, with a palpable pelvic mass on bimanual pelvic examination and ultrasonography would reveal a large ovarian cyst. Such patients should be managed in a hospital and they require emergency surgery, usually a laparotomy. Conservative surgery (cystectomy) is usually carried out, but sometimes ovarectomy is done.

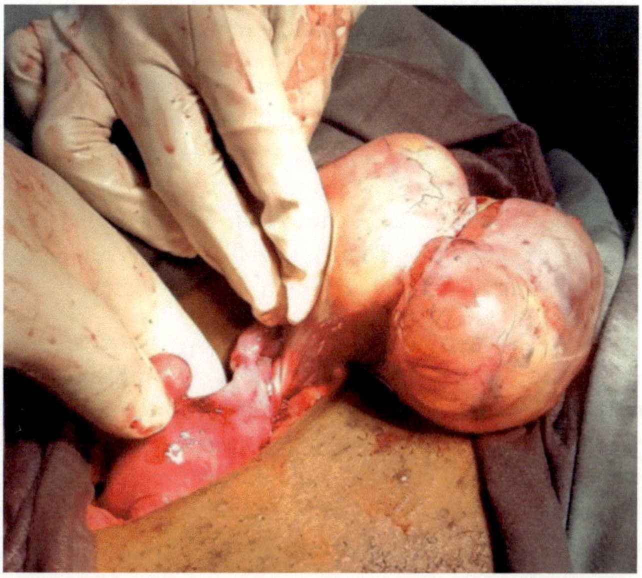

Figure 3. Torsion of left ovarian cyst (see torted stalk). This patient also had subserous uterine fibroids.

Ruptured ovarian cyst presents in a similar way to torsion of ovarian cyst. The patient may be known to have an ovarian cyst but this is no longer seen on ultrasonography. There may be evidence of peritonitis, including chemical peritonitis if the cyst was originally a dermoid cyst [29], and haemoperitonium. The patient would probably require a laparotomy if the condition worsens and so should be admitted to hospital urgently.

6. Uterine fibroids

Uterine leiomyomas or fibroids are benign tumours that arise from the myometrial smooth muscle fibres. They are the commonest tumours found in the human body. It is estimated that one-fifth of all women have one or more in the uterus at death [30]. Fibroids are present in 20-25% of women of reproductive age, commonly associated with nulliparity, and for some uncertain reasons are 3-9 times more common in blacks [30, 31]. Most uterine fibroids are symptomless but 35-50% of patients have symptoms [31], and these are dependent on their location, size, state of preservation and/ or degeneration, and whether or not the patient is pregnant.

Fibroids are usually not painful. Acute pain may arise under certain circumstances, such as torsion of pedunculated fibroids, degeneration (especially red degeneration), associated endometriosis/adenomyosis, and/or expulsion of pedunculated submucous fibroids through the cervix [32]. Fibroid also rarely causes acute pain when it outgrows its blood supply, thereby causing necrosis. Spasmodic dysmenorrhoea may result when expulsion of a pedunculated submucous fibroid stimulates uterine contraction [32]. Sarcomatous change, which occurs in 0.1-0.5% of cases [31], can result in pain as well. There is the need to look out for other co-morbid conditions in cases of fibroids associated with pains.

With respect to the treatment of fibroids the factor considered in this section is the pain, therefore the patient has to be thoroughly evaluated; history, examination, and investigations. Pain is generally managed with the use of analgesics, ranging from acetaminophen (paracetamol) to non-steroidal anti-inflammatory drugs and opioids. Definitive treatment would require surgery if analgesics alone, sometimes with antibiotics in cases associated with infection, fail to alleviate the symptoms. There is usually no room for use of medical treatment options for fibroids presenting with acute abdomen or severe pains.

Definitive surgical modalities for management of uterine fibroids include myomectomy, which leaves behind a functional uterus and thus preserving fertility, and hysterectomy, which is desirable for patients over 40 years of age and those not desirous of future fertility. Both procedures can be carried out via the abdominal route, vaginal route, or even laparoscopically. Hysteroscopic myomectomy is indicated for submucous fibroids complicated by abnormal bleeding with pain. Robotic surgery is employed in high technology medical facilities, especially in countries with advanced healthcare systems.

7. Acute Pelvic Inflammatory Disease

Pelvic inflammatory disease (PID) is a spectrum of inflammatory disorders of the upper female genital tract, including any combination of endometritis, salpingitis, oophoritis or tubo-ovarian abscess and pelvic peritonitis/cellulitis. Sexually transmitted organisms, particularly Neisseria gonorrhoeae and Chlamydia trachomatis, are implicated in many cases. Organisms of the vaginal flora however also cause PID, which is often polymicrobial.

There is a worldwide increase in the incidence of PID, and it is the most common infectious disease that affects young women and accounts for a significant percentage of the morbidity that is associated with sexually transmitted diseases (STDs). Although it does not usually constitute an emergency in the sense that immediate treatment is life-saving, urgent treatment is required to minimize the effect of the disease on subsequent fertility and reduces the risk of sequelae such as ectopic pregnancy and chronic pelvic pain. This applies to both mild and severe disease.

The diagnosis of PID is usually based on clinical features although clinical diagnosis is usually imprecise, and many cases of PID go unrecognized or are subclinical. These patients are usually young, sexually active, and complain of abdominal pain, with or without fever and vaginal discharge. Bimanual pelvic examination usually elicits extreme tenderness on movement of the cervix, uterus and parametria. On laboratory investigations, saline microscopy of vaginal discharge may show abundant leucocytic infiltration, complete blood count may reveal leucocytosis, and C-reactive protein and erythrocyte sedimentation rate may be raised.

Endocervical swab may be positive for infection with N. gonorrhoeae and C. trachomatis. The true significance of this is questionable and the results lack consistency. However all women who have acute PID should be tested for these organisms, and screened for other STDs [33].

Endometrial biopsy, though not often done in practice, is more specific and usually shows histopathologic evidence of endometritis. Imaging, most especially transvaginal ultrasonography, showing thickened fluid-filled tubes with or without free fluid in the pouch of Douglas or tubo-ovarian mass are quite specific for PID. In less complicated cases imaging may be normal.

Laparoscopy is the gold standard for diagnosis of PID. However limited access and attendant surgical risks preclude its universal use for this purpose. The criteria for diagnosis of PID using laparoscopy include visualizing an overt hyperaemia of the tubal surface, oedema of the tubal wall, and sticky exudates on the tubal surface and/or fimbrial ends. All 3 are required for diagnosis.

The treatment of PID is essentially empirical, with use of antibiotics (parenteral and oral) for 10-14 days. Based on the severity and response to treatment this can either be done on outpatient or inpatient basis. Goals of treatment are to alleviate the acute symptoms of inflammation, and prevent the long term sequelae associated with PID. There may be need for contact tracing and treatment of sexual partners. Follow up and education are necessary to prevent re-infection and complications.

For those complicated by tubo-ovarian abscess unresponsive to extended antibiotic therapy, surgical management involving exploratory laparotomy by an experienced gynaecologic surgeon may be required. The extent of the surgery depends on the extent of the disease, the patient's age and desire for future fertility. There is risk of injury to contiguous structures as a result of the inflammatory process, which may cause adhesions and a frozen pelvis.

8. Pelvic endometriosis

Endometriosis is the presence of endometrial stroma and glands outside of the uterine cavity. The pelvis is the commonest site, with the reproductive organs the most frequently affected [34]. The most common symptoms related to it are dysmenorrhoea, dyspareunia and low back pain which worsen during menstruation, and subfertility. It is a leading cause of disability in women of reproductive age, and the pain may be mild, or it may be severe enough to negatively affect health-related quality of life.

Endometriosis remains a difficult clinical problem and quite a number of patients are often referred to other specialists before seeing the gynaecologist [35]. Painful symptoms, especially when cyclical, may be caused by endometriosis, and it is the underlying cause of pelvic pain in 15% of cases [36]. The exact prevalence is unknown because surgery and/or histology is required for its diagnosis, but estimates of 3-10% of women in the reproductive age group, and 25-35% of infertile women have been made [37].

The symptoms of endometriosis and the laparoscopic findings do not always correlate [38]. The focus during management should be on the illness rather than the disease. There is no place for medical treatment of endometriosis with drugs in infertile women desirous of having babies [39]. Surgery can be done via laparotomy or laparoscopy [40, 41]. Analgesics are often required for symptomatic relief of pain. Unlike infection, endometriosis does not damage the luminal epithelium of the fallopian tube, and thus conservative surgery is more likely to be successful in restoring normal anatomic relations. However, endometriosis is also a well known cause of frozen pelvis.

9. Severe vaginal bleeding

Severe vaginal bleeding may or may not be related to menstruation. Common causes are dysfunctional uterine bleeding (DUB), uterine fibroids, adenomyosis and genital tract malignancy.

Normal menstrual cycles range from 21-35 days, with the estimated blood loss less than 80 ml, with flow not more than 7 days. Most women who complain of heavy periods have normal loss. Extremely heavy menstrual loss is uncommon and other causes such as a miscarriage or a genital tract malignancy like carcinoma of the cervix or endometrial carcinoma should be ruled out. If the patient is symptomatic after a heavy menstrual loss, like having dizziness or fainting spells, appears pale or has tachycardia, she should be admitted to hospital for treatment.

Patients with massive vaginal bleeding require resuscitation which includes securing of intravenous access with a wide bore cannula, obtaining blood samples for a complete blood count and infusing of crystalloids. Possible causes of the vaginal bleeding should be ruled out. There is the need to correct anaemia with haematinics and even blood transfusion.

Control of bleeding may be achieved by use of haemostatic drugs like tranexamic acid (an antifibrinolytic agent) and ethamsylate, or by hormonals like medroxyprogesterone, prior to definitive treatment of the cause. Mirena, a levonorgestrel-impregnated intrauterine system, and endometrial ablation techniques like the NovaSure system may also be employed [42] for control of bleeding.

The definitive treatment is dependent on the cause and emergency dilatation and curettage (D&C), myomectomy, and even a hysterectomy (Fig. 4) are possibilities. For those emanating from gynaecological cancers referral to oncology units with expertise in their management is required.

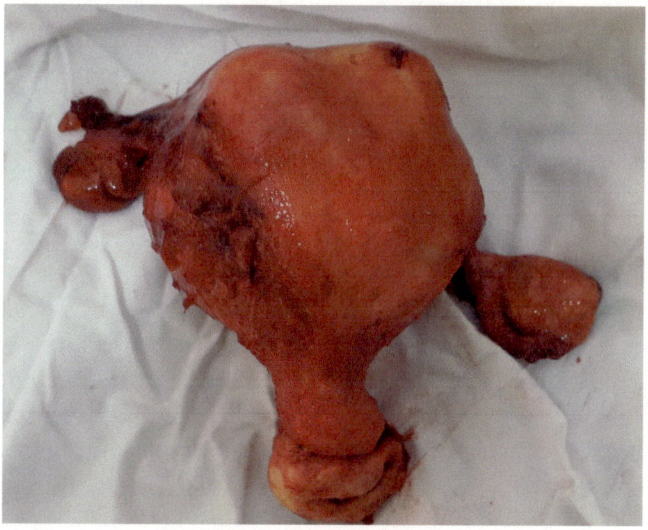

Figure 4. Hysterectomy specimen of a 50-year old woman who had total abdominal hysterectomy and bilateral salpingo-oophorectomy for uterine fibroids associated with menorrhagia.

10. Vulvar abscesses

Bartholin's cysts are the commonest cysts of the vulva, and they are of two types, a cyst of the duct and a cyst of the gland, with differentiation made on histology using the surface epithelium. The position of the swelling at the junction of the anterior two-third and the posterior one-third of the labia majora is diagnostic. Bartholin's abscesses are secondarily infected cysts. Organisms involved in the infection of the gland are similar to those responsible for PID [43, 44].

Drainage should be established whenever an abscess develops. Apart from the pains, which may be severe, there is the theoretical risk of ascending infection, with a more extreme inflammatory process, with systemic symptoms and signs of infection, and these may affect the quality of life. Cases of necrotizing fasciitis have been reported in immuno-compromised women, including those with diabetes mellitus. Septic shock and toxic shock-like syndrome can also complicate Bartholin's abscess [45], [46].

The treatment of Bartholin's abscess encompasses bed rest, use of antibiotics and analgesics, coupled with surgical drainage and warm sitz bath. The procedure of choice for surgical drainage is marsupialization, and this has the advantage of preserving the gland, which continues its secretory function and prevents recurrence by the creation of a new gland ostium or fistula to replace the function of the presumed damaged or obstructed duct. Simple incision and drainage (I&D) of the abscess is associated with a high recurrence rate.

Abscesses that rupture spontaneously are treated by warm sitz bath. Gland excision is not recommended for Bartholin's abscess because of the risk of spread of infection which may result following surgery in an inflamed hyperaemic tissue environment [47].

Another less common vulvar abscess is that involving the Skene's gland. Treatment basically follows the same principles as that for Barthoin's abscess.

11. Toxic shock syndrome

Toxic shock syndrome is a rare entity primarily occurring in menstruating women and caused by exotoxins produced by penicillinase-producing non invasive Staphylococcus aureus of phage type 1. It is associated with use of super absorbent tampons, especially if left in place for long. Tampon use may also excoriate the cervical and vaginal mucous membranes, thereby encouraging absorption of the exotoxin.

Non-menstrual toxic shock syndrome has been reported with prolonged use of contraceptive diaphragm or sponge [48], after delivery, laser therapy for condylomata acuminatum [49] and non-gynaecological surgery.

Toxic shock syndrome can also be caused by some streptococcus species, including Streptococcus viridans which causes a more fulminant disease with high mortality.

The clinical manifestations of toxic shock syndrome are diverse and these often develop rapidly in otherwise healthy persons. These include sudden onset of high fever, hypotension, and associated symptoms like vomiting, diarrhoea, myalgia, abdominal pain, and headache. A characteristic "sunburn-like" rash, a diffuse maculopapular erythroderma, appears over the face, trunk and proximal extremities over a period of 5-14 days, which later desquamates, especially over the palms and soles during convalescence. Multi-systemic involvement is typical and these include coagulopathy, renal, hepatic, muscular, cardiovascular, neurological and respiratory systems.

On taking a history, ask the patient if she is menstruating or using tampons. A vaginal examination should be performed and any foreign body in the vagina such as tampon or contraceptive device should be removed.

The diagnosis of toxic shock syndrome is usually clinical. A full septic and biochemical screen should be done to exclude multiorgan failure. Isolation of the exotoxin for Staphylococcus aureus is pathognomonic.

Treatment entails aggressive supportive therapy, preferably in an intensive care unit. Fluid resuscitation is necessary, and vasopressors, packed red cells and coagulation factors, mechanical ventilation and haemodialysis may be required. Antibiotics, given intravenously, are used for 10-14 days to eradicate the organism. Protein synthesis inhibitors such as clindamycin which suppress toxin production are more effective than cell wall active agents like beta-lactams. Cephalosporins or beta-lactamase-resistant penicillins like nafcillin or oxacillin, and vancomycin (for penicillin-allergic patients) may also be used. Since toxic shock syndrome is toxin related, antibiotic treatment is not directly effective, but it reduces the bacterial load and ultimately prevents further toxin production.

12. Sexual violence

Rape definitions vary from country to country, but generally regarded as the physically forced entry or the otherwise coerced penetration of the mouth, vulva, vagina or anus with a penis, other body part or object. It is an act of sexual violence. It can result in serious short and long-term physical, mental, sexual and reproductive health problems for victims and their families and can lead to social and economic costs.

Health consequences may include headache, back pain, abdominal pain, gastrointestinal disorders, limited mobility and poor overall health. Non fatal and fatal injuries can also result.

Rape can result in unwanted pregnancies, gynaecological problems, induced abortions, sexually transmitted infections, including human immunodeficiency virus (HIV) and hepatitis B infections. Mental disorders like post-traumatic stress disorder, sleep difficulties, depression, suicidal tendencies and drug and alcohol abuse can arise.

Some gynaecologists hardly receive proper orientation or training in managing intimate partner violence as part of their medical training and therefore tend to underestimate the extent of the problem and feel insufficiently skilled to deal with it [50]. Treatment here typically involves dealing with coital lacerations, STDs, including HIV and hepatitis-B post-exposure prophylaxis, tetanus prophylaxis, and emergency contraception to prevent unwanted pregnancy. Due to the extent of coital injuries, especially when foreign objects are used, emergency laparotomy may be required.

It is crucial that advice is sought from the police or sexual assault referral centre before undertaking any examination for forensic reasons, unless it is life-saving. Pictures of the victim, multiple swabs and aspirations from body cavities and parts, and a whole lot more may need to be taken. A checklist may be required to follow due process on the management of such cases, as well as employing the services of a clinical psychologist or psychiatrist for long-term management.

Author details

Dagogo Sementitari Abam*

Address all correspondence to: dagabam@yahoo.com

Department of Obstetrics and Gynaecology, Faculty of Clinical Sciences, College of Health Sciences, University of Port Harcourt, Nigeria

References

[1] Varma R, Mascarenhas L. Evidence based mangement of ectopic pregnancy. Current Obstet Gynaecol (2002) 12, 191-199.

[2] Olarewaju RS, Ujah IAO, Otubu JAM. Trends in ectopic pregnancy in the Jos University Teaching Hospital, Jos, Nigeria. Nig J Med 1994, 26:57-60.

[3] Grimes DA. The morbidity and mortality of pregnancy. Still risky business. Am J Obstet Gynecol 1994:170:1489-1494.

[4] Pisarka MD, Carson SA, Buster JE. Ectopic pregnancy. Lancet 1998; 351:115-20.

[5] Nair U. Acute abdomen and abdominal pain in pregnancy. Current Obstet Gynaecol (2003) 13, 14-20.

[6] Strandell A, Thorbum J, Hamberger L. Risk factors for ectopic pregnancy in assisted reproduction. Fertil Steril 1999; 71(2);282-6.

[7] Tay JI, Moore J, Walker JJ. Ectopic pregnancy. Regular review. BMJ. 2000, 300:916-9.

[8] Jimenez-Caraballo A, Rodriguez-Donoso G. A 6-year clinical trial of methotrexate therapy in the treatment of ectopic pregnancy. Eur J Obstet Gynaecol Reprod Bio 1998, 79:167-71.

[9] Abam DS, Ojule JD, Oriji VK. A three year review of management of ectopic pregnancy at the University of Port Harcourt Teaching Hospital. The Nigeria Health Journal Vol 7 No. 3&4 2007, 480-84.

[10] Okunlola MA, Adesina OA, Adekunle AO. Repeat ipsilateral ectopic gestation: a series of 3 cases. Afr J Med Sc 2006, Jun, 35(2):173-5.

[11] Orji EO, Fasubaa OB, Adeyemi B, Dare FO Onwudiegwu U, Ogunniyi SO. Mortality and morbidity associated with misdiagnosis of ectopic pregnancy in a defined Nigerian population. J Obstet Gynecol 2002, Sep 22(5): 548-50.

[12] Baffoe S, Nkyekyer K. Ectopic Pregnancy in Korle Bu Teaching Hospital, Ghana: a three-year review. Trop Doct 1999 Jan; 29 (1) 18-22.

[13] Saxena R. Early Pregnancy bleeding due to miscarriage. In: Saxena R. Bedside Obstetrics and Gynaecology 2nd edition. Jaypee Brothers Medical Publishers, New Delhi, 2014, 161-86.

[14] World Health Organization. Maternal mortality in 1995. Estimates developed by WHO, UNICEF and UNFPA. WHO/RHR/01.9. Geneva, WHO, 2001.

[15] World Health Organization. Safe abortion. Technical and Policy Guidance for Health Systems. Geneva, WHO, 2003.

[16] Sedgh G, Henshaw S, Singh S, Ahman E, Shah I. Induced abortion: estimated rates and trends worldwide. Lancet, 2007, 370(9595): 1338-45.

[17] World Health Organization. Unsafe abortion: global and regional estimates of incidence of unsafe abortion and associated mortality in 2008. Sixth edition. Geneva, WHO, 2011.

[18] Fawole AA, Aboyeji AP. Complications of unsafe abortion: presentations at Ilorin, Nigeria. Niger J Med 11(2) 2002; 77-80.

[19] Darney PD, Atkinson E, Hirabayashi K. Uterine perforation during second trimester abortion by cervical dilation and instrumental extraction: a review of 15 cases. Obstet Gynecol 1990, Mar; 75 (3Pt1). 441-4.

[20] Unuigbe JA, Oronsanye AU, Orhue AA. Abortion related morbidity and mortality in Benin City, Nigeria: 1973-1985. Int. J. Gynaecol Obstet. 1988 June; 26 (3) 435-39.

[21] Kay B, Katzenellenbogen J, Fawcus S, Karim SA. An analysis of the cost of incomplete abortion to the public health sector in South African-1994. South Afr Med J. 87, 442-7, 1997.

[22] Johnson BR, Benson J, Bradley J, Robago Ordonez A. Costs and resource utilization for the treatment of incomplete abortion in Kenya and Mexico. Social Sciences and Medicine, 36 (11) 1443-53, 1993.

[23] Cotran RS, Kumar V, Collins T. Ovarian tumours. Robbins Pathological basis of disease. 1999, 6th edition. 1065-1079.

[24] Russel P, Bannatyne P. Surgical pathology of the ovaries. Churchill Livingstone, Edinburgh, 1989.

[25] Serov SF, Scully RE, Sobin LH. International histological classification of tumours. No 9. Histological typing of ovarian tumours, WHO, Geneva, 1973.

[26] Bhatia N. Tumours of the ovary. In: Jeffcoates Principles of Gynaecology. International Edition (5th). 2001 Arnold. 503-540.

[27] Briggs ND. Common gynaecological tumours. Trop J Obstet Gynaecol. 1995; 12(12): 62-71.

[28] Caruso PA, Marsh MR, Minkowitz S, Karten G. An intense clinicopathologic study of 305 teratomas of the ovary. Cancer. 1971; 27(2):343-348.

[29] Climie AR, Heath LP. "Malignant degeneration of benign cystic teratomas of the ovary. Review of the literature and report of a chondrosarcoma and carcinoid tumor". Cancer 22:824-32, 1968.

[30] Whitefield CR, Benign tumours of the uterus. In: Whitefield CR ed. Dewhurst's Textbook of Obstetrics and Gynaecology for Postgraduate, 5th ed. Blackwell science, 736-746.

[31] Memarzadeh S, Broder MS, Wexler AS. Benign disorders of the uterine corpus. In: Decherney AH, Nathan L, Eds. Current Obstetrics and Gynecology Diagnosis and Treatment. International Edition. 9th ed. 2003. Lange. 693-707.

[32] Saxena R. Menorrhagia due to leiomyomas. In: Saxena R. Bedside Obstetrics and Gynaecology, 2nd edition Jaypee Brothers Medical Publishers, New Delhi, 2014, 691-737.

[33] Mackay G. Sexually transmitted diseases and pelvic infections. In: Decherney AH, Nathan L, Laufer N, Roman AS. Eds. Current Obstetrics and Gynnecology Diagnosis and Treatment. International edition. 11th ed. 2013, McGraw-Hill, Lange. 691-737.

[34] John CT, Ikimalo JI, Anya SE. Endometriosis. In: Comprehensive Gynaecology in the Tropics. Kwawukume EY, Emuveyan EE eds. 2005. Graphic Parkaging Limited. 158-67.

[35] Prentice A. Endometriosis. Regular review. BMJ. 2001; 323(7304):93-5.

[36] Mahmood TA, Templeton A. Prevalence and genesis of endometriosis. Hum Reprod. 1991; 6(4): 544-9.

[37] Memarzadeh S, Muse KN, Fox MD. Endometriosis, In: Current Obstetrics and Gynaecology Diagnosis and Treatment. Decherney AH, Nathan L. eds. International Edition. 9th ed, 2003, Lange 767-775.

[38] Vercellini P, Trespidi L, De Giorgi O, Cortesi I, Parazzini F, Crosignani PG. Endometriosis and pelvic pain: relation to disease stage and localization. Fertil Steril. 1996; 56:299-304.

[39] Hughes F, Fedorkow D, Collins J, Vandekerckhove P. Ovulation suppression for endometriosis. Cochrane Database Sys Rev. 2003(3):CD000155.

[40] Marcoux S, Maheux R, Berube S. Laparoscopic surgery in infertile women with minimal or mild endometriosis. Canadian Collaborative Group on Endometriosis. N Engl J Med, 1997; 337(4):217-22.

[41] Royal College of Obstetricians and Gynaecologists. The investigation and management of endometriosis. RCOG. 2006; Green-top Guideline No. 24.

[42] Lethaby A, Penninx J, Hicky M, et al. Endometrial resection and ablation techniques for heavy menstrual bleeding. Cochrane Database Syst Rev. 2013;8 CD 001501.

[43] Brook I. Aerobic and anaerobic microbiology of Bartholin's abscess. Surg Gynecol Obstet 1989: 169:32-4.

[44] Lee YH, Rankin JS, Alpert S, Daly AK, McCormack WM. Microbiological investigations of Bartholin's gland abscesses and cysts. Am J Obstet Gynecol 1977; 129:150-4.

[45] Carson GD, Smith LP. Escherichia coli endotoxic shock complicating Bartholin's gland abscess. Can Med Assoc J. 1980, 122(12): 1397-8.

[46] Lopez-Zeno JA, Ross AE, O'Grady JP. Septic shock complicating drainage of a Bartholin gland abscess. Obstet Gynecol 1990. 76(Pt. 2):76:915-6.

[47] Danso KA. Bartholin's gland cyst and abscess In: Kwawukume EY, Emuveyan EE. Comprehensive Gynaecology in the Tropics; 2005. Graphic packaging Limited, 112-113.

[48] Faich G, Pearson K, Fleming D, et al. Toxic shock syndrome and the vaginal contraceptive sponge. JAMA 255; 216, 1986.

[49] Bowen LW, Sand PK, Ostergard DR. Toxic shock syndrome following carbon dioxide laser treatment of genital condyloma acuminatum. Am J Obstet Gynecol 154:145, 1986.

[50] Gutmanis I, Beynon C, Tutty L, Wathen CN, MacMillan HL. Factors influencing identification of and response to intimate partner violence – a survey of physicians and nurses. BMC Public Health, 2007;7:12.

Chapter 3

Biomarkers of Ectopic Pregnancy-Present and Future

Soundravally Rajendiren and Pooja Dhiman

Additional information is available at the end of the chapter

http://dx.doi.org/10.5772/58954

1. Introduction

One of the most common complications of pregnancy is early pregnancy failure, of which 25% result in miscarriages and 1-2% ends in ectopic pregnancy. Both these entities can present with similar symptoms of abdominal pain and/or vaginal bleeding [1]. The most common site of ectopic pregnancy is fallopian tube. As tubal ectopic pregnancy (EP) is associated with high morbidity and mortality, early and accurate diagnosis of this condition is warranted. Present protocols for diagnosis of ectopic pregnancy utilize serial serum human chorionic gonadotropin (β-hCG) levels and pelvic ultrasound [2]. However, distinction between an intrauterine or extrauterine pregnancy may not be possible in 8-31% of cases at the first visit, even with sophisticated transvaginal ultrasound [3]. As a result, multiple visits for serial β-hCG and ultrasound monitoring are required before a diagnosis can be established and management initiated. This interim period of uncertainty may lead to potential life threatening complications like intra-abdominal bleed and future infertility because of compromised tubal integrity. Therefore, early diagnosis of tubal ectopic not only prevents the added mortality in patients, but also plays an important role in preventing future infertility. Also, the optimal management strategies for ectopic pregnancy and other abnormal intrauterine pregnancy (IUP) like miscarriages differ, and these two distinct clinical entities need to be differentiated at the early stages of pregnancy. A circulating serum biomarker may aid in predicting early pregnancy outcome (viable intrauterine pregnancy, miscarriage or tubal ectopic pregnancy), and may guide in deciding the best management strategy (conservative, medical or surgical) for the patient. Numerous groups have focussed their attention on this issue, and have reported many potential candidate biomarkers. The present chapter discuss the recent status of these candidate biomarkers in diagnosing tubal ectopic pregnancy, along with our experience, and attempt to foresee the future diagnostic trend of this clinically significant entity.

1.1. Problem statement

Tubal ectopic pregnancy is an important cause of early pregnancy failure attributing significantly to morbidity and mortality, in absence of expeditious diagnosis. Currently, the diagnosis of ectopic pregnancy is based on combined ultrasonograhic findings and serial β-hCG levels. However, low positivity rates in early gestational age and a need for repeated testing are major limitations of these diagnostic procedures, leading to added risk of tubal rupture and intra-abdominal bleed. Therefore, a circulating serum based biomarker, which could differentiate tubal ectopic from viable intrauterine pregnancy and other abnormal gestation (miscarriages) at the first visit of the patient, is the need of the hour.

1.2. Application area

A circulating serum based biomarker which could accurately predict the outcome of pregnancy such as ectopic pregnancy, miscarriage and viable intrauterine pregnancy. This may be used to diagnose tubal ectopic, decide the course of management (medical or surgical), and may aid in monitoring the prognosis and response to treatment in patients. This advancement in clinical diagnostic may help in significantly bringing down the maternal morbidity and mortality associated with early pregnancy failure.

1.3. Research course

Due to paucity of suitable animal models of tubal ectopic pregnancy, biomarker researches have mainly been carried out in cohorts of women with tubal ectopic, miscarriages and viable intrauterine pregnancy (IUP).

1.4. Method used

Comprehensive literature search was carried out for identifying studies on women with gestational age of less than 12 weeks in which serum markers were used to predict the outcome of pregnancy. The databases used were Medline, Embase, CINAHIL and Cochrane library, using key work search ectopic pregnancy", "tubal pregnancy" alone and in combination with "diagnosis", "screening" and "biomarkers". Only the articles published in English were included and references of all selected articles were also thoroughly searched. All the studies that assessed diagnostic accuracy were included.

1.5. Status

The factors deciding the fate of first trimester pregnancy, and hence the potential biomarkers for tubal ectopic pregnancy can be systematically categorized into two groups-Markers related to implantation site & milieu and Markers related to embryo (Fig 1). Important biomarkers in both these categories are described

http://dx.doi.org/10.5772/58954

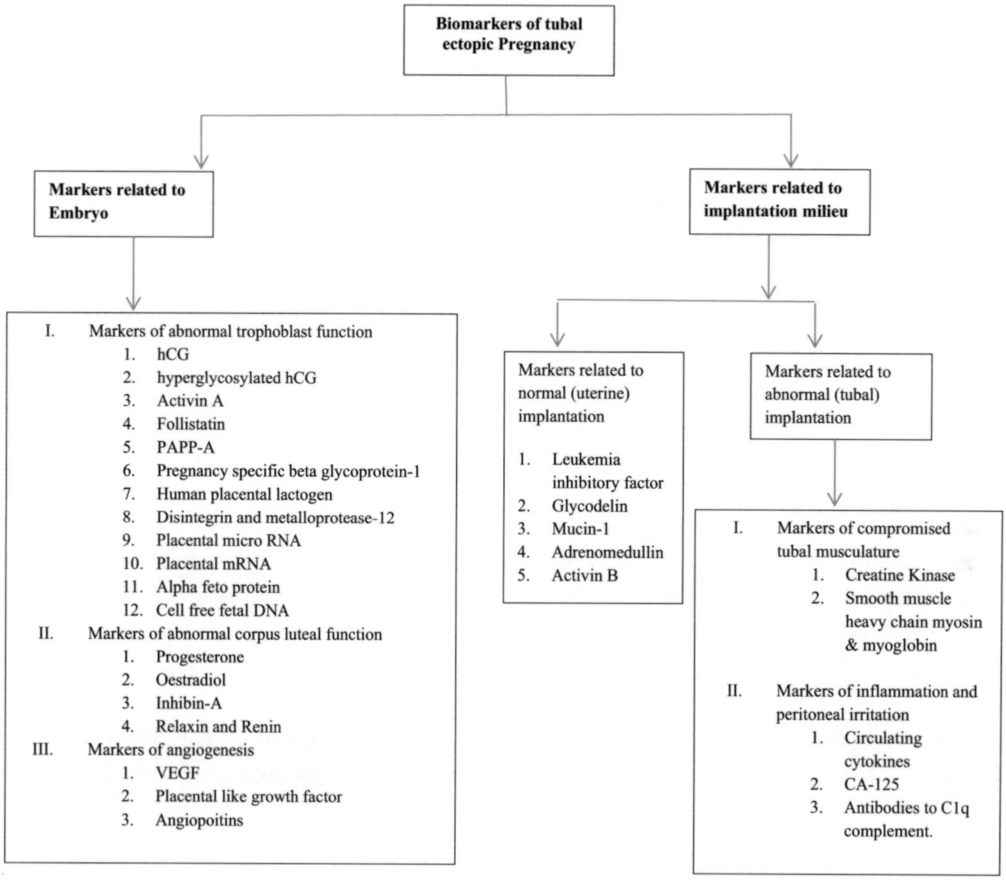

Figure 1. Candidate biomarkers for Ectopic Pregnancy

2. Markers related to embryo

2.1. Markers of abnormal trophoblast function

Theses are the molecules secreted from the conceptus. It would be probable that the pregnancy implanted in the ectopic environment will have abnormal growth kinetics that can be reflected in disarrayed trophoblast function. The following markers have been described in this section:

1. Beta-human chorionic gonadotropin (β-hCG)

It is a glycoprotein hormone produced by trophoblast which maintains corpus luteum. Currently, β-hCG is the only biomarker used clinically in the diagnosis of ectopic pregnancy[4]. A doubling of serum β-hCG over 48 hours is suggestive of viable intrauterine pregnancy [5]. If the levels remain static or fall, it is suggestive of early pregnancy failure, and the diagnosis need to be confirmed by more invasive procedures like endometrial curettage or laproscopy. To prevent unnecessary invasive procedures, studies suggested that the minimum rise of β-hCG over 48 hours to predict normal viable intrauterine pregnancy can be reduced to 53% [6] or 35% [7,8]. Another important concept in serum β-hCG estimation is the discriminatory zone, that is the minimum β-hCG concentration at which an intrauterine gestational sac could be reliably identified on ultrasound. The current discriminatory zone lies between 1500-3000 mIU/L [9]. Recently, a series of mathematical models incorporating β-hCG ratio (serum β-hCG at 48 hours/ serum β-hCG at 0 hours) have been developed to predict early pregnancy outcome, although it has not been sufficiently validated [10-13]. Another retrospective cohort study observed that in addition to the two values of serum β-hCG at 0 and 48 hours, third β-hCG evaluation on day 4 improved the accuracy of ectopic pregnancy prediction by 9.3% [14]. The role of β-hCG has also been studied to predict response to therapy. A cut-off value of 2121 mIU/L of the initial serum β-hCG, has shown a specificity of 76.4% and a sensitivity of 80.56% in predicting response to methotrexate therapy, with poor response below the cut-off [15]. Similarly, a cut-off of more than 1790mIU/ml was found to predict methotrexate treatment failure by another group [16]. Presently, serial monitoring of β-hCG is in use for the diagnostic triage of first trimester bleeding, but further studies are being conducted to use it in the prognostic protocol of EP.

2. Hyperglycosylated hCG

Hyperglycosylated hCG (hCG-H) is a variant of hCG with four instead of two oligosaccharides. The site of production is first trimester invading extravillous cytotrophoblast, where it prevents trophoblast cell apoptosis [17,18]. Low proportions of hCG-H (< 50% of total hCG) was shown to predict failed pregnancy [19,20]. Another study identified a cut-off of 13μg/L for identifying failed pregnancy with 73% sensitivity and 98% specificity [21]. On the other hand, Butler et al did not find a role of hCG-H in the diagnostic algorithm for EP [22]. Recent study explored the role of hCG-H in predicting ongoing pregnancies after in vitro fertilization and found that day 9 level of hCG-H > 110pg/ml was 96% specific for ongoing pregnancy [23]. Conflicting results regarding the use of hCG-H as a marker of preeclampsia have also been reported [24,25]. Since, there is paucity of data on use of either concentration or proportion in distinguishing ectopic pregnancy from miscarriage, further studies are required to validate its usefulness as a biomarker for EP.

3. Activin A

Activin A is a dimeric glycoprotein of TGF-β superfamily, with a role in cytotrophoblast invasion [26]. A study by Florio et al found Activin A level at a cut-off of ≤0.37ng/mL to have 100% sensitivity and 99.6% specificity for the diagnosis of EP [27]. Rausch et al found Activin A to have 80% sensitivity and 72% specificity as a single marker in a cohort of patients with EP [28]. Daponte et al also observed activin A concentrations to be significantly lower in women with EP and women with missed abortion, compared to IUP, and reported that at a threshold value of 505 pg/mL, activin A had 87.9% sensitivity and 100% specificity for discriminating an ectopic pregnancy from viable pregnancies [29]. On the contrary, Activin-A was not found useful in diagnosing EP [30, 31]. Similarly, Elito et al demonstrated that serum activin A levels could not discriminate between an EP from a normal intrauterine pregnancy when an adnexal mass was found by transvaginal scan [32]. Therefore, A validation of this biomarker in a larger cohort would be encouraged before makes it a tool for diagnostics.

4. Follistatin (FS)

Follistatin is a circulating protein produced from human placenta, with rising serum concentration throughout pregnancy [33, 34]. Follistatin is primarily involved in modulating the biological activity of activin by binding to activin by high-affinity, which can neutralize the majority of the actions of activin [35]. Daponte et al reported that the concentration of FS was significantly lower in EP and MA compared to women with a viable IUP, and found that FS was able to discriminate IUP from EP, But not miscarriage from EP [29].

5. Pregnancy associated plasma protein-A (PAPPA)

PAPPA is a glycoprotein produced by trophoblast. Normally, PAPPA is up-regulated by progesterone, which promotes the adhesion and proliferation potential of trophoblastic cells [36]. It has been extensively studied and used as a marker of screening for first trimester aneuploidy [37]. Mueller et al found decreased levels of PAPPA in patients with ectopic pregnancy when compared to normal viable intrauterine pregnancy [38]. Dumps et al found a cut-off of <14.3 ng/ml to have a sensitivity of 64.5% with a 99% specificity for pregnancy failure [39] But the levels were found to be lower in miscarriages making the discrimination between EP and other abnormal intrauterine pregnancy dissatisfactory. On the other hand Ugurlu et al and Daponte et al observed that PAPPA can differentiate abnormal pregnancy from the viable normal IUP [40, 41]. Inconsistency in these results prompts us to study this marker in greater details.

6. Pregnancy specific beta glycoprotein-1 (SP-1)

Pregnancy specific beta glycoprotein-1 (SP-1) is a secreted protein produced from syncytiotrophoblast, thought to be involved in immunomodulation [42]. In addition, recently it has been observed that SP-1 induce transforming growth factor beta 1 (TGFB1), which among its other diverse functions inhibits T-cell function and has proangiogenic properties [43]. SP1 has also been reported as a first trimester maternal serum marker of small for gestational age (SGA) and preterm delivery [44]. For early pregnancy failure, Tornehave et al found lower levels of SP-1 to be suggestive of ectopic pregnancy [45]. Witt et al found a sensitivity of 65 % and a specificity of 74 % by taking a cut-off of 103.3μg/ml [46]. Further studies are needed to validate the use of SP-1 in EP.

7. Human placental lactogen (hPL)

Human placental lactogen is a circulating protein produced by the trophoblasts. Mueller et al found hPL levels to be decreased in ectopic pregnancy [38], but Rausch et al and Daponte et al found no difference in hPL levels between Ectopic pregnancy, abnormal IUP and normal viable IUP [28,41]. hPL as a biomarker of EP has to be evaluated in larger cohort of patients.

8. A disintegrin and metalloprotease-12 (ADAM-12)

ADAM-12 is a glycoprotein primarily produced by syncytiotrophoblast, with a role in syncytial fusion [47]. ADAM-12 was found to be significantly decreased in patients with EP when compared to viable IUP in a cohort of 199 patients [48]. Horne et al observed that when measured in isolation, ADAM-12 levels had limited value as a diagnostic biomarker for EP [49], whereas Yang et al observed low levels of ADAM12 in complete spontaneous abortion and ectopic pregnancy compared to normal pregnancies [50]. Overall, this promising new marker still requires large prospective cohorts for validation.

9. Placental micro-RNA

At least 31micro-RNA expressed from placenta have been isolated with various functions in gene regulation[51,52]. Zhao et al found that microRNA miR-323-3p was found to be lower in patients with EP as compared to those with normal IUP, yielding a sensitivity of 30% and a specificity of 90% in the diagnosis of ectopic pregnancy [53]. This is another promising area of biomarker discovery with further studies being conducted.

10. Placental mRNA

Placental mRNAs secreted by trophoblasts can be altered in early pregnancy failure, and therefore have been studied recently for their diagnostic potential in EP. A recent case-control study conducted by Takacs et al demonstrated that patients with EP have significantly lower copy numbers of hCG and hPL mRNA in plasma compared to viable IUP [54]. Placental mRNA have also been studied for viability and chromosomal aneuploidy [55,56]. Evaluation of changes in placental mRNA expression may serve as a potential biomarker in future for detecting early pregnancy failures.

11. Alpha feto protein (AFP)

AFP is a produced from both yolk sac and fetal liver with a role analogous to adult albumin [57]. Grosskinsky et al found AFP to be elevated in EP, whereas Kuscu et al study contradicted these findings [58, 59]. In our experience, we observed AFP concentration to be elevated in women with miscarriages when compared to normal IUP, but found it to be decreased in women with tubal ectopic compared to both IUP and miscarriages. ROC analysis in our study revealed that AFP was able to discriminate between miscarriage and ectopic, as well as between IUP and ectopic [Unpublished data].

12. Cell free fetal DNA

Cell free fetal DNA escaping into the maternal circulation has also been evaluated as a marker of early pregnancy failure. Lazar et al estimated the cell-free foetal DNA of the Sry gene, and observed its concentration to be significantly higher in those with a tubal ectopic pregnancy. At a cut-off of more than 80 GE/ml, cell free fetal DNA was able to differentiate a tubal ectopic from an intrauterine pregnancy with sensitivity of 84%, a specificity of 76% [60]. As the technology at present is cumbersome, its utility as a useful serum biomarker in a clinical setup has been limited.

2.2. Markers of abnormal corpus luteal function

These are the markers for the evaluation of luteal function by measuring secreted products from the ovary. As the continuous function of the corpus luteum is essential for the maintenance of early pregnancy, these functions may be suboptimal in ectopic pregnancy, and can be measured for diagnostic usage.

1. Progesterone

Maternal progesterone is initially produced by corpus luteum followed by placenta, and ensures appropriate development of the endometrium, uterine growth, adequate uterine blood supply, and preparation of the uterus for labor [60]. Progesterone levels are found to be low in both ectopic pregnancy and other abnormal IUP, when compared to viable IUP [62]. Extensive studies have been performed for the use of progesterone both as a single marker and in multiple marker settings to diagnose EP. A recent meta-analysis of 26 cohort studies, including 9436 pregnant women observed that at a cut-off values from 3.2 to 6 ng/mL, progesterone predicted a non-viable pregnancy with sensitivity of 74.6% and a specificity of 98.4%, although it was not able to distinguish EP from other abnormal IUP [63]. Similar results were observed by the meta analysis performed by Mol et al with a progesterone cut-off of <5ng/ml [64]. In our experience of the cohort of women, progesterone concentration was significantly lower in woman with ectopic pregnancy and women with miscarriages compared to patients with normal IUP. We observed a cut-off of <4.6ng/ml, to have a sensitivity of 93.3% and a specificity of 96.7% in differentiating EP from viable IUP, and a a cut-off of <12ng/ml, to have a sensitivity of 92.8% and a specificity of 90% in differentiating miscarriages from viable IUP, but found progesterone to be unable to discriminate between EP and other abnormal IUP [Unpublished data]. Also, high progesterone does not rule out EP in a patient with inconclusive ultrasound findings. Therefore, further large scale studies are required to study the utility of progesterone as a single marker or as a part of multiple markers to diagnose EP with acceptable sensitivity and specificity.

2. Oestradiol

Oestradiol (E2) is another important steroid secreted from the corpus luteum of pregnancy in response to hCG and could serve as a marker of pregnancy dynamics. Guillaume at al observed in his preliminary study that all of the EP patients had an E2 level of less than 650 pg/ml giving a sensitivity of 100% and specificity of 99% [65]. Witt et al however, did not find any difference in serum E2 when women with EP were compared with those with nonviable intrauterine pregnancies [46]. Mantzavinos et al on the other hand reported that E2 concentrations rose continuously in viable pregnancies, whereas in EP the values plateaued after the sixth week and declined after the eighth week of gestation [66]. However, as the concentrations of serum oestradiol have a considerable overlap among various clinical studies, this marker has not been put into clinical use.

3. Inhibin A

Inhibin A is a dimeric protein produced from corpus luteum [67]. Seifer et al observed lower levels of inhibin-A in EP compared to normal viable IUP [68]. Further, Segel et reported that at a cut-off of 50 pg/mL, Inhibin-A had 100% sensitivity and specificity for diagnosing EP compared to viable IUPs, but found decrease in both sensitivity and specificity when patients of EP were compared with those of other abnormal IUP [69]. Similarly, Rausch et al found Inhibin A to have a sensitivity of 83% and a sensitivity of 79% at a lower cut-off of 23.67pg/ml in discriminating EP from viable IUP [28]. In contrast to the above findings, Chetty et al found Inhibin-A to be unable to discriminate EP from viable IUP in their cohort of 109 patients [70]. It can be concluded that although Inhibin-A is a promising marker for the early pregnancy viability, further studies need to be carried out to use it as a biomarker in the detection of EP.

4. Relaxin and renin

Relaxin is a peptide hormone produced by the corpus luteum of pregnancy, which is elevated shortly after conception and remain steady until the 15th week of gestation [71]. Garcia et al observed a lower levels of serum relaxin concentrations in patients with EP than that in those with a viable IUP [72]. On the other hand, Witt et al found relaxin to be poorly discriminatory as a biomarker of ectopic pregnancy [46].

Renin is another peptide produced by ovaries and the production rises after pregnancy [73]. Meunier et al reported that active renin was significantly decreased in women with EP when compared with those with an ongoing IUP or spontaneous miscarriage, however because of its low specificity and sensitivity, the use of renin in the clinical setting has been limited [74].

2.3. Markers of angiogenesis

1. Vascular Endothelial Growth Factor (VEGF)

VEGF plays an important role in the angiogenesis of the fetomaternal unit [75]. It has been reported that maternal serum VEGF concentrations are associated with depth of trophoblastic penetration into the tubal wall [76]. A case control study observed a cut-off of 200pg/ml had a sensitivity of 60% and a specificity of 90 % in predicting EP [77]. Similar findings were observed by Felemban et al [78]. Daponte et al observed a sensitivity of 78% and a specificity of 100 % in predicting EP at a cut-off of 174.5pg/ml. [41]. Recently Fernandes et al reported that serum level of VEGF was significantly higher in women with EP, and when threshold concentrations of serum VEGF level > 200 pg/ml were used, an EP could be distinguished from a normal pregnancy with a sensitivity of 51.4%, a specificity of 90.9% [79]. On the contrary, Rausch et al found no difference in the levels of VEGF between EP, abnormal IUP and viable IUP [28]. The variations in the study results of VEGF shows that further investigations are required to ascertain its suitability as a biomarker for EP.

2. Placental like growth factor (PlGF)

PIGF is a pro-angiogenic growth factor produced by the trophoblast at the site of implantation [80]. Horne et al reported the expression of PIGF m-RNA to be lower in trophoblastic cells in patients with EP as compared to those with viable IUP [81]. Daponte et al later observed that at a PIGF level of more than 15.73pg/ml could differentiate viable pregnancy from early pregnancy failures including EP and abnormal IUP with reasonable sensitivity and specificity, but could not differentiate among them [82]. Recent report by Martínez-Ruiz et al also didn't find significant differences for PlGF between EP and viable IUP [83]. Therefore, there is a need of validation of this marker in a larger cohort.

3. Angiopoietins

Angiopoietins are proteins which belong to the family of angiogenic proteins, which has been shown to be critically involved in the process of placental maturation and growth from early pregnancy. Angiopoietin-1 (Ang-1) and Ang-2 are two critical regulators with different functions of vascular development and angiogenesis [84, 85]. Daponte et al reported Ang-1 and Ang-2 concentrations and their ratio to be lower in EP compared to IUP. They also found the trophoblastic Ang-1 mRNA expression levels to be lower in EP compared to IUP, while Ang-2 mRNA was found to be higher in EP than in IUP [86]. Schneuer et al in their recent study suggested that the lower Ang-1/Ang-2 ratio in first trimester is associated with most adverse pregnancy outcomes, but do not predict outcomes any better than clinical and maternal risk factor information [87].

2.4. Markers related to normal uterine implantation

These biomarkers are released into the circulation as a result of normal interaction between the pregnancy and the uterine decidua. As the normal process is disrupted in EP, these surrogate markers can be used to diagnose EP.

1. Leukemia inhibitory factor (LIF)

LIF is a cytokine of interleukin-6 family with a key role in implantation [88]. Wegner et al observed that women with ectopic pregnancy had low serum concentrations of LIF and could diagnose it with moderate sensitivity and specificity [89]. However, Daponte et al failed to find any difference in LIF concentrations in patients with ectopic pregnancy and other abnormal intrauterine pregnancy [41]. A further attempt in validation of LIF has yielded conflicting results. Mueller et al found LIF levels to be undetectable in serum of patients with ectopic pregnancy and viable intrauterine pregnancy [38], whereas Iyibozkurt AC et al found increased levels of LIF in patients with EP compared to IUP [90]. Increased immunohistochemical expression of LIF in fallopian tube was found to be increased in EP compared to non –pregnant and healthy pregnant controls, indicating its role in ectopic implantation of embryo [91]. Similarly it was observed that LIF expression was increased in inflamed fallopian tube and might be one of the reasons of increased susceptibility of salphingitis patients to EP [92].

2. Glycodelin (Placental protein 14)

Glycodelin is secreted from endometrium and fallopian tube, with immunomodulatory role in implantation. Its serum concentration increases during early first trimester of pregnancy, till 8-10 weeks of gestation and then progressively declines [93, 94]. Foth et al found significantly lower levels of serum glycodelin in patients with ectopic pregnancy compared to IUP and incomplete abortion with a study population of 169 subjects [95]. Out of the three groups, who studied glycodelin in a multiple marker setting, two had found glycodelin levels to be decreased in EP, while one observed no significant difference between EP and abnormal IUP [28, 38, 41]. Further studies are required to validate the use of this marker in EP.

3. Mucin-1 (Muc-1)

Muc-1 is a glycoprotein expressed by endometrium and fallopian tube epithelium involved in implantation [96]. Muc-1 expression was observed to be lower in luminal epithelial of tubes with ectopic pregnancies [97]. Similar findings were observed by Reefaat et al [98]. However, the role of serum Muc-1 as a diagnostic modality has not been studied in much detail.

4. Adrenomedullin

Adrenomedullin is a peptide hormone belonging to calcitonin/calcitonin gene related peptide, and is thought be involved in endometrial angiogenesis. Liao et al found plasma and oviductal tissue adrenomedullin to be lower in EP and suggested that this decreases ciliary beating and muscle contraction leading to retained embryo and its implantation in the oviduct [99]. Similar findings were observed in nasal epithelium in patients of tEP by the same group [100]. Further studies are required to explore the possible role of serum adrenomedullin as a diagnostic marker for EP.

5. Activin B

Activins, dimeric proteins of transforming growth factor-beta (TGF-b), have recently been found in gonadal fluid with growth factor like actions [101]. It is produced by many organs including pituitary gland, gonads, placenta etc. It has been shown to promote decidualization of the endometrium during pregnancy [102]. Consequently low serum activin levels have been associated with ectopic pregnancy. Although recent studies have mainly focussed the role of serum activin A as a potential marker of ectopic pregnancy, limited literature is available regarding the role of activin B in-spite of the experimental evidence of differential effect of activin B on decidua. In our population, we observed that the concentration of activin B in maternal serum to be significantly lower in patients with tEP compared to those with normal IUP [Unpublished data]. Similar results were observed by Horne et al, who found decreased expression of activin B in endometrium along with decreased serum levels of activin B with normal levels of progesterone in 11 women with tEP [103]. Activin B is a new, though promising marker for EP diagnostic triage.

3. Markers related to tubal implantation

3.1. Markers of compromised tubal musculature markers

These markers reflect the disruption of the integrity of the tubal circular smooth muscle layer, which can happen in an ectopic implantation. These markers of muscle damage have been investigated as biomarkers for diagnosing EP.

1. Creatine Kinase (CK)

Creatine Kinase is the enzyme released from damaged muscles, which is currently used in the diagnosis of myocardial infarction. Lavie et al found serum CK levels to be significantly higher in patients with tEP as compared to those with missed abortion or normal IUP [104]. Similar findings were observed by Birkhahn et al and Duncan et al [105,106]. In a study conducted in our population, we found that the optimal cut-off for total CK, CK-MM and CPK-MB% as predictors of ruptured EP were 147 IU/L, 135 IU/L and 10%, respectively, with the former two having higher specificity, and latter high sensitivity [107]. On the contrary, several independent study groups found CK to be inadequate in diagnosing EP [108-112]. Recently, Safdarian et al studied the role of CK-1 as an indicator for differentiating between the successful and unsuccessful treatment groups in EP, but failed to find any relation between initial CPK serum levels [113].

2. Smooth muscle heavy-chain myosin (SMHC) & Myoglobin

Smooth muscle heavy chain myosin and myoglobin are markers of smooth muscle damage. As the ectopic pregnancy grows to invade the muscular layer of the fallopian tube, markers of muscle damage should also rise. Birkhahn et al studied serum myoglobin and smooth muscle heavy-chain myosin and observed a statistically significant elevation in the serum levels of SMHC, but did not find it useful in the screening for EP [105,114]. As there is paucity of data regarding the usefulness of these markers in the screening of EP, their clinical utility is limited.

3.2. Markers of inflammation and peritoneal irritation

EP can lead to inflammation and peritoneal irritation and the following biomarkers have been investigated as an potential biomarkers of the same process.

1. Circulating cytokines

Several cytokines as marker of peritoneal inflammation has been reported including IL-2R, IL-6, IL-8, IL-10, IL-11, IL-15 and TNF-α. Soriano et al observed increased concentration of IL-6, IL-8 and TNF-α in patients with EP compared with normal and abnormal IUP. IL-8 at a cut-off of >40 pg/ml was shown to have a sensitivity and specificity of 82.4% and 81.8 % respectively in diagnosing EP [115]. Experience in our population regarding IL-6 & IL-8 levels, we observed that the level of IL-6 shows a significant increase in the women with tubal ectopic pregnancy in comparison to intrauterine abortion and normal pregnancy. It was also seen that IL-8 levels decrease significantly in the tubal ectopic pregnancy cases and in intrauterine abortion patient when compared to the normal pregnancy group. ROC analysis revealed that at the cut-off of 26.48pg/ml of IL-6 level predict the probability of tubal ectopic pregnancy with 53.57% sensitivity, 80%specificity [Unpublished paper]. Similar observations were made by Rausch et al, who observed lower values of IL-8 and TNF-α in women with EP, whereas no significant difference was observed in the IL-6 levels between EP and viable IUP [28]. No difference has been observed in the levels of IL-10 and IL-11between EP and viable IUP [90]. IL-15 has also been studied as it is expressed by human placental tissue culture and it is maximally expressed during the implantation period in the deciduas. Daponte et al reported that IL-15 concentrations were significantly higher in women with EP compared to patients with IUP, and found IL-15 to have high diagnostic accuracy for the discrimination of a viable IUP from an EP with an area under the curve of 0.818 [116].

2. CA-125

Conflicting results have been reported by several groups regarding the status of circulating CA-125 in EP with some groups reporting an increase, some decrease and few found no difference between viable IUP and EP [117-121]. In our experience in the cohort of patients, we found CA125 concentration to be significantly higher in woman with miscarriages compared to patients with normal IUP, but not in women with ectopic compared to IUP [Unpublished paper]. Women with **IU** abortion were found to have significantly higher CA-125 levels, compared to the other two groups. Katsikis et al also reported that when using CA-125 concentration of more than 41.9 U/ml as a threshold for the diagnosis of IU abortive pregnancy, sensitivity was 80% and specificity was 87% for discriminating it from EP [122].

3. Antibodies to C1q complement

C1q complement has been shown to promote trophoblast invasion of deciduas, a crucial step in normal placental development. Animal models have demonstrated that the lack of C1q is characterized by poor trophoblast invasion and pregnancy failure [123,124]. Studies based on these observations have measured the levels of antibodies to C1q complement in early pregnancy failure have been conducted. Daponte et al failed to observe any difference between normal viable IUP, EP and other abnormal IUP [116]. As new studies would be undertaken by different groups, more information regarding this marker is likely to emerge.

The biomarkers studied in ectopic pregnancy with their current status are summarized in table 1.

Sl No	Biomarker	Cut-off	Sensitivity	Specificity	Reference
1	B-hCG				
	a. Single serum levels	<2000mIU/ml	87%	39%	Shaunik et al 2011
	b. 48 hours rise	<53% rise	91%	66.6%	Barnhart 2004
		<35% rise	83.2%	70.8%	Morse 2012
	c. Mathematical models				
	M1	0.21	83%	88%	Condous 2004
	M4	-	92%	91%	Condous 2007
			31%	98%	Kirk 2006
			81%	89%	Barnhart 2010
2	Hyperglycosylated hCG	13μg/L	73%	98.1%	Sutton-Riley 2006
3	Pregnancy associated plasma protein-A (PAPPA)	0.53 ng/ml	81%	54%	Rausch 2011
4	Pregnancy specific beta glycoprotein-1 (SP-1)	103.3μg/ml	65%	74%	Witt 1990

http://dx.doi.org/10.5772/58954

Sl No	Biomarker	Cut-off	Sensitivity	Specificity	Reference
5	ADAM-12	48.49ng/ml	97%	37%	Rausch 2011
6	Activin A	0.37ng/ml	100%	99.6%	Florio 2007
		0.38 ng/ml	80%	72%	Rausch 2011
		0.26 ng/ml	59.6%	69%	Warrick 2012
		505 pg/ml	87.9%	100%	Daponte 2013
7	Progesterone	3.2-6 ng/ml	74.6%	98.4%	Verhaegen 2012
		5ng/ml	95%	40%	Mol 1998
		10.75 ng/ml	85%	85%	Katsikis 2006
8	Oestradiol	650 pg/ml	100%	90%	Guillaume 1990
9	Inhibin A	50 pg/ml	100%	100%	Segel 2008
		28.67 pg/ml	83%	79%	Rausch 2011
10	VEGF	200 pg/ml	60%	90%	Daniel 1999
		174.5 pg/ml	78%	100%	Daponte 2005
		200 pg/ml	88%	100%	Felemban 2002
		28.24 pg/ml	95%	50%	Rausch 2011
11	PIGF	15.7 pg/ml	86%	73%	Daponte 2011
12	LIF	6.2pg/ml	73%	72%	Wegener 2001
13	Interleukin-8	40 pg/ml	82.4%	81.8%	Soriano 2003
14	Interleukin-15	16.1 pg/ml	92%	68%	Daponte 2013

Table 1. Current status of biomarkers of tubal Ectopic pregnancy

4. Further research

Since the factors and their interplay involved in maintenance of normal viable pregnancy are not completely understood, various approaches have been explored in biomarker discovery including unbiased proteomics, shotgun proteomics [125,126]. The challenges in biomarker discovery include the variability of biomarkers with gestational age, impact of coexistent morbidities like hypertension, diabetes, chromosomal anomalies on biomarker levels and their interpretation. Other emerging markers studied in ectopic pregnancy include: Endocannibinoid system abnormalities in the form of high anandamide levels and reduced receptor expression have been implicated, in women with ectopic pregnancy [127,128].

Brown et al conducted a proteomics study and identified fibronectin has ability to discriminate EP from other pregnancy outcomes suggesting its diagnostic potential and its use as an adjunct to future multiplex EP diagnostic tests [129].

Serum Macrophage Inhibitory Cytokine-1 levels were found to be lower in women with histologically confirmed EP compared to women with definite viable intra-uterine pregnancy by Skubisz et al [130].

Another recent study by Beer et al that screened the proteome of a small group of women with EP and controls identified potential novel biomarkers, including ADAM-12 and ISM2 (Isthmin 2) as well as five specific isoforms of pregnancy-specific beta-1-glycoprotein 131].

5. Use of multiple biomarkers in ectopic pregnancy

As maintenance of a viable pregnancy requires an interplay of multiple factors, no single marker has been used successfully as a biomarker for EP. It seems prudent, therefore, to combine these markers and use them in the multiple marker setting. Rausch et al demonstrated that a four-marker test including Progesterone, VEGF, Inhibin A, and Activin A could predict EP with 100% accuracy in those with an hCG<1500 mIU/mL [28]. Further studies are necessary to fully assess the discriminatory capacity of such a test. Similarly, Feng et al found a combination of Δβ-hCG, Progesterone and Oestradiol to be helpful in distinguishing EPs and normal IUPs, facilitating earlier diagnosis and the timely implementation of medical treatment to prevent tubal rupture [132].

Soriano et al found that the combination of inflammatory cytokines IL-6, IL-8, and TNF-alpha was able to predict EP with specificity of 100%, but sensitivity of 52.9% [115].

Another group in Switzerland developed a multiple marker test, the "triple marker analysis" [VEGF/(PAPP-A X P)] had a sensitivity of 97.7% with a specificity of 92.4% in diagnosing EP [38].

In another study, investigators studied serum levels of 17β-estradiol (E2), progesterone (P4), testosterone (T), beta-human chorionic gonadotropin (β-hCG), vascular endothelial growth factor-A (VEGF-A), placental growth factor (PIGF), and a distintegrin and metalloprotease protein 12 (ADAM12) in different patient groups with no definite results [133].

6. Conclusion

Novel biomarker of ectopic pregnancy with adequate sensitivity and specificity could assist in early diagnosis and hence timely intervention, thereby dramatically reducing the morbidity and mortality. There are number of potential molecules for use as biomarkers in women at risk for EP. As no single biomarker is ready for use in clinical setting, more prospective cohorts including ectopic pregnancy, normal and abnormal IUPs are required to validate these markers. Also, it would be prudent to concentrate the efforts on developing a panel of markers which include markers of viability, location of implantation and fetal milieu. Recent times have witnessed positive developments in this field, but lot of validation is required before a marker can be used independently in clinical setting.

http://dx.doi.org/10.5772/58954

Author details

Soundravally Rajendiren* and Pooja Dhiman

*Address all correspondence to: soundy27@yahoo.co.in

Department of Biochemistry, JIPMER, Puducherry, India

References

[1] Hasan R, Baird DD, Herring AH, Olshan AF, Johnsson Funk ML, Hartmann KE. Pattern and predictors of vaginal bleeding in the first trimester of pregnancy. Ann Epidemiol 2010;20 (7):524-31.

[2] Barnhart KT. Clinical practice-Ectopic pregnancy. N Engl J Med 2009; 361:379-87.

[3] Condous G, Okaro E, Bourne T. The conservative management of early pregnancy complication: a review of literature. Ultrasound Obstet Gynecol 2003; 22: 420-30.

[4] Shaunik A, Kulp J, Appleby DH, Sammel MD, Barnhart KT. Utility of dilation and curettage in the diagnosis of pregnancy of unknown location. Am J Obstet Gynecol 2011;204:130–136.

[5] Lenton EA, Neal LM, Sulaiman R. Plasma concentrations of human chorionic gonadotropin from the time of implantation until the second week of pregnancy. Fertil Steril 1982;37(6):773-8.

[6] Barnhart KT, Sammel MD, Rinaudo PF, Zhou L, Hummel AC, Guo W. Symptomatic patients with an early viable intrauterine pregnancy: hCG curves redefined. Obstetrics and Gynecology 2004;104:50-55.

[7] Seeber BE, Sammel MD, Guo W, Zhou L, Hummel A, Barnhart KT. Application of redefined of human chorionic gonadotropin curves for the diagnosis of women at risk for ectopic pregnancy. Fertility and sterility 2006; 86:454-9.

[8] Morse CB, Sammel MD, Shaukina A, Allen-Taylor L, Oberfoell NL, Takacas P, Chung K et al. Performance of human chorionic gonadotropin curves in women at risk for ectopic pregnancy: exceptions to the rules. Fertili Steril 2012;97(1):101-6.

[9] Desai D, Lu J, Wyness SP, Greene DN, Olson KN, Wiley CL, Grenache DG. Human chorionic gonadotropin discriminatory zone in ectopic pregnancy: does assay harmonization matter? Fertil Steril. 2014;101(6):1671-4.

[10] Condous G, Okaro E, Khalid A, Timmerman D, Lu C, Zhou Y et al. The use of a new logistic regression model for predicting the outcome of pregnancies of unknown location. Hum Reprod 2004; 19: 1900-10.

[11] Kirk E, Condous G, Haid Z, Lu C, Van Huffel S, Timmerman D, Bourne T. The practical application of a mathematical model to predict the outcome of pregnancies of unknown location. Ultrasound Obstet Gynecol 2006; 27(3): 311-5.

[12] Barnhart KT, Sammel MD, Appleby D, Rausch M, Molinaro T, Van Calster B et al. Does a prediction model for pregnancy of unknown location developed in the UK validate on a US population? Hum Reprod 2010; 25:2434-40.

[13] Condous G, Van Calster B, Kirk E, Haider Z, Timmerman D, Van Huffel S, Bourne T. Prediction of ectopic pregnancy in women with a pregnancy of unknown location. Ultrasound Obstet Gynecol 2007b;29:680–687.

[14] Zee J, Sammel MD, Chung K, Takacs P, Bourne T, Barnhart KT. Ectopic pregnancy prediction in women with a pregnancy of unknown location: data beyond 48 hour are necessary. Hum Reprod 2014;29(3):441-7.

[15] Helmy S, Bader Y, Pablik E, Tiringer D, Pils S, Lami T, Koblik H et al. Cut-off value of initial serum β-hCG level predicting a successful methotrexate therapy in tubal ectopic pregnancy: a retrospective cohort study. Eur J Obstet Gynecol Reprod Biol 2014;179C:175-80.

[16] Nowak-Markwitz E, Michalak M, Olejnik M, Spaczynski M. Cut-off value of human chorionic gonadotropin in relation to the number of methotrexate cycles in the successful treatment of ectopic pregnancy. Fertil Steril 2009;92(4):1203-7.

[17] Cole LA, Butler SA. Hyperglycosylated human chorionic gonadotropin and human chorionic gonadotropin free beta-subunit: tumor markers and tumor promoters. J Reprod Med 2008;53:499-512.

[18] Guibourdenche J, Handschuh K, Tsatsaris V, Gerbaud P, Leguy MC, Muller F, Brion DE, Fournier T. Hyperglycosylated hCG is a marker of early human trophoblast invasion. J Clin Endocrinol Metab 2010; 95:E240-244.

[19] Sasaki Y, Ladner DG, Cole LA. Hyperglycosylated human chorionic gonadotropin and the source of pregnancy failures. Fertil Steril 2008;89(6):1781-6.

[20] Cole LA. Hyperglycosylated hCG and pregnancy failures. J Reprod Immunol 2012;93(2):119-22.

[21] Sutton-Riley JM, Khanlian SA, Byrn FW, Cole LA. A single serum test for measuring early pregnancy outcome with high predictive value. Clin Biochem 2006;39:682-7.

[22] Butler SA, Abban TK, Borrelli PT, Luttoo JM, Kemp B, Iles RK. Single point biochemical measurement algorithm for early diagnosis of ectopic pregnancy. Clin Biochem. 2013 ;46(13-14):1257-63.

[23] Chuan S, Homer M, Pandian R, Conway D, Garzo G, Yeo L, Su HI. Hyperglycosylated human chorionic gonadotropin as an early predictor of pregnancy outcomes after in vitro fertilization. Fertil Steril. 2014;101(2):392-8.

[24] Keikkala E, Ranta JK, Vuorela P, Leinonen R, Laivuori H, Väisänen S, Marttala J, Romppanen J, Pulkki K, Stenman UH, Heinonen S. Serum hyperglycosylated human chorionic gonadotrophin at 14-17 weeks of gestation does not predict preeclampsia. Prenat Diagn. 2014;34(7):699-705.

[25] Keikkala E, Vuorela P, Laivuori H, Romppanen J, Heinonen S, Stenman UH. First trimester hyperglycosylated human chorionic gonadotrophin in serum-a marker of early-onset preeclampsia. Placenta. 2013;34(11):1059-65.

[26] Bearfield C, Jauniaux E, Groome N, Sargent IL, Muttukrishna S. The secretion and effect of inhibin A, activin A and follistatin on first-trimester trophoblasts in vitro. Eur J Endocrinol. 2005; 152(6):909-16.

[27] Florio P, Severi FM, Bocchi C, Luisi S, Mazzini M, Danero S, Torricelli M, Petraglia F. Single serum activin a testing to predict ectopic pregnancy. J Clin Endocrinol Metab. 2007; 92(5):1748-53.

[28] Rausch ME, Sammel MD, Takacs P, Chung K, Shaunik A, Barnhart KT. Development of a multiple marker test for ectopic pregnancy. Obstet Gynecol. 2011; 117(3):573-82.

[29] Daponte A, Deligeoroglou E, Garas A, Pournaras S, Hadjichristodoulou C, Messinis IE. Activin A and follistatin as biomarkers for ectopic pregnancy and missed abortion. Dis Markers. 2013;35(5):497-503.

[30] Warrick J, Gronowski A, Moffett C, Zhao Q, Bishop E, Woodworth A. Serum activin A does not predict ectopic pregnancy as a single measurement test, alone or as part of a multi-marker panel including progesterone and hCG. Clin Chim Acta. 2012; 413(7-8):707-11.

[31] Kirk E, Papageorghiou AT, Van Calster B, Condous G, Cowans N, Van Huffel S, Timmerman D, Spencer K, Bourne T. The use of serum inhibin A and activin A levels in predicting the outcome of 'pregnancies of unknown location'. Hum Reprod. 2009; 24(10):2451-6.

[32] Elito Júnior J, Gustavo Oliveira L, Octávio Fernandes Silva M, Araujo Júnior E, Camano L. Serum activin A levels and tubal ectopic pregnancy. Iran J Reprod Med. 2014;12(3):227-8.

[33] de Kretser, DM, Foulds, LM, Hancock, M, Robertson DM. Partial characterization of inhibin, activin, and follistatin in the term human placenta. J. Clin. Endocrinol. Metab 1994;79:502–507.

[34] Woodruff, T.K., Sluss, P., Wang, E, Janssen I, Mersol-Barg MS. Activin A and follistatin are dynamically regulated during human pregnancy. J. Endocrinol 1997;152:167–175.

[35] Nakamura, T, Takio K., Eto Y, Shibai H, Titani K, Sugino H. Activin-binding protein from rat ovary is follistatin. Science 1990;247:836–838.

[36] Wang J, Liu S, Qin HM, Zhao Y, Wang XQ, Yan Q. Pregnancy-associated plasma protein A up-regulated by progesterone promotes adhesion and proliferation of trophoblastic cells. Int J Clin Exp Pathol. 2014;7(4):1427-37.

[37] Nicolaides KH, Spencer K, Avgidou K, Faiola S, Falcon O. Multicenter study of first-trimester screening for trisomy 21 in 75 821 pregnancies: results and estimation of the potential impact of individual risk-orientated two-stage first-trimester screening. Ultrasound Obstet Gynecol. 2005; 25(3):221-6.

[38] Mueller MD, Raio L, Spoerri S, Ghezzi F, Dreher E, Bersinger NA. Novel placental and non-placental serum markers in ectopic versus normal intrauterine pregnancy. Fertil Steril 2004;81(4):1106-11.

[39] Dumps P, Meisser A, Pons D, Morales MA, Anguenot JL, Campana A, Bischof P. Accuracy of single measurements of pregnancy-associated plasma protein-A, human chorionic gonadotropin and progesterone in the diagnosis of early pregnancy failure. Eur J Obstet Gynecol Reprod Biol. 2002; 100(2):174-80.

[40] Ugurlu EN, Ozaksit G, Karaer A, Zulfikaroglu E, Atalay A, Ugur M. The value of vascular endothelial growth factor, pregnancy-associated plasma protein-A, and progesterone for early differentiation of ectopic pregnancies, normal intrauterine pregnancies, and spontaneous miscarriages. Fertil Steril. 2009;91:1657–61.

[41] Daponte A, Pournaras S, Zintzaras E, Kallitsaris A, Lialios G, Maniatis AN, et al. The value of a single combined measurement of VEGF, glycodelin, progesterone, PAPP-A, HPL and LIF for differentiating between ectopic and abnormal intrauterine pregnancy. Hum Reprod. 2005;20:3163–6.

[42] Horne CH, Towler CM, Pugh-Humphreys RG, Thomson AW, Bohn H. Pregnancy specific beta1-glycoprotein--a product of the syncytiotrophoblast. Experientia. 1976; 32(9):1197.

[43] Ha CT, Wu JA, Irmak S, Lisboa FA, Dizon AM, Warren JW, Ergun S, Dveksler GS. Human pregnancy specific beta-1-glycoprotein 1 (PSG1) has a potential role in placental vascular morphogenesis. Biol Reprod. 2010 ;83(1):27-35.

[44] Pihl K, Larsen T, Laursen I, Krebs L, Christiansen M. First trimester maternal serum pregnancy-specific beta-1-glycoprotein (SP1) as a marker of adverse pregnancy outcome. Prenat Diagn. 2009;29(13):1256-61.

[45] Tornehave D, Chemnitz J, Westergaard JG, Teisner B, Poulsen HK, Bolton AE, Grudzinskas JG. Placental proteins in peripheral blood and tissues of ectopic pregnancies. Gynecol Obstet Invest. 1987; 23(2):97-102.

[46] Witt BR, Wolf GC, Wainwright CJ, Johnston PD, Thorneycroft IH. Relaxin, CA-125, progesterone, estradiol, Schwangerschaft protein, and human chorionic gonadotropin as predictors of outcome in threatened and non-threatened pregnancies. Fertil Steril. 1990; 53(6):1029-36.

[47] Huppertz B, Bartz C, Kokozidou M. Trophoblast fusion: fusogenic proteins, syncytins and ADAMs, and other prerequisites for syncytial fusion. Micron. 2006; 37(6): 509-17.

[48] Rausch ME, Beer L, Sammel MD, Takacs P, Chung, Shaunik A, Speicher D, Barnhart KT. A disintegrin and metalloprotease protein-12 as a novel marker for the diagnosis of ectopic pregnancy. Fertil Steril. 2011;95(4):1373-8.

[49] Horne AW, Brown JK, Tong S, Kaitu'u-Lino T. Evaluation of ADAM-12 as a diagnostic biomarker of ectopic pregnancy in women with a pregnancy of unknown location. PLoS One. 2012;7(8):e41442.

[50] Yang J, Wu J, Guo F, Wang D, Chen K, Li J, Du L, Yin A. Maternal serum disintegrin and metalloprotease protein-12 in early pregnancy as a potential marker of adverse pregnancy outcomes. PLoS One. 2014;9(5):e97284.

[51] Lagos-Quintana M, Rauhut R, Lendeckel W, Tuschl T. Identification of novel genes coding for small expressed RNAs. Science. 2001; 294:853–8.

[52] Lee RC, Ambros V. An extensive class of small RNAs in Caenorhabditis elegans. Science. 2001;294:862–4.

[53] Zhao Z, Zhao Q, Warrick J, Lockwood CM, Woodworth A, Moley KH, Gronowski AM. Circulating microRNA miR-323-3p as a biomarker of ectopic pregnancy. Clin Chem. 2012; 58:896–905.

[54] Takacs P, Jaramillo S, Datar R, Williams A, Olczyk J, Barnhart K. Placental mRNA in maternal plasma as a predictor of ectopic pregnancy. Int J Gynaecol Obstet. 2012;117:131–3.

[55] Lo YM, Tsui NB, Chiu RW, Lau TK, Leung TN, Heung MM, Gerovassili A et al. Plasma placental RNA allelic ratio permits noninvasive prenatal chromosomal aneuploidy detection. Nat Med.2007;13:218–23.

[56] Ng EK, Tsui NB, Lau TK, Leung TN, Chiu RW, Panesar NS, Lit LC et al. mRNA of placental origin is readily detectable in maternal plasma. Proc Natl Acad Sci U S A. 2003;100:4748–53.

[57] Jones EA, Clement-Jones M, James OF & Wilson DI. Differences between human and mouse alpha-fetoprotein expression during early development. Journal of Anatomy 2001;198:555–559.

[58] Grosskinsky CM, Hage ML, Tyrey L, Christakos AC & Hughes CL. hCG, progesterone, alpha-fetoprotein, and estradiol in the identification of ectopic pregnancy. Obstetrics and Gynecology 1993; 81:705–709.

[59] Kuscu E, Vicdan K, Turhan NO, Oguz S, Zorlu G &Gokmen O. The hormonal profile in ectopic pregnancies. Materia Medica Polona 1993; 25:149–152.

[60] Lazar L, Nagy B, Ban Z, Nagy GR & Papp Z. Presence of cell-free fetal DNA in plasma of women with ectopic pregnancies. Clinical Chemistry 2006;52: 1599–1601.

[61] Arck P, Hansen PJ, Mulac Jericevic B, Piccinni MP, Szekeres-Bartho J. Progesterone during pregnancy: endocrine-immune cross talk in mammalian species and the role of stress. Am J Reprod Immunol. 2007; 58(3):268-79.

[62] Hinshaw K, Fayyad A, Munjuluri P. The management of early pregnancy loss. Royal College of Obstetricians and Gynaecologists, 2006. (Green-top guideline No 25).

[63] Verhaegen J, Gallos ID, van Mello NM, Abdel-Aziz M, Takwoingi Y, Harb H, Deeks JJ, Mol BWJ, Coomarasamy A. Accuracy of single progesterone test to predict early pregnancy outcome in women with pain or bleeding: meta-analysis of cohort studies. BMJ 2012;345:e6077.

[64] Mol BW, Lijmer JG, Ankum WM, van der Veen F, Bossuyt PM. The accuracy of single serum progesterone measurement in the diagnosis of ectopic pregnancy: a meta-analysis. Hum Reprod. 1998; 13:3220–7.

[65] Guillaume J, Benjamin F, Sicuranza BJ, Deutsch S, Seltzer VL &Tores W. Serum estradiol as an aid in the diagnosis of ectopic pregnancy. Obstetrics and Gynecology 1990;76: 1126–1129.

[66] Mantzavinos T, Phocas I, Chrelias H, Sarandakou A&Zourlas PA.Serum levels of steroid and placental protein hormones in ectopic pregnancy. European Journal of Obstetrics, Gynecology, and Reproductive Biology 1991;39:117–122.

[67] Treetampinich C, O'Connor AE, MacLachlan V, Groome NP, de Kretser DM. Maternal serum inhibin A concentrations in early pregnancy after IVF and embryo transfer reflect the corpus luteum contribution and pregnancy outcome. Hum Reprod. 2000; 15:2028–32.

[68] Seifer DB, Lambert-Messerlian GM, Canick JA, Frishman GN, Schneyer AL. Serum inhibin levels are lower in ectopic than intrauterine spontaneously conceived pregnancies. Fertil Steril. 1996;65:667–9.

[69] Segal S, Gor H, Correa N, Mercado R, Veenstra K, Rivnay B. Inhibin A: marker for diagnosis of ectopic and early abnormal pregnancies. Reprod Biomed Online. 2008; 17:789–94.

[70] Chetty M, Sawyer E, Dew T, Chapman AJ, Elson J. The use of novel biochemical markers in predicting spontaneously resolving 'pregnancies of unknown location'. Hum Reprod. 2011;26:1318–23.

[71] Weiss G, O'Byrne EM &Steinetz BG. Relaxin: a product of the human corpus luteum in pregnancy. Science 1976;194:948–949.

http://dx.doi.org/10.5772/58954

[72] Garcia A, Skurnick JH, Goldsmith LT, Emmi A & Weiss G. Human chorionic gonadotropin and relaxin concentrations in early ectopic and normal pregnancies. Obstetrics and Gynecology 1990;75:779–783.

[73] Sealey JE, Cholst I, Glorioso N, Troffa C, Weintraub ID, James G &Laragh JH. Sequential changes in plasma luteinising hormone and plasma prorenin during the menstrual cycle. Journal of Clinical Endocrinology and Metabolism1987;65: 1.

[74] Meunier K, Mignot TM, Maria B, Guichard A, Zorn JR &Cedard L. Predictive value of renin assay for the diagnosis of ectopic pregnancy. Fertility and Sterility 1991;55:432–435.

[75] Carmeliet P, Ferreira V, Breier G, Pollefeyt S, Kieckens L, Gertsenstein M, Fahriq M et al. Abnormal blood vessel development and lethality in embryos lacking a single VEGF allele. Nature 1996; 380:435–9.

[76] Cabar FR, Pereira PP, Schultz R, Francisco RP, Zugaib M. Vascular endothelial growth factor and β-human chorionic gonadotropin are associated with trophoblastic invasion into the tubal wall in ectopic pregnancy. Fertil Steril. 2010;94(5):1595-600.

[77] Daniel Y, Geva E, Lerner-Geva L, Eshed-Englender T, Gamzu R, Lessing JB, et al. Levels of vascular endothelial growth factor are elevated in patients with ectopic pregnancy: is this a novel marker? Fertil Steril. 1999; 72:1013–7.

[78] Felemban A, Sammour A, Tulandi T. Serum vascular endothelial growth factor as a possible marker for early ectopic pregnancy. Hum Reprod. 2002; 17:490–2.

[79] Fernandes da Silva MO, Elito J Jr, Daher S, Camano L, Fernandes Moron A. Association of serum levels of vascular endothelial growth factor and early ectopic pregnancy. Clin Exp Obstet Gynecol. 2013;40(4):489-91.

[80] Plaisier M, Rodrigues S, Willems F, Koolwijk P, van Hinsbergh VW, Helmerhorst FM. Different degrees of vascularization and their relationship to the expression of vascular endothelial growth factor, placental growth factor, angiopoietins, and their receptors in first-trimester decidual tissues. Fertil Steril. 2007; 88(1):176-87.

[81] Horne AW, Shaw JL, Murdoch A, McDonald SE, Williams AR, Jabbour HN, Duncan WC, Critchley HO. Placental growth factor: a promising diagnostic biomarker for tubal ectopic pregnancy. J Clin Endocrinol Metab. 2011; 96(1):E104-8.

[82] Daponte A, Pournaras S, Polyzos NP, Tsezou A, Skentou H, Anastasiadou F, Lialios G, Messinis IE. Soluble FMS-like tyrosine kinase-1 (sFlt-1) and serum placental growth factor (PlGF) as biomarkers for ectopic pregnancy and missed abortion. J Clin Endocrinol Metab. 2011; 96(9):E1444-51.

[83] Martínez-Ruiz A, Sarabia-Meseguer MD, Pérez-Fornieles J, Vílchez JA, Tovar-Zapata I, Noguera-Velasco JA. Placental growth factor, soluble fms-like tyrosine kinase 1 and progesterone as diagnostic biomarkers for ectopic pregnancy and missed abortion. Clin Biochem. 2014 ;47(9):844-7.

[84] Woolnough C, Wang Y, Kan CY, Morris JM, Tasevski V, Ashton AW. Source of angiopoietin-2 in the sera of women during pregnancy. Microvasc Res 2012;84: 367–374.

[85] Seval Y, Sati L, Celik-Ozenci C, Taskin O, Demir R. The distribution of angiopoietin-1, angiopoietin-2 and their receptors tie-1 and tie-2 in the very early human placenta. Placenta 2008;29: 809–815.

[86] Daponte A, Deligeoroglou E, Pournaras S, Tsezou A, Garas A, Anastasiadou F, Hadjichristodoulou C, Messinis IE. Angiopoietin-1 and angiopoietin-2 as serum biomarkers for ectopic pregnancy and missed abortion: a case-control study. Clin Chim Acta. 2013;415:145-51.

[87] Schneuer FJ, Roberts CL, Ashton AW, Guilbert C, Tasevski V, Morris JM, Nassar N. Angiopoietin 1 and 2 serum concentrations in first trimester of pregnancy as biomarkers of adverse pregnancy outcomes. Am J Obstet Gynecol. 2014;210(4):345.e1-9.

[88] Senturk LM, Arici A. Leukemia inhibitory factor in human reproduction. American journal of Reproductive Immunology 1998;39:137-143.

[89] Wegener NT, Mershon JL. Evaluation of leukemia inhibitory factors as a marker of ectopic pregnancy. American journal of Obstetrics and Gynaecology 2001;184:1074-76.

[90] Iyibozkurt AC, Kalelioglu I, Gursoy S, Corbacioglu A, Gurelpolat N, Karahan GE, Saygili H, Bengisu E. Evaluation of serum levels of IL-10, IL-11 and LIF in differentiation of eutopic and tubal ectopic pregnancy. Clin Exp Obstet Gynecol 2010;37(3): 217-20.

[91] Guney M, Erdemoglu E, Oral B, Karahan N, Mungan T. Leukemia inhibitory factor is immunohistochemically localized in tubal ectopic pregnancy. Acta Histochem 2008;110(4):319-23.

[92] Ji YF, Chen LY, Xu KH, Yao JF, Shi YF. Locally elevated leukemia inhibitory factor in the inflamed fallopian tube resembles that found in tubal pregnancy. Fertil Steril 2009;91(6):2308-14.

[93] Ruge S, Sorensen S, Vegtorp M, Vejerslev LO. The secretory endometrial protein, placental protein 14, in women with ectopic gestation. Fertility &Sterlity 1992;57:102-6.

[94] Vigne JL, Hornung D, Mueller MD, Taylor RN. Purification and characterization of an immunomodulatory endometrial protein glycodelin. J Biol Chem 2001;276:17101-5.

[95] Foth D, Romer T. Glycodelin serum levels in women with ectopic pregnancy. Eur J Obstet Gynecol Reprod Biol 2003;108(2):199-202.

[96] Aplin JD, Hey NA. MUC1, endometrium and embryo implantation. Biochem Soc Trans 1995;23:826-31.

[97] Savaris RF, da Silva LC, Moraes Gda S, Edelweiss MI. Expression of MUC1 in tubal pregnancy. Fertil Steril 2008;89(4):1015-17.

[98] Refaat B, Simpson H, Britton E, Biswas J, Wells M, Aplin JD, Ledger W. Why does the fallopian tube fail in ectopic pregnancy? The role of activins, inducible nitric oxide synthase and MUC 1 in ectopic implantation. Fertil Steril 2012;97(5):1115-23.

[99] Liao SB, Li HW, Ho JC, Yeung WS, Ng EH, Cheung AN, Tang F, O WS. Possible role of adrenomedullin in the pathogenesis of tubal ectopic pregnancy. J Clin Endocrinol Metab 2012;97(6):2105-12.

[100] O WS, Li HW, Liao SB, Cheung AN, Ng EH, Yeung WS, Ho JC, Tang F. Decreases in adrenomedullin expression and ciliary beat frequency in the nasal epithelium in tubal pregnancy. Fertil Steril. 2013;100(2):459-63.e1.

[101] Luisi S, Florio P, Reis FM, Petraglia F. Expression and secretion of activin A: Possible physiological and clinical implications. Eur J Endocrinol. 2001;145:225–36.

[102] Jones RL, Salamonsen LA, Zhao YC, Ethier JF, Drummond AE, Findlay JK. Expression of activin receptors, follistatin and betaglycan by human endometrial stromal cells; consistent with a role for activins during decidualization. Mol Hum Reprod 2002; 8:363–374.

[103] Horne AW, van den Driesche S, King AE, Burgess S, Myers M, Ludlow H, Lourenco P, Ghazal P, Williams AR, Critchley HO, Duncan WC. Endometrial inhibin/activin beta-B subunit expression is related to decidualization and is reduced in tubal ectopic pregnancy. J Clin Endocrinol Metab. 2008;93(6):2375-82.

[104] Lavie O, Beller U, Neuman M, Ben-Chetrit A, Gottcshalk-Sabag S and Diamant Y. Maternal serum CK: a possible predictor of tubal pregnancy. American Journal of Obstetrics and Gynaecology 1993;169:1149-50.

[105] Birkhahn RH, Gaeta TJ, Leo PJ, Bove JJ. The utility of maternal creatine kinase in the evaluation of ectopic pregnancy. Am J Emerg Med. 2000;18:695–7.

[106] Duncan WC, Sweeting VM, Cawood P, Illingworth PJ. Measurement of creatine kinase activity and diagnosis of ectopic pregnancy. Br J Obstet Gynaecol. 1995;102:233–7.

[107] Soundravally R, Krishna Latha T, Soundara Raghavan S, Ananthanarayanan PH, Srilatha K. Diagnostic significance of total creatine kinase and its isoform in tubal ectopic pregnancy. J Obstet Gynaecol Res. 2013;39(12):1587-91.

[108] Korhonen J, Alfthan H, Stenman UH, Ylostalo P. Failure of creatine kinase to predict ectopic pregnancy. Fertil Steril. 1996;65:922–4.

[109] Lincoln SR, Dockery JR, Long CA, Rock WA, Jr, Cowan BD. Maternal serum creatine kinase does not predict tubal pregnancy. J Assist Reprod Genet. 1996;13:702–4.

[110] Plewa MC, Ledrick D, Buderer NF, King RW. Serum creatine kinase is an unreliable predictor of ectopic pregnancy. Acad Emerg Med. 1998;5:300–3.

[111] Qasim SM, Trias A, Sachdev R, Kemmann E. Evaluation of serum creatine kinase levels in ectopic pregnancy. Fertil Steril. 1996;65:443–5.

[112] Vandermolen DT, Borzelleca JF. Serum creatine kinase does not predict ectopic pregnancy. Fertil Steril. 1996;65:916–21.

[113] Safdarian L, Aghahosseini M, Alleyassin A, Kohbodi M. Evaluation of Plasma Creatine Phosphokinase (CPK) Level Following a Single Injection of Methotrexate as a Predicator of Treatment Success in Ectopic Pregnancy. J Family Reprod Health. 2013;7(4):151-5.

[114] Birkhahn RH, Gaeta TJ, Paraschiv D, Bove JJ, Suzuki T, Katoh H, Nagai R. Serum levels of myoglobin, creatine phosphokinase, and smooth muscle heavy-chain myosin in patients with ectopic pregnancy. Ann Emerg Med. 2001; 38(6):628-32.

[115] Soriano D, Hugol D, Quang NT, Darai E. Serum concentrations of interleukin-2R (IL-2R), IL-6, IL-8, and tumor necrosis factor alpha in patients with ectopic pregnancy. Fertil Steril. 2003; 79(4):975-80.

[116] Daponte A, Deligeoroglou E, Pournaras S, Hadjichristodoulou C, Garas A, Anastasiadou F, Messinis IE. Interleukin-15 (IL-15) and anti-C1q antibodies as serum biomarkers for ectopic pregnancy and missed abortion. Clin Dev Immunol. 2013;2013:637513.

[117] Sadovsky Y, Pineda J, Collins JL. Serum CA-125 levels in women with ectopic and intrauterine pregnancies. J Reprod Med. 1999; 36(12):875-8.

[118] Brumsted JR, Nakajima ST, Badger G, Riddick DH, Gibson M. Serum concentration of CA-125 during the first trimester of normal and abnormal pregnancies. J Reprod Med. 1990; 35(5):499-502.

[119] Condous G, Kirk E, Syed A, Van Calster B, Van Huffel S, Timmerman D, et al. Do levels of serum cancer antigen 125 and creatine kinase predict the outcome in pregnancies of unknown location? Hum Reprod. 2005;20:3348–54.

[120] Kuscu E, Vicdan K, Turhan NO, Oguz S, Zorlu G, Gokmen O. The hormonal profile in ectopic pregnancies. Mater Med Pol. 1993;25:149–52.

[121] Schmidt T, Rein DT, Foth D, Eibach HW, Kurbacher CM, Mallmann P, et al. Prognostic value of repeated serum CA 125 measurements in first trimester pregnancy. Eur J Obstet Gynecol Reprod Biol. 2001;97:168–73.

[122] Katsikis I, Rousso D, Farmakiotis D, Kourtis A, Diamanti-Kandarakis E, Panidis D. Receiver operator characteristics and diagnostic value of progesterone and CA-125 in the prediction of ectopic and abortive intrauterine gestations. Eur J Obstet Gynecol Reprod Biol. 2006;125(2):226-32.

[123] Girardi G, Prohászka Z, Bulla R, Tedesco F, Scherjon S. Complement activation in animal and human pregnancies as a model for immunological recognition. Mol Immunol. 2011; 48(14):1621-30.

[124] Agostinis C, Bulla R, Tripodo C, Gismondi A, Stabile H, Bossi F, Guarnotta C, Garlanda C, De Seta F, Spessotto P, Santoni A, Ghebrehiwet B, Girardi G, Tedesco F. An alternative role of C1q in cell migration and tissue remodeling: contribution to trophoblast invasion and placental development. J Immunol. 2010; 185(7):4420-9.

[125] Echan LA, Tang HY, Ali-Khan N, Lee K, Speicher DW. Depletion of multiple high-abundance proteins improves protein profiling capacities of human serum and plasma. Proteomics. 2005;5:3292–303.

[126] Boschetti E, Righetti PG. The ProteoMiner in the proteomic arena: a non-depleting tool for discovering low-abundance species. J Proteomics. 2008;71:255–64.

[127] Gebeh AK, Willets JM, Marczylo EL, Taylor AH, Konje JC. Ectopic Pregnancy Is Associated with High Anandamide Levels and Aberrant Expression of FAAH and CB1 in Fallopian Tubes. J Clin Endocrinol Metab. 2012;97:2827–35.

[128] Horne AW, Phillips JA, 3rd, Kane N, Lourenco PC, McDonald SE, Williams AR, et al. CB1 expression is attenuated in Fallopian tube and decidua of women with ectopic pregnancy. PLoS One. 2008;3:e3969.

[129] Brown JK, Lauer KB, Ironmonger EL, Inglis NF, Bourne TH, Critchley HO, Horne AW. Shotgun proteomics identifies serum fibronectin as a candidate diagnostic biomarker for inclusion in future multiplex tests for ectopic pregnancy. PLoS One. 2013;8(6):e66974.

[130] Skubisz MM, Brown JK, Tong S, Kaitu'u-Lino T, Horne AW. Maternal Serum Macrophage Inhibitory Cytokine-1 as a Biomarker for Ectopic Pregnancy in Women with a Pregnancy of Unknown Location. PLoS One. 2013;8(6):e66339.

[131] Beer LA, Tang HY, Sriswasdi S, Barnhart KT, Speicher DW. Systematic discovery of ectopic pregnancy serum biomarkers using 3-D protein profiling coupled with label-free quantitation. J Proteome Res. 2011; 10(3):1126-38.

[132] Feng C, Chen ZY, Zhang J, Xu H, Zhang XM, Huang XF. Clinical utility of serum reproductive hormones for the early diagnosis of ectopic pregnancy in the first trimester. J Obstet Gynaecol Res. 2013 ;39(2):528-35.

[133] Zou S, Li X, Feng Y, Sun S, Li J, Egecioglu E, Billig H, Shao R. Comparison of the diagnostic values of circulating steroid hormones, VEGF-A, PIGF, and ADAM12 in women with ectopic pregnancy. J Transl Med. 2013;11:44.

Section 3

Endocrinal Problems

Chapter 4

Polycystic Ovary Syndrome

Fahimeh Ramezani Tehrani and
Samira Behboudi-Gandevani

Additional information is available at the end of the chapter

http://dx.doi.org/10.5772/59591

1. Introduction

Polycystic ovary syndrome (PCOS) is a common endocrinophaty disorder that affecting reproductive aged women [1]; it becomes frequently manifest during early reproductive age [2]. It is a heterogeneous disorder, with multiple reproductive, cosmetic and metabolic complexities which is characterized by dysfunction in ovulation and clinical or biochemical hyperandrogenism and the presence of polycystic ovarian morphology. It is the most common endocrine cause of infertility and increased the risk of adverse pregnancy outcome, metabolic syndrome, type 2 diabetes mellitus, and some carcinoma [2-5]. However, there is not a consensus on its definition [6]. At the first time, PCOS was described by Stein and Leventhal in 1935 [6] as the presence of bilaterally enlarged ovaries with multiple cysts in seven women with infertility, menstrual irregularity and hyperandrogenism [7]. The National Institutes of Health (NIH) in 1990 introduced NIH standard criteria in PCOS for applying in researches and clinics [3]. This definition relied on clinical or biochemical evidence of hyperandrogenaemia (in the absence of adrenal hyperplasia and hyperprolactinemia and thyroid dysfunction) in combination of oligomenorrhoea or amenorrhea. Therefore, PCOS was diagnosed in the absence of an ultrasound appearance of polycystic ovaries morphology [8]. In 2003, a consensus workshop in Rotterdam in the Netherlands presented new diagnostic criteria [3]. Rotterdam criteria describe PCOS as persistence of PCO and hyperandrogenism in women with normal menstrual cycles and especially women presenting with PCO and ovulatory disturbance without hyperandrogenism [9].

In 2009, the Androgen Excess and PCOS Society (AE-PCOS Society) introduced criteria for PCOS. Based on AE-PCOS Society criteria, PCOS should be define by the presence of hyperandrogenism (clinical and /or biochemical), ovarian dysfunction (ovulation disturbance and or polycystic ovary morphology), and the exclusion of other androgen excess or related disorders [10]. These criteria reflected differences in defining PCOS which could affect reporting, diagnosis and treatment of it.

1.1. Epidemiology

Despite PCOS being considered the most common endocrine disorder, the estimation of its prevalence is highly variable, ranging from 2.2% to 26.7% [11-13], due to differences in the presentation of PCOS phenotype methods [12]. In a study in Iran, a total of 646 reproductive-age women were assessed by Rotterdam, Androgen Excess Society, and NIH criteria, the prevalence of PCOS were 14.1%, 12%, and 4.8% respectively [14]. In a study from china, levels of luteinizing hormone and higher luteinizing hormone/follicle-stimulating hormone ratios were used for defining PCOS for 915 women in reproductive age, the results demonstrated 2.2 % prevalence [14]. In a study from china, levels of luteinizing hormone and higher luteinizing hormone/follicle-stimulating hormone ratios were used for defining PCOS for 915 women in reproductive age, the results demonstrated 2.2 % prevalence [11]. The prevalence based on NIH criteria in an unselected population black and white women in the southeastern United States were 3.4% and 4.7% respectively [15]. Using same criteria, the prevalence of PCOS was almost 6.5% between Caucasian and Greek women [16, 17].

2. Pathogenesis

The pathogenesis of PCOS are not fully understood, it seems that there are many different factors are associated with PCOS.

2.1. Gene's role

Some studies suggest that genetic plays an important role in pathogenesis of PCOS. The high prevalence of women with PCOS and the wide range of phenotypes can be explained by the interaction of key genes with environmental factors [18, 19]. There are some evidences showed that there are association between cytochrome P450 17-hydroxylase/17, 20-desmolase (CYP17) and PCOS. Cytochrome P450 side-chain cleavage enzyme (CYP11A) is another candidate gene that some studies find a role for it in PCOS. This gene encodes the cholesterol side-chain cleavage enzyme. Mutation in cytochrome P450 21-hydroxylase (CYP21) gene has found to have a role in PCOS in studies. This gene encodes 21-hydroxylase, which is responsible for most cases of congenital adrenal hyperplasia (CAH) [20].

2.2. Obesity-insulin

Approximately 50% of women with PCOS are overweight or obese and most of them have the android obesity. Obesity may play a pathogenetic role in the development of the PCOS in women through disturbances in insulin and androgenesis.

Accumulation of adipose tissue mass around abdomen increases the availability of metabolites, which are able to affect the secretion, the metabolism, and peripheral action of insulin.

http://dx.doi.org/10.5772/59591

Insulin, together with liver, adipose tissue and muscles, plays a role in the regulation of ovary. At ovarian level, insulin stimulates ovarian steroidogenesis by interacting with insulin and insulin growth factor type I receptors, in granulosa, thecal and stromal cells. Insulin increases 17-hydroxylase and 17-20 lyase activity and stimulates the expression of 3-hydroxysteroid dehydrogenase in granulosa cells. In addition, insulin seems to increase the sensitivity of pituitary cells to gonadotropin releasing hormone (GnRH) action and by increase the number of the luteinizing hormone (LH) receptor, increase the ovarian steroidogenic response to gonadotropins. Also, insulin is able to reduce sex hormone binding globulin (SHBG) synthesis in liver and ovary. IGFBP-1 regulates ovarian growth and cyst formation and adrenal steroidogenesis [21].

2.3. IGFs

IGF-I and IGF-II may be involved in the pathogenesis of the hyperandrogenism in the women with PCOS. IGFs are able to stimulate ovarian progesterone and estrogen secretion and increase the aromatase activity. In normal weight PCOS women, IGF bioavailability seems to be increased. But, in obese women with PCOS, IGF-1 bioavailability has been reduced. It could be suggested that insulin resistance and hyperinsulinemia may play a central role in obese PCOS patients; however disturbance of the IGF-IGFBP system may be important in normal-weight PCOS women [21-23].

2.4. SHBG

Sex hormone binding globulin (SHBG) is a glycoprotein that regulate circulating concentrations of free sexual steroid hormones and their transport to target tissues [24]. The concentrations of SHBG are regulated by a number of factors such as cortisol, estrogens, iodothyronines and growth factors, and decreased by androgens, insulin, prolactin and IGF-I [25]. SHBG concentration reduced specially in women with PCOS influence by hyperinsulinemia. Therefore, the free androgens increase at the level of peripheral tissues [21].

3. Androgens-estrogens-pituitary secretion

Hyperandrogenism play an important role in process of anovulation. In in-vitro study, the ovarian theca cells could increase steroidogenic activity in women with PCOS. Androgens levels originate from both ovarian and adrenal glands in PCOS. LH, ACTH, insulin and IGFs regulate production of androgen by affecting P450c17 enzyme at ovarian theca-interstitial cells and in the adrenal gland. Therefore, hyperactivity of the P450c17 enzyme represents the main mechanism resulting to ovarian hyperandrogenism that manifest in the great majority of women with PCOS. However, it is not cleared that hyperactivity of the P450c17 enzyme is a primary event or secondary to peripheral or central factors [21, 26]. Insulin is involved in hyperandrogenism from three ways. First, insulin in association with free IGF stimulates ovarian androgenesis. Second, hyperinsulinemia lead to reduce production of SHBG from liver, as a result lead to increase in free androgen level. Third, insulin may affect ovarian follicle maturation, lead to ateresia, and increase level of androgen [22].

Decrease in SHBG level affected the concentration of estron and free estradiol in women with PCOS. Due to none fluctuated production of estrogen, pituitary receive both positive feedback for LH secretion and negative feedback for secretion of FSH. As a result, the LH-FSH ratio increases. LH has pulsatile pattern. In women with PCOS, the frequency of LH secretion is increase. This change happens in response to receiving stmilution by GnRH and increase bioavailabilty of LH. The high level of LH, lead to ovarian hyperplasia and production of androgen from ovarian stromal and tecal cells. This condition fixes the chronic anovulation. It is not clear that the impairment in hypothalamic-pituitary-ovarian axis leads to PCOS or this disturbance happen as an outcome of PCOS [21, 22, 27-29].

4. Metabolic syndrome and polycystic ovary syndrome

The metabolic syndrome (MetS) is a cluster of cardiovascular risk factors, including impaired fasting glucose, central obesity, dyslipidaemia and raised blood pressure [30]. Ever since the metabolic syndrome was described by Reaven in 1988 [31], at least six diagnostic definitions have been published by different organizations. In this respect, although there is a general agreement regarding the main components of the MetS including abnormalities in glucose metabolism (insulin resistance, hyperinsulinemia, glucose intolerance, diabetes mellitus), central obesity, and cardiovascular risk factors (hypertension, increased triglyceride, decreased HDL cholesterol), this variation requires different cut-off points and inclusion criteria [30]. Table 1 shows most important definition of MetS according to World Health Organization (WHO) [32], and International Diabetes Federation (IDF) [33] criteria.

It has been shown that the combination of different components of MetS may predict a higher risk for cardiovascular than individuals and insulin resistance plays as a common link between these coexisting abnormalities [34].

The MetS affects roughly 25% of adults over the age of 20 y and up to 45% over age 50 y [35-37]. Some studies reported that during the last decade, the prevalence of MetS has increased in the general population, especially among young women [38]. However, this incremental trend may be attributable not only to anthropometric differences between diverse ethnicity, but also to differences in the criteria used for MetS diagnosis. Mechanisms underlying the metabolic syndrome are not completely clear. There is no single etiology of the MetS. Hyperinsulinemia, the most accepted and unifying hypothesis and a cornerstone of the syndrome [30],, results from interplay between environmental and genetic factors. Excess caloric intake and lack of physical exercise, combined with a predisposition to visceral adiposity, play a key role in the development of a pro-inflammatory insulin-resistant state that generates the clinical features of the MetS [37, 39]. However, the relationship between PCOS and MS is possibly mutual [34]. Majority of women with PCOS present clinically with at least one component of the metabolic syndrome [40]. In this respect, the prevalence of MetS among PCOS women is 43%-53%; approximately 2-fold higher that general women population [40]. However, the pathophysi-

http://dx.doi.org/10.5772/59591

ology that may link are not fully understood. Possible hypothesis regarding the association include: (I) insulin resistance underlies the pathogenesis of both the metabolic syndrome and PCOS; (II) obesity and related adipose tissue factors, independently of insulin resistance, are the major pathogenic contributors to both conditions; and (III) vascular and coagulation abnormalities are the primary pathogenic contributors to both conditions.

WHO	T2D or IFG or IGT or insulin resistance plus ≥ 2 of the following: • BMI > 30 kg/m² or WHR > 0.85 • HDL < 1.0 mmol/L (< 40 mg/dL) • TG ≥ 1.7 mmol/L (150 mg/dL) • BP ≥ 140/90 mmHg or use of blood pressure medication • microalbuminuria > 20 pg/min • Alb/Crea ratio ≥ 30 mg/g
rNCEP ATP III	≥ 3 of the following: • WC ≥ 88 cm • HDL < 1.3 mmol/L (< 50 mg/dL), or on drug treatment for lipid abnormality • TG ≥ 1.7 mmol/L (≥150 mg/dL), or on drug treatment for this lipid abnormality • FBS ≥100 mg/dl (≥5.6mmol/L) • systemic hypertension ≥ 135/85 mmHg or use of blood pressure medication
IDF	Central obesity defined as WC above the ethnicity-specific cut-off plus ≥ 2 of the following: • TG ≥ 1.7 mmol/L (150 mg/dL) or specific treatment • HDL < 1.3 mmol/L (< 50 mg/dL) or specific treatment • BP ≥ 135/85 mmHg or use of blood pressure medication f• asting plasma glucose ≥ 5.6 mmol/L (100 mg/dL) or previously diagnosed T2D

Table 1. Definitions of MBS for women, according to WHO, NCEP ATP III and IDF criteria

Insulin resistance is the major underlying pathophysiologic abnormality linking the metabolic syndrome and PCOS. Indeed, the co-morbidities associated with insulin resistance are well-known to be common to both conditions [41, 42]. Nevertheless, it is likely that a combination of various factors interacts with or results from insulin resistance to manifest the metabolic abnormalities of the metabolic syndrome and PCOS. In addition, genetic susceptibilities and genetic polymorphisms or mutations likely contribute to the expression of these manifestations [43].

Although PCOS and MetS often coexist, several factors have been shown to predict the risk of metabolic syndrome among women with PCOS. Among these factors fasting insulin, obesity and family history of diabetes have the capacity for prediction of metabolic syndrome in women with PCOS [44, 45].

It seems that it is reasonable to assess the components of MetS in women with PCOS; however there is no consensus on the methods and interval of these assessments [43]. Assessments of blood pressure, waist circumference and/ BMI, fasting lipid profile, Fasting glucose and glucose tolerance by a 2-hour oral glucose tolerance test have been suggested and aboratory studies for cardiovascular risk markers such as C-reactive protein and homocysteine are recommend [46, 47]. There were therapeutic overlap between PCOS and MetS. *Weight loss with life-style modification* is the safest and cheapest therapy that has shown benefit both in MetS and PCOS.

Reduction of insulin resistance is the primary goal for Weight loss in women with PCOS. Life-style modification through increased physical activity and reduction in body weight, especially waist circumference, represents the first-line therapy for MetS in PCOS. Successful maintenance of exercise and weight loss can lower blood pressure, central adiposity, and very low density lipoprotein cholesterol while improving lipid profile and insulin sensitivity [21, 48]. *Medical therapies for insulin resistance* with pharmacological approaches like metformin improve insulin sensitivity, glucose control and even reproductive abnormalities. Also metformin could decreases weight and BMI, blood pressure and LDL cholesterol [49, 50].

However, evidence has demonstrated that a combination of metformin and lifestyle modification improves the metabolic profile in women with PCOS to a greater degree than either measure alone [51].

5. Obesity and PCOS

The prevalence of obesity has increased worldwide in the last few decades [52]. Obesity status is defined according to the body mass index (BMI=body weight in kilograms divided by height in meters ^{2}) of 30 kg/m^2 or more. BMI of 25 to 29.9 kg/m^2 is defined as 'overweight', while BMI of less than 25 kg/m^2 is considered normal [53]. This had significant impact on the development of chronic diseases such as the metabolic syndrome, coronary heart disease and type 2 diabetes. Also, central obesity can be diagnosed clinically by measuring the waist circumference (WC) larger than 88 cm or waist-to-hip circumference ratio (WHR) greater than 0.85, confer high risk for metabolic complications in obese individuals with BMI between 25.0 and 34.9 kg/m^2.

However, obesity is a common finding in women with PCOS and between 40–80% of women with this condition is reported to be overweight, obese or centrally obese depending on the setting of the study and the ethnical background of the subjects [53-55]. Obesity has a worse additive effect on features of PCOS such as insulin resistance, hyperandrogenism, infertility, hirsutism and pregnancy complications [56].

The relationship between PCOS and obesity is complex, and most likely involves interaction of genetic and environmental factors [57]. Obesity in PCOS is usually of the central variety. It is shown that central obesity is associated with increased risk for diabetes, hyperlipidemia, hypertension, atherosclerosis, and insulin resistance [58]. Fat localized in the upper body is correlated with significantly reduced overall clearance of insulin, which contributes to hyperinsulinemia [59]. The mechanisms underlying obesity causes insulin resistance are not fully understood, the 2 main pathogenetic hypotheses that have been proposed focus on the

http://dx.doi.org/10.5772/59591

roles of free fatty acids (FFAs) and tumor necrosis factor-α (TNF-α). FFAs, which are released from adipose tissue triglycerides via lipolysis, as mediators of impaired insulin sensitivity, elevate in PCOS patients. Increased FFA flux into the liver, irrespective of its source, decreases hepatic insulin extraction, increases gluconeogenesis, and produces hyperinsulinemia [60]. Additionally, high circulating FFA concentrations lead to peripheral insulin resistance by reducing glucose uptake by the skeletal muscle [61].

TNF-α is produced by adipose tissue has been increasing in hyperandrogenic PCOS women. It leads to insulin resistance by stimulating the phosphorylation of serine residues of the insulin receptor substrate-1. Consequently, tyrosine kinase activity of the insulin receptor β-subunit, the rate-limiting component of the insulin receptor signaling cascade, is inhibited [62].

However, obese and non-obese PCOS patients may have differences in clinical manifestations. The differences in biochemical and clinical features between obese and non-obese PCOS patients allow determining, to some degree, the contributions of obesity to the clinical manifestations of PCOS. Differences in menstrual function have been reported, with obese patients exhibiting a greater prevalence of oligoamenorrhea and anovulation than non-obese women, And the prevalence of infertility has been increasing in obese PCOS patient [63]. Also, it is known that obesity has a direct relationship with the degree of hirsutism in PCOS patients. Obese women with PCOS had a greater prevalence of hirsutism, acanthosis nigricans, than non-obese patients, reflecting a higher prevalence and magnitude of insulin resistance and hyperinsulinemia among obese PCOS patients [64]. Impaired glucose tolerance, type 2 diabetes mellitus and the dyslipidemia has highest risk in obese PCOS patients. Overall, given the prevalence of risk factors for atherosclerosis in women with PCOS, a higher prevalence of cardiovascular events in these patients can be expected [65]. In addition, obese PCOS patients have higher prevalence of endometrial carcinoma than non-obese PCOS women. Anovulation, unopposed estrogen stimulation, and hyperinsulinemia may play a role in the increased risk of this gynecologic carcinoma in PCOS patients [66]. Also, it is reported that obstructive sleep apnea, pregnancy complications such as preeclampsia, gestational induced hypertension and gestational diabetes are more prevalent in obese PCOS patient [67, 68].

However, the impact of obesity on PCOS therapy is very important. Therapeutic modalities directed at the reduction of hyperinsulinemia (weight loss or insulin-sensitizing agents) appear to ameliorate symptoms of PCOS and restore normal ovarian function in obese women with PCOS.

Weight loss, especially more than 5% of the baseline weight, is the first-line therapy in treatment of these women. It leads to hormonal, menstrual, and metabolic improvement with increased serum concentrations of SHBG and reduced serum concentrations of free testosterone in obese women with PCOS. The mechanism by which weight loss leads to a reduction of hyperandrogenism appears to involve improved insulin sensitivity with a resultant decline in circulating insulin levels [69]. *Metformin* can be suggested as a second-line treatment for most obese women with PCOS [70].

6. Poly cystic ovarian syndrome and cancers

Since 1940s, there is emerging evidence of increased risk of gynecological cancer including endometrial, breast and ovary cancer among women with PCOS [71, 72]. Any association with malignant disease would be highly important from a public health perspective in view of the high prevalence of PCOS. The lack of appropriate recognition of risks takes these patients at highest risk of delayed diagnosis of pre-malignant or malignant disease [70]. At a cellular level there are numerous potential mechanisms which could promote neoplastic disease in women with PCOS, including the prolonged anovulatory state and associated hyperandrogenism with unopposed estrogen action [73]. These could increase the risk of cancer through the effect of these hormones on various tissue and organs [74].

6.1. Endometrial carcinoma and PCOS

Endometrial carcinoma (EC) is the second most frequent gynecological malignancy among women [74]. The number of reported cases of EC makes it the leading cause of cancer-related deaths across the globe [75]. Major EC-related symptoms include dysfunctional uterine bleeding, hyper-menorrhea, irregular menstruation, and sterility. The two main types of EC are estrogen-dependent type I (the most prevalent type) and estrogen-independent type II carcinomas. Among numerous risk factors, PCOS is commonly considered to be a significant and causative risk factor for the development and progression of type I EC [76]. The prevalence of endometrial hyperplasia with and without atypia in women with PCOS varies from 1 to 48.8% [77]. The prevalence of EC is three times higher among women with PCOS than among women without PCOS [71]. The mechanisms underlying EC and PCOS are also unclear, but it is widely assumed that chronic anovulation, which results in continuous estrogen stimulation of the endometrium unopposed by progesterone, is a major factor. Obesity, hyperinsulinemia, and hyperandrogenism state in PCOS, results in increased bioavailability of unopposed estrogens by progesterone due to the increased peripheral conversion of endogenous androgens such as testosterone and androstenedione into estrogen. Also, Insulin up-regulates aromatase activity in endometrial glands and stroma, endogenous estrogen production is enhanced in women with high circulating insulin. Estrogens act as proliferative factors in the endometrial tissue. Continuous exposure of the endometrium to estrogens with persistent progesterone deficiency, lead to endometrial overgrowth and hyperplasia or cancer [78]. The exact molecular mechanisms linking hyperinsulinaemia as found in PCOS and EC are uncertain. It is however thought that it may be modulated by a direct effect of insulin and IGF on endometrial cells or alterations in the P13K-mTOR-AKT signaling pathway with the loss of PTEN expression which have mitogenic effect on endometrial cells [79] and activation of insulin/IGF-1 signaling through overexpression of INSR and/or IGF-1R.

Overlay, the evidences suggest that interplay between hyperinsulinaemia and estrogen may mediate the mitogenic effect of the hyperinsulinaemia in PCOS.

Other potential risk factors for EC such as androgens and LH are also present in PCOS. Hypersecretion of luteinising hormone, a feature of PCOS, has also been implicated in the development of endometrial cancer in women with PCOS. Receptors for luteinising hormone and human chorionic gonadotropin are over expressed at both mRNA and protein levels in endometrial adenocarcinomas. Over expression of receptors for both these hormones in endometrial hyperplasia (with stronger staining in complex or atypical hyperplasia), and endometrial carcinoma were detected [80]. Insulin levels reduce the amount of IGFBP which in turn increases the amount of circulating IGF. IGF has been shown to induce LH receptors increasing LH levels, again suggesting an interaction between insulin resistance, LH and EC [81]. It should be noted that the triad of obesity, insulin resistance and diabetes in metabolic syndrome carried significant risks of EC [82]. However, the evidence for impact of PCOS on prognosis of endometrial carcinoma is incomplete and contradictory. Jafari et al. suggested that the presence of PCOS was associated with a favorable prognosis [83]. Insulin has also been found to accelerate the proliferation of cancer cell in the endometrium in an in-vitro study [82], and the concentration of IGF-1 was correlated well to the malignant cells differentiation [79], but, There is not enough knowledge supporting that mortality from endometrial cancer is differ in women with the syndrome.

However, it has been clearly shown in both animal and human studies that *metformin* is valuable insulin sensitizer agent in reversing endometrial hyperplasia. Metformin has exerted a chemo-protective and anti-proliferative effect on EC. It does this by a reduction in cell growth, which is modulated partly via insulin and non-insulin relevant path-ways. In the context of the links between EC and hyperproloferation of endometrium in PCOS, Metformin may therefore prevent EC in PCOS or treatment of EC.

6.2. Ovarian carcinoma and PCOS

Ovarian cancer accounts for 5% of all cancers among women and is the fourth most common cause of cancer deaths in developed countries, causing more deaths than any other female genital tract cancer [84]. Ovarian cancer typically presents late, with symptoms such as pelvic pain, abnormal vaginal bleeding, or involuntary weight loss, and has an overall 5-year survival of 30% after diagnosis. However, if detected early, at stage I, the 5-year survival is as high as 90%. It is, therefore, imperative that high-risk groups are identified so that appropriate screening is undertaken to detect early ovarian malignancy [85].

The majority of malignant ovarian tumors including epithelial malignancies appear to have steroid receptors for estrogen, progesterone and androgen. Cytokines may also play a role in malignant transformation. The various interactions of altered local ovarian factors and environmental factors have been associated with OC, as many of these factors are altered in PCOS.

Epidemiology studies showed that women with PCOS had a 2.5-fold increased risk of developing ovarian cancer, with a 95% confidence interval of 1.1–5.9 [86]. Also, clomiphene citrate and gonadotropin therapy or ovulation induction was found to increase the relative risk of ovarian tumors in women with PCOS around 4.1 [87]. The pathophysiological mechanisms that may be involved in ovarian oncogenesis in women with PCOS are not completely understood. Perhaps the high local steroid and growth factor concentrations that are frequently observed in women with PCOS may be implicated [88]. In addition, ovulation inducing drugs potentially which are used for infertility treatment, may have effect on ovarian cancer

[89]. Some researchers suggest that oral contraceptive use in some anovulatory women with PCOS may protect against ovarian cancer through gonadotropin suppression rather than the prevention of ''incessant ovulation'', with its putative dangers of inclusion cyst formation, epithelial proliferation, genetic damage and ovarian carcinogenesis [89].

6.3. Breast cancer and PCOS

Obesity, hyperandrogenism and infertility occur frequently in PCOS, and are feature known to be associated with the development of breast carcinoma [89]. In this respect, meta analysis about the association between PCOS and breast cancer showed that the risk of breast cancer was not significantly increased overall [90]. However, some studies showed that women with PCOS independently of age, age at menarche or menopause, parity, using oral contraceptive pill, BMI and family history of breast cancer, have 1.8 times as likely to report benign breast disease [91]. In this regard there is a need for more research.

7. Polycystic ovary syndrome and pregnancy

Normal pregnancy is characterized by induction of insulin resistance associated with compensatory hyperinsulinemia in second and third trimesters [49]. This insulin resistance of normal pregnancy is a physiologically advantageous adaptation designed to restrict maternal glucose uptake and to ensure shunting of nutrients to the growing fetus. It is probably mediated by increases in hormonal levels of estradiol, progesterone, prolactin, cortisol, human chorionic gonadotropin, placental growth hormone (PGH), and human placental lactogen (HPL) [33]. HPL and PGH are the hormones mainly responsible for insulin resistance in pregnancy. HPL is responsible for adaptive increase in insulin secretion necessary for pregnancy and for diversion of maternal carbohydrate metabolism to fat metabolism in the third trimester. PGH seems to be a paracrine growth factor probably regulating the metabolic and growth needs of the fetus partially [92]. There is approximately 200 to 250% increase in insulin secretion in lean women with normal glucose tolerance with advancing gestation [93]. However, there is comparatively less robust increase in insulin levels of obese women with normal glucose tolerance.

As we state before, hyperandrogenism and insulin resistance are the metabolic hallmark of PCOS women. In these patients, the baseline insulin resistance seems to be exacerbated with entry into pregnancy. There is an increased risk of pregnancy complications in PCOS women [94]. Nowadays a growing body of evidence points to a high prevalence of pregnancy complications in PCOS women. PCOS was strongly associated increased risk of early pregnancy loss, gestational diabetes (GDM), pregnancy-induced hypertension, preeclampsia, preterm birth, small for gestational age, large for gestational age, caesarean section, operative vaginal delivery, neonatal meconium aspiration and having a low Apgar score (<7) at five minutes and admission to an NICU [95-98].

It should be noted that there were the close link between PCOS and obesity and the association of obesity with poor pregnancy outcome, so, it might be possible that possible confounding effect of BMI play a role in adverse effect of PCOS on pregnancies.

7.1. PCOS and abortion

Abortion is the spontaneous loss of a fetus before the 20th week of pregnancy. Women with PCOS most probably have an increased risk of spontaneous Abortion [95]. It occurs in 30 to 50% of PCOS women compared with 10 to 15% of normal women [99]. Several mechanisms underlying the increased risk of abortion in women with PCOS have been proposed. Treatment with ovulation-inducing agents is associated with a higher incidence of abortion in PCOS women [95]. Obesity has been conclusively associated with an increased prevalence of miscarriage and obesity is obviously more common in PCOS patients than in the normal population. Also, elevated LH levels in women with PCOS and hyperandrogenemia play important role in increased risk of abortion. High androgen levels antagonize estrogen, which may adversely affect endometrial development and implantation [100]. Researchers showed that sex steroids regulate uterine receptivity for embryo implantation by controlling the expression of HOXA10 gene, which is spatially and temporally regulated during embryonic development. Elevated testosterone in PCOS down-regulates the expression of HOXA10 gene, thereby decreasing the uterine receptivity and implantation [100]. In addition high plasminogen activator inhibitor-1(PAI-1) activity which has been found to be associated with unexplained recurrent abortion, is significantly higher in women with PCOS, possibly due to impaired fibrinolysis, which results in placental insufficiency through increased thrombosis of the placental bed [101]. It is suggested that *metformin* therapies before and throughout pregnancy, could decrease the risk of early abortion, but more studies are needed [102].

7.2. PCOS and gestational diabetes mellitus

Gestational diabetes mellitus (GDM), defined as carbohydrate intolerance at onset of pregnancy (or first recognition), affects 4–7% of pregnancies overall [103]. There are 2.4-fold increased risks of GDM among PCOS women, independent of age, race/ethnicity, and multiple gestations. It means that GDM complicates 40 to 50% of PCOS pregnancies. The increased odds of GDM among women with PCOS symptoms are consistent with the overlap of metabolic perturbation and reproductive abnormalities and the possibility that some women actually had PCOS. It intervenes in pregnancy when pancreatic β cells cannot overcome the superimposed insulin resistance of pregnancy on intrinsic insulin resistance of PCOS women. It is too suggested that metformin may decrease of GDM among GDM, but recent meta-analysis, strictly, showed that metformin did not significantly effect on GDM with PCOS, though more multi-centers RCTs still need to be investigated [104].

7.3. PCOS and hypertensive disorders in pregnancy

Hypertensive disorders of pregnancy include: i. new onset of hypertension during pregnancy (or gestational hypertension which is defined as new-onset hypertension in pregnancy after 20 weeks of gestation), ii. Preeclampsia (defined as defined as gestational hypertension with proteinuria due to endothelial dysfunction and damage), iii. Pre-existing hypertension, and iv. exacerbation of pre-existing hypertension. The etiology of hypertensive pregnancy is uncertain and includes immune, genetic, and placental abnormalities. Three main hypotheses have been proposed regarding the metabolic alterations involved in the etiology of hypertensive disorders in pregnancy, namely endothelial dysfunction and activation, oxidative stress and insulin resistance [105]. Hypertensive disorders occurs in 8% of PCOS pregnancies [106]. Increased levels of androgens in PCOS have been associated with the development of preeclampsia [107]. Various studies have documented hyperinsulinemia and/ or hyperglycemia in early or mid pregnancy, before the development of preeclampsia, gestational hypertension, or both [108]. Hyperinsulinemia may directly predispose to hypertension by increased renal sodium re-absorption and stimulation of the sympathetic nervous system. Insulin resistance and/or associated hyperglycemia may impair endothelial function.

Two other factors, obesity and physical inactivity, are closely associated with insulin resistance, and are predictive of hypertensive pregnancy. A higher body mass index before pregnancy or early in pregnancy is associated with increased risk for both gestational hypertension and preeclampsia. Furthermore, it has been suggested that gestational diabetes, which itself is associated with underlying insulin resistance, is a risk factor for the development of hypertensive pregnancy. This association persists even after adjusting for obesity and maternal age. Also, a higher prevalence of preeclampsia and gestational diabetes may account for increased fetal stress leading to preterm birth, low Apgar scores at five minutes, and meconium aspiration.

7.4. PCOS and preterm birth

There was evidence of a significant positive association between PCOS and preterm births (<37weeks) [109]. It complicates 6 to 15% of pregnancies of PCOS women [110]. Although preterm birth may be higher in this group of women, PCOS by itself may not be an independent risk factor. Patients who have received ovulation induction agents are more likely to be at higher risk of preterm births, because these medications, together with the increased chance of multiple pregnancies related to them, will increase the risk of preterm birth or delivery [111]. Preeclampsia itself is a risk factor for preterm deliveries. Also, Obstetric intervention may be responsible for iatrogenic prematurity [110].

7.5. PCOS and Small for Gestational Age (SGA) and Large for Gestational Age (LGA)

There is still some controversy as to whether women diagnosed as having PCOS were more likely to have been born small for SGA and LGA, and whether theses baby is more prone to develop the symptoms of PCOS later in life. Whereas the probable association of higher maternal body weight, increased weight gain during pregnancy, and increased prevalence of gestational diabetes in women with PCOS would be expected to produce birth weights higher than the mean. Also, the prevalence of SGA offspring seems to be increased in women with PCOS. Insulin resistance resulting in impaired insulin-mediated growth and the fetal programming hypothesis are the possible explanations for this higher prevalence of SGA infants in mothers with PCOS [33].

http://dx.doi.org/10.5772/59591

8. Management of women with PCOS

The medical management of PCOS can be broken down into four components, three of which are "acute" issues (control of irregular menses, treatment of hirsutism and management of infertility) and one that is more "chronic." This latter issue may be the most important but least remembered by patients and providers alike–management of the IR syndrome. "Acute" issues that need management may change; however, a continuous life-long management approach is important for the IR of PCOS.

8.1. Weight reduction

As mentioned above the central obesity related to PCOS hyperandrogenism and anovulation. Also, obesity reduces the treatment effect in women with PCOS [112]. Weight lose can modified the hormonal profile, and androgen level therefore has good effect on ovulation and treatment of infertility. It is showed that 5 % weight reduction can modify menstruation cycle and ovulation. However, weight reduction is effective for women, who are overweight, a BMI 25-27 kg/m2. It includes change in life style with diet, exercise and surgery. Low carbohydrate and fat diets is recommended for obese PCOS women. Bariatric surgery may be recommended for morbidly obese women [112].

8.2. Induction ovulation

In PCOS, patient complaints of menstrual disturbance, that often related to chronic anovulation. It can increase risk of endometrial hyerplegisa and carcinoma. Therefore, this complication needs treatment. Low FSH concentration, high LH, androgen and insulin have roles in anovulation. Medications and another option apply for correct these underlying disturbance [112]. Treatments options are explained further in the following sections.

8.3. Clomiphene citrate

The first line medication for treatment of anovulation is clomiphene citrate (CC). CC is a nonsteroidal triphenylethylene with both estrogenic agonist and antagonist properties. CC bind to estrogen receptors by structural similarity with it. Improvement in ovulation happens with the CC effect at hypothalamic level. Reduction of hypothalamic estrogen receptor leads to mis interpretation of blood level estrogen. Therefore, estrogen feedback reduces and pulsatile GnRH secretion modify. As a result, FSH and LH secretion from pituitary normalized, in turn, improve follicular activity in ovarian. CC is administered for 5 days with doses of 50–150 mg, starting on days third or fifth days of mensural cycle or a progestin-induced menss. Most pregnancies occurred within the first six cycles with ovulation following the application of 50 mg CC. Higher doses may be required in patients with greater BMI. The rates of multiple pregnancies are under 10%, and ovaraian hyper stimulation syndrome is rare [112].

8.4. Metformin

Metformin is a biguanide, insulin-lowering effects, which are used for treatment of type 2 diabetes mellitus. Metformin has several benefits to manage PCOS complication. It improves ovulation, menstrual irregularity and reduces concentration of androgen. Also metformin help to weight reduction. Metformin has more effect in obese PCOS women [115]. Serious side effects of metformin are rare. Hypoglycemia is a rare side effect. For reducing common complication with metformin, it is start at 500 mg daily after food. The week after increase to achieved 1000 mg daily. After one week, the dose is increase to 1500 mg daily. The target is 1500–2550 mg/day. Usually, treatment effect appears at 1000 mg/day [113].

8.5. Aromatase inhibitors

The third generation aromatase inhibitors available include anastrozole and letrozole. They block production of estrogen from ovarian, conversion of androgen in referral fat cells, and suppress locally estrogen produced in brain. Therefore, this condition acts as positive feedback for hypothalamous to secrete GnRH, in turn, increase gonadotropin secretion. Also, reduction in estrogen concentration leads to increase activin that is a positive stimulation for FSH secretion. This positive feedback helps to growth of ovarian follicles. Usually Letrozole is used as anaromatase inhibitor for ovulation induction in women with PCOS. The administration dose is between 2.5–7.5 mg daily for 5 days starting on third day of the menstrual cycle. The main advantage of letrozole is antiestrogenic effect on endometrium, despite of stimulating follicle growth [113].

8.6. Gonadotropins

After resistance to CC, gonadotropins are another option for induction ovulation. Gonadotropins induce ovulation, and help to achieve a capable follicle for fertilization. The serious side effect of gonadotropins is ovarian hyperstimulation syndrome (OHSS) that result from simultaneous growth of multiple follicles. Several treatment protocols have been developed, one of the low-dose gonadotropin protocols regimen starts with a 37.5–50 IU/day, which increases, if confirm the lack of follicle response. Control is made by ultrasound. HCG is act as LH surge; leading to maturation of the oocyte, rupture of the follicle, and formation of the corpus luteum [112].

8.7. Laparoscopic ovarian diathermy

In clomiphene resistant condition, and when gonadotropin is not useful, laparoscopic ovarian diathermy is an acceptable treatment. The mechanism of action of ovarian diathermy is correction of hypersecretion of LH via modification in ovarian pituitary feedback. To assess the efficacy of unilateral laparoscopic ovarian diathermy in the induction of ovulation, researchers find unilateral ovarian diathermy resulted in ovulation from both ovaries [112, 113].

http://dx.doi.org/10.5772/59591

8.8. Treatment of menstrual dysfunction

In patient complaints of menstrual irregularity, often there is chronic anovulation that associated with risk of endometrial hyperplasia and carcinoma. Thus, treatment of menstrual dysfunction is important. Endometrial biopsy is recommended for PCOS women, who have not menstrual bleeding for a long time (m0re than 6 months). In women, who does not intent to be pregnant, oral contraceptive pills (OCPs) or cyclic progestin are recommended. OCPs increase production of SHBG at liver, thus reduce androgen concentration, and improved LH secretion. It is important to consider the androgenic effect of progestin component of OCPs. New OCPs have less androgenic effects [112].

8.9. Treatment of androgen-related symptoms

Hirsutism, acne, alopecia are the androgen-related symptoms that appeared in patients with PCOS. Antiandrogens such as spironolactone, cyproterone acetate (CPA), or flutamide act by competitive inhibition of androgen-binding receptors or by decreasing androgen production.

Spironolactone is a specific antagonist of aldosterone, acting through blocks androgen receptors. Its treatment effect is dosage-dependent: low dosages are less effective than other antiandrogens, whereas high dosages (200 mg/day) are very effective but have several adverse effects such as dysfunctional uterine bleeding but the concurrent use of OCPs may prevent from it. Spironolactone have feminizing effect on male fetus, therefore concomitant use of OCPs with spironolactone is useful for sexually active women [112]. Cyproterone acetate (CPA) is a progestin agent. This drug inhibits gonadotropin secretion and suppresses androgen action. CPA is recommended in 50-100mg (high dose) for ten days of cycle with 20-50 μg Ethinyl Estradiol. CPA is effective for management of hirsutism and acne. It may leads to nausea, headaches, and breast tenderness, reduce libido, and weight gain. CPA rarely appears hepatotoxicity effects. This drug has feminizing effect such as Spironolactone. Finasteride restrain 5α-reductase and inhibit androgen production, therefore, it is useful for management of hirsitism. In a study that patients treated with finasteride, reduction in hirsutism occurred after 6 months. Concomitant use of OCPs with 5 mg Finasteride was shown to be more effective than OCPs alone. It has feminizing effect, thus risks and benefits of treatment must be carefully considered and discussed with the patient. In conclusion, at least 6 months is required to see benefit from medication and prolong treatment is often necessary for maintain benefit. Pregnancy must be avoided during treatment with all antiandrogens [112, 113].

Author details

Fahimeh Ramezani Tehrani* and Samira Behboudi-Gandevani

*Address all correspondence to: ramezani@endocrine.ac.ir

Reproductive Endocrinology Research Center, Research Institute for Endocrine Sciences, Shahid Beheshti University of Medical Sciences, Tehran, Iran

References

[1] Zacur HA. Epidemiology, clinical manifestations and pathophysiology of polycystic ovary syndrome. Adv Stud Med. 2003;3:S733-S9.

[2] Buggs C, Rosenfield RL. Polycystic Ovary Syndrome in Adolescence. Endocrinology and Metabolism Clinics of North America. 2005;34(3):677-705.

[3] NIH. Evidence-based Methodology Workshop on Polycystic Ovary Syndrome: National Institutes of Health 2012.

[4] Vutyavanich T, Khaniyao V, Wongtra-ngan S, Sreshthaputra O, Sreshthaputra R, Piromlertamorn W. Clinical, endocrine and ultrasonographic features of polycystic ovary syndrome in Thai women. Journal of Obstetrics and Gynaecology Research. 2007;33(5):677-80.

[5] Fauser BC, Tarlatzis BC, Rebar RW, Legro RS, Balen AH, Lobo R, et al. Consensus on women's health aspects of polycystic ovary syndrome (PCOS): the Amsterdam ESHRE/ASRM-Sponsored 3rd PCOS Consensus Workshop Group. Fertility and sterility. 2012;97(1):28-38. e25.

[6] Balen A, Michelmore K. What is polycystic ovary syndrome? Are national views important? Human Reproduction. 2002;17(9):2219-27.

[7] Atiomo WU, Pearson S, Shaw S, Prentice A, Dubbins P. Ultrasound criteria in the diagnosis of polycystic ovary syndrome (PCOS). Ultrasound in Medicine & Biology. 2000;26(6):977-80.

[8] Hart R, Hickey M, Franks S. Definitions, prevalence and symptoms of polycystic ovaries and polycystic ovary syndrome. Best Practice & Research Clinical Obstetrics & Gynaecology. 2004;18(5):671-83.

[9] Broekmans F, Knauff E, Valkenburg O, Laven J, Eijkemans M, Fauser B. PCOS according to the Rotterdam consensus criteria: change in prevalence among WHO-II anovulation and association with metabolic factors. BJOG: An International Journal of Obstetrics & Gynaecology. 2006;113(10):1210-7.

[10] Azziz R, Carmina E, Dewailly D, Diamanti-Kandarakis E, Escobar-Morreale HF, Futterweit W, et al. The Androgen Excess and PCOS Society criteria for the polycystic ovary syndrome: the complete task force report. Fertility and sterility. 2009;91(2): 456-88.

[11] Chen X, Yang D, Mo Y, Li L, Chen Y, Huang Y. Prevalence of polycystic ovary syndrome in unselected women from southern China. European Journal of Obstetrics & Gynecology and Reproductive Biology. 2008;139(1):59-64.

[12] March WA, Moore VM, Willson KJ, Phillips DI, Norman RJ, Davies MJ. The prevalence of polycystic ovary syndrome in a community sample assessed under contrasting diagnostic criteria. Human Reproduction. 2010;25(2):544-51.

[13] Peppard HR, Marfori J, Iuorno MJ, Nestler JE. Prevalence of polycystic ovary syndrome among premenopausal women with type 2 diabetes. Diabetes care. 2001;24(6): 1050-2.

[14] Rashidi H, Ramezani Tehrani F, Bahri Khomami M, Tohidi M, Azizi F. To what extent does the use of the Rotterdam criteria affect the prevalence of polycystic ovary syndrome? A community-based study from the Southwest of Iran. European Journal of Obstetrics & Gynecology and Reproductive Biology. 2014;174:100-5.

[15] Knochenhauer E, Key T, Kahsar-Miller M, Waggoner W, Boots L, Azziz R. Prevalence of the Polycystic Ovary Syndrome in Unselected Black and White Women of the Southeastern United States: A Prospective Study 1. The Journal of Clinical Endocrinology & Metabolism. 1998;83(9):3078-82.

[16] Asunción M, Calvo RM, San Millán JL, Sancho J, Avila S, Escobar-Morreale HF. A Prospective Study of the Prevalence of the Polycystic Ovary Syndrome in Unselected Caucasian Women from Spain 1. The Journal of Clinical Endocrinology & Metabolism. 2000;85(7):2434-8.

[17] Diamanti-Kandarakis E, Kouli CR, Bergiele AT, Filandra FA, Tsianateli TC, Spina GG, et al. A survey of the polycystic ovary syndrome in the Greek island of Lesbos: hormonal and metabolic profile. The Journal of Clinical Endocrinology & Metabolism. 1999;84(11):4006-11.

[18] Crosignani P, Nicolosi A. Polycystic ovarian disease: heritability and heterogeneity. Human reproduction update. 2001;7(1):3-7.

[19] Urbanek M. The genetics of the polycystic ovary syndrome. Nature Clinical Practice Endocrinology & Metabolism. 2007;3(2):103-11.

[20] Amato P, Simpson JL. The genetics of polycystic ovary syndrome. Best Practice & Research Clinical Obstetrics & Gynaecology. 2004;18(5):707-18.

[21] Gambineri A, Pelusi C, Vicennati V, Pagotto U, Pasquali R. Obesity and the polycystic ovary syndrome. International journal of obesity and related metabolic disorders: journal of the International Association for the Study of Obesity. 2002;26(7):883-96.

[22] Poretsky L, Cataldo NA, Rosenwaks Z, Giudice LC. The insulin-related ovarian regulatory system in health and disease. Endocrine reviews. 1999;20(4):535-82.

[23] Voutilainen R, Franks S, Mason HD, Martikainen H. Expression of insulin-like growth factor (IGF), IGF-binding protein, and IGF receptor messenger ribonucleic acids in normal and polycystic ovaries. The Journal of Clinical Endocrinology & Metabolism. 1996;81(3):1003-8.

[24] Wallace IR, McKinley MC, Bell PM, Hunter SJ. Sex hormone binding globulin and insulin resistance. Clinical endocrinology. 2013;78(3):321-9.

[25] Von Schoultz B, Carlström K. On the regulation of sex-hormone-binding globulin—a challenge of an old dogma and outlines of an alternative mechanism. Journal of steroid biochemistry. 1989;32(2):327-34.

[26] Rosenfield RL. Ovarian and adrenal function in polycystic ovary syndrome. Endocrinology and Metabolism Clinics of North America. 1999;28(2):265-93.

[27] Fauser BC, Pache TD, Hop WC, Jong FH, Dahl KD. The significance of a single serum LH measurement in women with cycle disturbances: discrepancies between immunoreactive and bioactive hormone estimates*. Clinical endocrinology. 1992;37(5): 445-52.

[28] Hautanen A. Synthesis and regulation of sex hormone-binding globulin in obesity. International journal of obesity and related metabolic disorders: journal of the International Association for the Study of Obesity. 2000;24:S64-70.

[29] Taylor AE, McCourt B, Martin KA, Anderson EJ, Adams JM, Schoenfeld D, et al. Determinants of Abnormal Gonadotropin Secretion in Clinically Defined Women with Polycystic Ovary Syndrome 1. The Journal of Clinical Endocrinology & Metabolism. 1997;82(7):2248-56.

[30] Day C. Metabolic syndrome, or What you will: definitions and epidemiology. Diabetes and Vascular Disease Research. 2007;4(1):32-8.

[31] Reaven G. Metabolic syndrome pathophysiology and implications for management of cardiovascular disease. Circulation. 2002;106(3):286-8.

[32] Consultation W. Definition, diagnosis and classification of diabetes mellitus and its complications: Part; 1999.

[33] Altieri P, Gambineri A, Prontera O, Cionci G, Franchina M, Pasquali R. Maternal polycystic ovary syndrome may be associated with adverse pregnancy outcomes. European Journal of Obstetrics & Gynecology and Reproductive Biology. 2010;149(1):31-6.

[34] Kandaraki E, Christakou C, Diamanti-Kandarakis E. Metabolic syndrome and polycystic ovary syndrome... and vice versa. Arquivos Brasileiros de Endocrinologia & Metabologia. 2009;53(2):227-37.

[35] Aekplakorn W, Chongsuvivatwong V, Tatsanavivat P, Suriyawongpaisal P. Prevalence of metabolic syndrome defined by the International Diabetes Federation and National Cholesterol Education Program criteria among Thai adults. Asia-Pacific Journal of Public Health. 2011;23(5):792-800.

[36] McCullough AJ. Epidemiology of the metabolic syndrome in the USA. Journal of digestive diseases. 2011;12(5):333-40.

[37] Mehta NN, Reilly MP. Mechanisms of the metabolic syndrome. Drug Discovery Today: Disease Mechanisms. 2004;1(2):187-94.

[38] Ramos RG, Olden K. The prevalence of metabolic syndrome among US women of childbearing age. American journal of public health. 2008;98(6):1122.

[39] Eckel RH, Grundy SM, Zimmet PZ. The metabolic syndrome. The Lancet. 2005;365(9468):1415-28.

[40] Apridonidze T, Essah PA, Iuorno MJ, Nestler JE. Prevalence and characteristics of the metabolic syndrome in women with polycystic ovary syndrome. The Journal of Clinical Endocrinology & Metabolism. 2005;90(4):1929-35.

[41] Kadowaki T, Yamauchi T, Kubota N, Hara K, Ueki K, Tobe K. Adiponectin and adiponectin receptors in insulin resistance, diabetes, and the metabolic syndrome. The Journal of clinical investigation. 2006;116(7):1784-92.

[42] Wijeyaratne CN, Balen AH, Barth JH, Belchetz PE. Clinical manifestations and insulin resistance (IR) in polycystic ovary syndrome (PCOS) among South Asians and Caucasians: is there a difference? Clinical endocrinology. 2002;57(3):343-50.

[43] Essah P, Nestler J. The metabolic syndrome in polycystic ovary syndrome. Journal of endocrinological investigation. 2006;29(3):270-80.

[44] Coviello AD, Legro RS, Dunaif A. Adolescent girls with polycystic ovary syndrome have an increased risk of the metabolic syndrome associated with increasing androgen levels independent of obesity and insulin resistance. The Journal of Clinical Endocrinology & Metabolism. 2006;91(2):492-7.

[45] Ehrmann DA, Liljenquist DR, Kasza K, Azziz R, Legro RS, Ghazzi MN. Prevalence and predictors of the metabolic syndrome in women with polycystic ovary syndrome. The Journal of Clinical Endocrinology & Metabolism. 2006;91(1):48-53.

[46] Bickerton A, Clark N, Meeking D, Shaw K, Crook M, Lumb P, et al. Cardiovascular risk in women with polycystic ovarian syndrome (PCOS). Journal of clinical pathology. 2005;58(2):151-4.

[47] Boulman N, Levy Y, Leiba R, Shachar S, Linn R, Zinder O, et al. Increased C-reactive protein levels in the polycystic ovary syndrome: a marker of cardiovascular disease. The Journal of Clinical Endocrinology & Metabolism. 2004;89(5):2160-5.

[48] Moran LJ, Lombard CB, Lim S, Noakes M, Teede HJ. Polycystic ovary syndrome and weight management. Women's Health. 2010;6(2):271-83.

[49] ASRM-Sponsored P. Consensus on infertility treatment related to polycystic ovary syndrome. Fertility and sterility. 2008;89(3):505.

[50] Moghetti P, Castello R, Negri C, Tosi F, Perrone F, Caputo M, et al. Metformin Effects on Clinical Features, Endocrine and Metabolic Profiles, and Insulin Sensitivity in Polycystic Ovary Syndrome: A Randomized, Double-Blind, Placebo-Controlled 6-Month

Trial, followed by Open, Long-Term Clinical Evaluation 1. The Journal of Clinical Endocrinology & Metabolism. 2000;85(1):139-46.

[51] Hoeger KM, Kochman L, Wixom N, Craig K, Miller RK, Guzick DS. A randomized, 48-week, placebo-controlled trial of intensive lifestyle modification and/or metformin therapy in overweight women with polycystic ovary syndrome: a pilot study. Fertility and sterility. 2004;82(2):421-9.

[52] Finkelstein EA, Khavjou OA, Thompson H, Trogdon JG, Pan L, Sherry B, et al. Obesity and severe obesity forecasts through 2030. American journal of preventive medicine. 2012;42(6):563-70.

[53] Melmed S, Polonsky KS, Larsen PR, Kronenberg HM. Williams textbook of endocrinology: Expert consult: Elsevier Health Sciences; 2011.

[54] Cupisti S, Kajaia N, Dittrich R, Duezenli H, Beckmann MW, Mueller A. Body mass index and ovarian function are associated with endocrine and metabolic abnormalities in women with hyperandrogenic syndrome. European Journal of Endocrinology. 2008;158(5):711-9.

[55] Vrbikova J, Hainer V. Obesity and polycystic ovary syndrome. Obesity facts. 2009;2(1):26-35.

[56] Qin JZ, Pang LH, Li MJ, Fan XJ, Huang RD, Chen HY. Obstetric complications in women with polycystic ovary syndrome: a systematic review and meta-analysis. Reprod Biol Endocrinol. 2013;11:56.

[57] Lim SS, Norman RJ, Davies MJ, Moran LJ. The effect of obesity on polycystic ovary syndrome: a systematic review and meta-analysis. Obesity Reviews. 2013;14(2): 95-109.

[58] Tehrani FR, Solaymani-Dodaran M, Hedayati M, Azizi F. Is polycystic ovary syndrome an exception for reproductive aging? Human Reproduction. 2010:deq088.

[59] Peiris A, Struve M, Kissebah A. Relationship of body fat distribution to the metabolic clearance of insulin in premenopausal women. International journal of obesity. 1986;11(6):581-9.

[60] Salehi M, Bravo-Vera R, Sheikh A, Gouller A, Poretsky L. Pathogenesis of polycystic ovary syndrome: what is the role of obesity? Metabolism. 2004;53(3):358-76.

[61] Kelley DE, Goodpaster BH. Skeletal muscle triglyceride an aspect of regional adiposity and insulin resistance. Diabetes Care. 2001;24(5):933-41.

[62] Martyn JJ, Kaneki M, Yasuhara S. Obesity-Induced Insulin Resistance and Hyperglycemia: Etiological Factors and Molecular Mechanisms. Anesthesiology. 2008;109(1): 137.

[63] Chen L, Xu WM, Zhang D. The association of abdominal obesity, insulin resistance, and oxidative stress in adipose tissue in women with polycystic ovary syndrome. Fertility and Sterility. 2014(0).

[64] Maiti NN, Kanungo S, Bhattacharya SM. O427 Acanthosis Nigricans in Adolescents with Polycystic Ovary Syndrome. International Journal of Gynecology & Obstetrics. 2012;119, Supplement 3(0):S412.

[65] Cussons AJ, Stuckey BGA, Watts GF. Cardiovascular disease in the polycystic ovary syndrome: New insights and perspectives. Atherosclerosis. 2006;185(2):227-39.

[66] Lou X-f, Lin J-f, Fang S-p, Wang F-l. Analysis on Reverse of Atypical Endometrial Hyperplasia by Drugs in Patients with Polycystic Ovary Syndrome. Journal of Reproduction and Contraception. 2013;24(4):205-14.

[67] Nitsche K, Ehrmann DA. Obstructive sleep apnea and metabolic dysfunction in polycystic ovary syndrome. Best Practice & Research Clinical Endocrinology & Metabolism. 2010;24(5):717-30.

[68] Thatcher SS, Jackson EM. Pregnancy outcome in infertile patients with polycystic ovary syndrome who were treated with metformin. Fertility and Sterility. 2006;85(4): 1002-9.

[69] Pelletier L, Baillargeon J-P. Clinically significant and sustained weight loss is achievable in obese women with polycystic ovary syndrome followed in a regular medical practice. Fertility and Sterility. 2010;94(7):2665-9.

[70] Al-Nozha O, Habib F, Mojaddidi M, El-Bab MF. Body weight reduction and metformin: Roles in polycystic ovary syndrome. Pathophysiology. 2013;20(2):131-7.

[71] Chittenden B, Fullerton G, Maheshwari A, Bhattacharya S. Polycystic ovary syndrome and the risk of gynaecological cancer: a systematic review. Reproductive biomedicine online. 2009;19(3):398-405.

[72] Legro RS. Long-Term Sequelae of Polycystic Ovary Syndrome. Insulin Resistance and Polycystic Ovarian Syndrome: Springer; 2007. p. 335-48.

[73] Brinton LA, Moghissi KS, Westhoff CL, Lamb EJ, Scoccia B. Cancer risk among infertile women with androgen excess or menstrual disorders (including polycystic ovary syndrome). Fertility and sterility. 2010;94(5):1787-92.

[74] Hardiman P, Pillay OS, Atiomo W. Polycystic ovary syndrome and endometrial carcinoma. The lancet. 2003;361(9371):1810-2.

[75] Leslie KK, Thiel KW, Yang S. Endometrial cancer: potential treatment and prevention with progestin-containing intrauterine devices. Obstetrics & Gynecology. 2012;119(Part 2):419-20.

[76] Chittenden BG, Fullerton G, Maheshwari A, Bhattacharya S. Polycystic ovary syndrome and the risk of gynaecological cancer: a systematic review. Reproductive biomedicine online. 2009;19(3):398-405.

[77] Tingthanatikul Y, Choktanasiri W, Rochanawutanon M, Weerakeit S. Prevalence and clinical predictors of endometrial hyperplasiain anovulatory women presenting with amenorrhea. Gynecological endocrinology. 2006;22(2):101-5.

[78] Horn L-C, Meinel A, Handzel R, Einenkel J. Histopathology of endometrial hyperplasia and endometrial carcinoma: an update. Annals of diagnostic pathology. 2007;11(4):297-311.

[79] Nagamani M, Stuart CA, Dunhardt PA, Doherty MG. Specific binding sites for insulin and insulin-like growth factor I in human endometrial cancer. American journal of obstetrics and gynecology. 1991;165(6):1865-71.

[80] Konishi I, Koshiyama M, Mandai M, Kuroda H, Yamamoto S, Nanbu K, et al. Increased expression of LH/hCG receptors in endometrial hyperplasia and carcinoma in anovulatory women. Gynecologic oncology. 1997;65(2):273-80.

[81] Shafiee MN, Chapman C, Barrett D, Abu J, Atiomo W. Reviewing the molecular mechanisms which increase endometrial cancer (EC) risk in women with polycystic ovarian syndrome (PCOS): Time for paradigm shift? Gynecologic oncology. 2013;131(2):489-92.

[82] Lathi RB, Hess A, Tulac S, Nayak N, Conti M, Giudice L. Dose-dependent insulin regulation of insulin-like growth factor binding protein-1 in human endometrial stromal cells is mediated by distinct signaling pathways. The Journal of Clinical Endocrinology & Metabolism. 2005;90(3):1599-606.

[83] Jafari K, Javaheri G, Ruiz G. Endometrial adenocarcinoma and the Stein-Leventhal syndrome. Obstetrics & Gynecology. 1978;51(1):97-100.

[84] Hennessy BT, Coleman RL, Markman M. Ovarian cancer. The lancet. 2009;374(9698): 1371-82.

[85] Galazis N, Olaleye O, Haoula Z, Layfield R, Atiomo W. Proteomic biomarkers for ovarian cancer risk in women with polycystic ovary syndrome: a systematic review and biomarker database integration. Fertility and sterility. 2012;98(6):1590-601. e1.

[86] Schildkraut JM, Schwingl PJ, Bastos E, Evanoff A, Hughes C. Epithelial ovarian cancer risk among women with polycystic ovary syndrome. Obstetrics & Gynecology. 1996;88(4, Part 1):554-9.

[87] Ron E, Lunenfeld B, Menczer J, Blumstein T, Katz L, Oelsner G, et al. Cancer incidence in a cohort of infertile women. American journal of epidemiology. 1987;125(5): 780-90.

[88] Balen A. Polycystic ovary syndrome and cancer. Human reproduction update. 2001;7(6):522-5.

[89] Dumesic DA, Lobo RA. Cancer risk and PCOS. Steroids. 2013;78(8):782-5.

[90] Barry JA, Azizia MM, Hardiman PJ. Risk of endometrial, ovarian and breast cancer in women with polycystic ovary syndrome: a systematic review and meta-analysis. Human reproduction update. 2014:dmu012.

[91] Vink J, Sadrzadeh S, Lambalk C, Boomsma D. Heritability of polycystic ovary syndrome in a Dutch twin-family study. The Journal of Clinical Endocrinology & Metabolism. 2006;91(6):2100-4.

[92] Barbour LA, Shao J, Qiao L, Pulawa LK, Jensen DR, Bartke A, et al. Human placental growth hormone causes severe insulin resistance in transgenic mice. American journal of obstetrics and gynecology. 2002;186(3):512-7.

[93] Catalano PM, Huston L, Amini SB, Kalhan SC. Longitudinal changes in glucose metabolism during pregnancy in obese women with normal glucose tolerance and gestational diabetes mellitus. American journal of obstetrics and gynecology. 1999;180(4):903-16.

[94] Palomba S, Falbo A, Russo T, Tolino A, Orio F, Zullo F. Pregnancy in women with polycystic ovary syndrome: the effect of different phenotypes and features on obstetric and neonatal outcomes. Fertility and sterility. 2010;94(5):1805-11.

[95] Homburg R. Pregnancy complications in PCOS. Best Practice & Research Clinical Endocrinology & Metabolism. 2006;20(2):281-92.

[96] Kjerulff LE, Sanchez-Ramos L, Duffy D. Pregnancy outcomes in women with polycystic ovary syndrome: a metaanalysis. American journal of obstetrics and gynecology. 2011;204(6):558. e1-. e6.

[97] Roos N, Kieler H, Sahlin L, Ekman-Ordeberg G, Falconer H, Stephansson O. Risk of adverse pregnancy outcomes in women with polycystic ovary syndrome: population based cohort study. BmJ. 2011;343.

[98] Toulis KA, Goulis DG, Kolibianakis EM, Venetis CA, Tarlatzis BC, Papadimas I. Risk of gestational diabetes mellitus in women with polycystic ovary syndrome: a systematic review and a meta-analysis. Fertility and sterility. 2009;92(2):667-77.

[99] Jakubowicz DJ, Iuorno MJ, Jakubowicz S, Roberts KA, Nestler JE. Effects of metformin on early pregnancy loss in the polycystic ovary syndrome. The Journal of Clinical Endocrinology & Metabolism. 2002;87(2):524-9.

[100] Apparao K, Lovely LP, Gui Y, Lininger RA, Lessey BA. Elevated endometrial androgen receptor expression in women with polycystic ovarian syndrome. Biology of reproduction. 2002;66(2):297-304.

[101] Glueck C, Wang P, Fontaine RN, Sieve-Smith L, Tracy T, Moore SK. Plasminogen activator inhibitor activity: an independent risk factor for the high miscarriage rate dur-

ing pregnancy in women with polycystic ovary syndrome. Metabolism. 1999;48(12): 1589-95.

[102] Palomba S, Orio Jr F, Falbo A, Manguso F, Russo T, Cascella T, et al. Prospective parallel randomized, double-blind, double-dummy controlled clinical trial comparing clomiphene citrate and metformin as the first-line treatment for ovulation induction in nonobese anovulatory women with polycystic ovary syndrome. The Journal of Clinical Endocrinology & Metabolism. 2005;90(7):4068-74.

[103] Lo JC, Feigenbaum SL, Escobar GJ, Yang J, Crites YM, Ferrara A. Increased Prevalence of Gestational Diabetes Mellitus Among Women With Diagnosed Polycystic Ovary Syndrome A population-based study. Diabetes care. 2006;29(8):1915-7.

[104] Zhuo Z, Wang A, Yu H. Effect of Metformin Intervention during Pregnancy on the Gestational Diabetes Mellitus in Women with Polycystic Ovary Syndrome: A Systematic Review and Meta-Analysis. Journal of Diabetes Research. 2014;2014.

[105] Katsikis I, Kita M, Karkanaki A, Prapas N, Panidis D. Late pregnancy complications in polycystic ovarian syndrome. Hippokratia. 2006;10(3):105.

[106] Roberts JM, Pearson G, Cutler J, Lindheimer M. Summary of the NHLBI working group on research on hypertension during pregnancy. Hypertension. 2003;41(3): 437-45.

[107] Troisi R, Potischman N, Johnson CN, Roberts JM, Lykins D, Harger G, et al. Estrogen and androgen concentrations are not lower in the umbilical cord serum of preeclamptic pregnancies. Cancer Epidemiology Biomarkers & Prevention. 2003;12(11): 1268-70.

[108] Innes KE, Wimsatt JH, McDuffie R. Relative glucose tolerance and subsequent development of hypertension in pregnancy. Obstetrics & Gynecology. 2001;97(6):905-10.

[109] Boomsma C, Eijkemans M, Hughes E, Visser G, Fauser B, Macklon N. A meta-analysis of pregnancy outcomes in women with polycystic ovary syndrome. Human reproduction update. 2006;12(6):673-83.

[110] Ghazeeri GS, Nassar AH, Younes Z, Awwad JT. Pregnancy outcomes and the effect of metformin treatment in women with polycystic ovary syndrome: an overview. Acta obstetricia et gynecologica Scandinavica. 2012;91(6):658-78.

[111] Mikola M, Hiilesmaa V, Halttunen M, Suhonen L, Tiitinen A. Obstetric outcome in women with polycystic ovarian syndrome. Human reproduction. 2001;16(2):226-9.

[112] Badawy A, Elnashar A. Treatment options for polycystic ovary syndrome. International journal of women's health. 2011;3:25.

[113] Sirmans SM, Pate KA. Epidemiology, diagnosis, and management of polycystic ovary syndrome. Clinical epidemiology. 2014;6:1.

Chapter 5

Treatment of Congenital Adrenal Hyperplasia by Reducing Insulin Resistance and Cysticercosis Induced Polycystic Ovarian Syndrome

Alan Sacerdote and Gül Bahtiyar

Additional information is available at the end of the chapter

http://dx.doi.org/10.5772/58953

1. Introduction

Among the most common causes of female infertility, anovulation, menstrual irregularity, hirsutism, acne, and alopecia are congenital adrenal hyperplasia (CAH) and polycystic ovarian syndrome (PCOS). These two conditions resemble one another quite a bit, especially the non-classic forms of CAH (NCAH). Another common cause of such problems is hyperprolactinemia, which results in increased androgen synthesis by both the ovaries and the adrenal cortex, while suppressing gonadotrophin-releasing hormone, gonadotrophin, and estrogen synthesis. Hyperprolactinemia, in turn, may be caused by primary hypothyroidism, prolactinomas, stalk effects of other pituitary and hypothalamic neoplasia, as well as a host of prescription and recreational drugs; it may also be idiopathic. Other, less frequently encountered causes of these problems include Cushing's syndrome and virilizing tumors (ovarian, adrenal, or ectopic). A growing worldwide problem in this sphere is androgen doping to improve athletic performance.

Additional causes of menstrual irregularity include uterine leiomyomata, puberty, perimenopause, chronic illnesses eg. poorly controlled diabetes mellitus and sickle cell disease, elite athletics and dancing, eating disorders, endometriosis, and Asherman's syndrome.

Infertility may also be caused by stress, tubal factors, Asherman's syndrome, immune response to spermatozoa, luteal phase inadequacy, and male factors.

In this chapter we shall focus on 3 novel concepts:

- The treatment of the congenital adrenal hyperplasias and the acquired/unmasked adrenal hyperplasias by interventions which reduce insulin resistance.

- The induction of PCOS and enhanced 1-α-hydroxylation of 25-OH-vitamin D by parasite endocrine disruption.
- The amelioration of the latter by alteration of the hormonal milieu.

2. Insulin resistance in CAH

2.1. Recognition of insulin resistance in CAH

The first report of insulin resistance in CAH was published by Speiser et al. in female patients with non-classic 21-hydroxylase deficiency [1].

In 1994 Andersson et al. reported that women with type 2 Diabetes Mellitus (T2DM), the archetypal insulin-resistant condition, had higher mean free testosterone levels, higher waist/hip ratios, lower sex hormone-binding globulin (SHBG) levels, and higher plasma insulin levels than gender/BMI matched controls [2]. In commenting on the report of Andersson et al., Sacerdote reported a sample of 57 consecutive male and female T2DMs, all of whom had adrenal hyperandrogenism [3].

In 2005 Saygili et al. reported that women with non-classic 21-hydroxylase deficiency were both insulin and leptin resistant compared BMI-matched controls [4].

Several groups have reported insulin resistance as a common feature of both classic 21-hydroxylase deficiency and classic 11-hydroxylase activity [5-14]. Importantly, in most of these studies, the insulin resistance was independent of the corticosteroid dosage, suggesting that it is intrinsic to CAH, rather than a result of exogenous corticosteroid. Glucocorticoid receptor polymorphism (BclI GR variant) may contribute to the insulin resistance as reported by Moreira et al [14].

In 2006 we reported additional endocrine disrupter effects of two classes of drugs used in anti-retroviral therapy that were already known to cause insulin resistance, protease inhibitors and nucleoside analogues-the induction/unmasking of adrenal hyperplasia [15].

Despite the slowly growing recognition that insulin resistance is an intrinsic feature of both CAH and acquired/unmasked CAH, just at is in PCOS, the medical community has been very slow in exploring treatment approaches based on improving insulin sensitivity analogous to the treatment approaches now used so successfully in PCOS. This is despite the widely recognized limitations of mainstream corticosteroid replacement therapy, which, as excellent as it is, often cannot normalize androgen levels without producing adverse effects of glucocorticoid excess, such as decreased bone mineral density, hyperglycemia, soft-tissue changes, and affective changes. The respective advantages and disadvantages of corticosteroid replacement therapy, including the latest advances are discussed extensively in our earlier chapter [16].

http://dx.doi.org/10.5772/58953

2.2. Treating CAH by reducing insulin resistance

In 2000 we reported the first series of patients with T2DM/pre-diabetes and non-classic CAH (NCAH) in whom the biochemical and clinical features of NCAH were ameliorated by treatment with metformin and/or troglitazone [17], from 2 different classes of insulin sensitizers, biguanides and thiazolidinediones.

In 2003 we reported that the biochemical/phenotypic expression of NCAH, including 21-hydroxylase deficiency, 3-β-ol dehydrogenase deficiency, 11-hydroxylase deficiency, and aldosterone synthase deficiency could be ameliorated with the thiazolidinedione insulin sensitizer, rosiglitazone [18]. An example of this is shown in Figure 1. Of note, in this patient, the observed sharp drop in serum 17-OH-progesterone occurred within 24 hours of initiating rosiglitazone, consistent with an effect on DNA transcription/ mRNA translation.

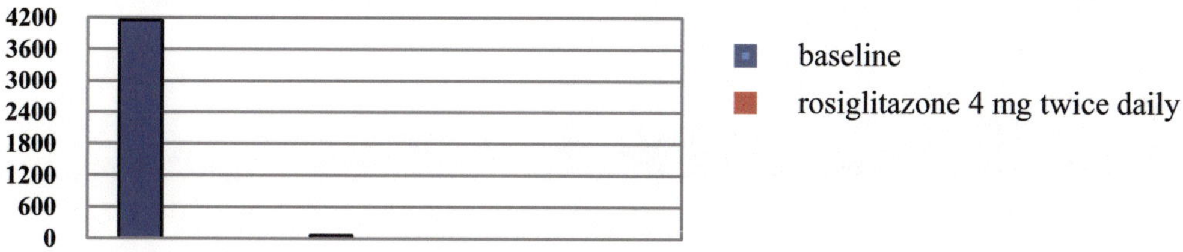

Figure 1. Response of a 43 year old male's 17-OH-Progesterone (ng/dl) to rosiglitazone 4mg bid.

In 2004 we reported that the biochemical/phenotypic expression of NCAH is ameliorated by pioglitazone [19]. An example of the combined effect of metformin and pioglitazone compared with standard glucocorticoid/mineralocorticoid replacement therapy in a patient with non-classical 21-hydroxylase deficiency is shown in Figure 2. Note that the response of the patient's serum 17-OH-progesterone to the insulin sensitizers, metformin and pioglitazone is more complete than to the standard of care therapy with glucocorticoid and mineralocorticoid.

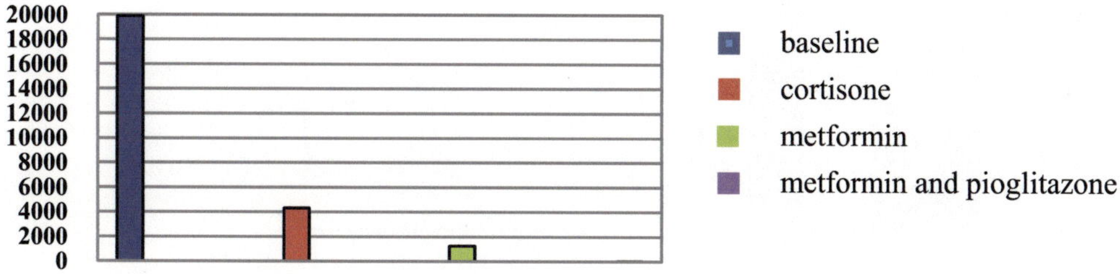

Figure 2. Response of a 57 year old female's 17-OH-Progesterone (ng/dl) to cortisone acetate, metformin, & pioglitazone

Arslanian et al. reported that metformin therapy in obese teen-agers with PCOS and impaired glucose tolerance (IGT) attenuated the exaggerated adrenocortical response to ACTH with a reduction in hyperinsulinemia/insulin resistance [20]..

In 2007 we reported that the anti-psychotic drugs and valproate, which were already known to cause insulin resistance and, in the case of the latter, PCOS, also induced and/or unmasked adrenal hyperplasia [21]. This endocrine disrupter effect of these drugs was reversible with the insulin sensitizers metformin (Figure 3) or rosiglitazone (Figure 4).

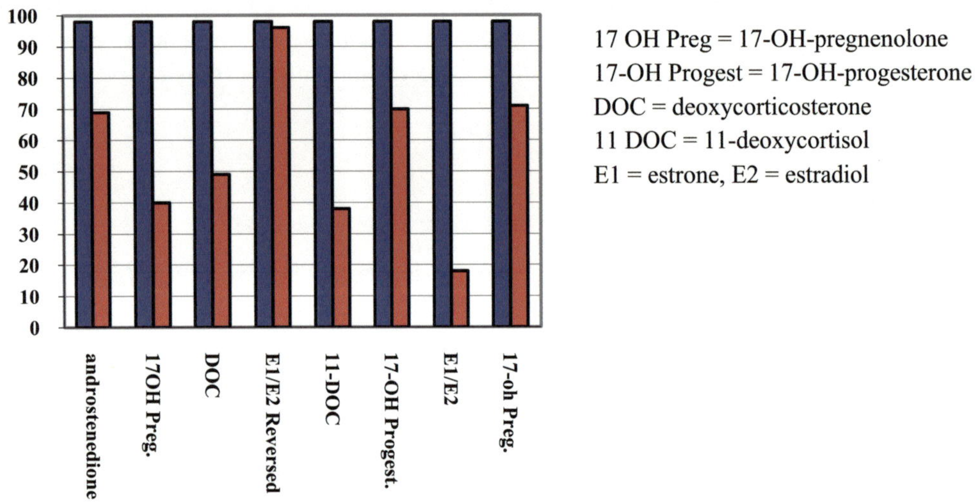

Figure 3. Effect of metformin on elevated steroid metabolites in 8 patients (represented as % of baseline)

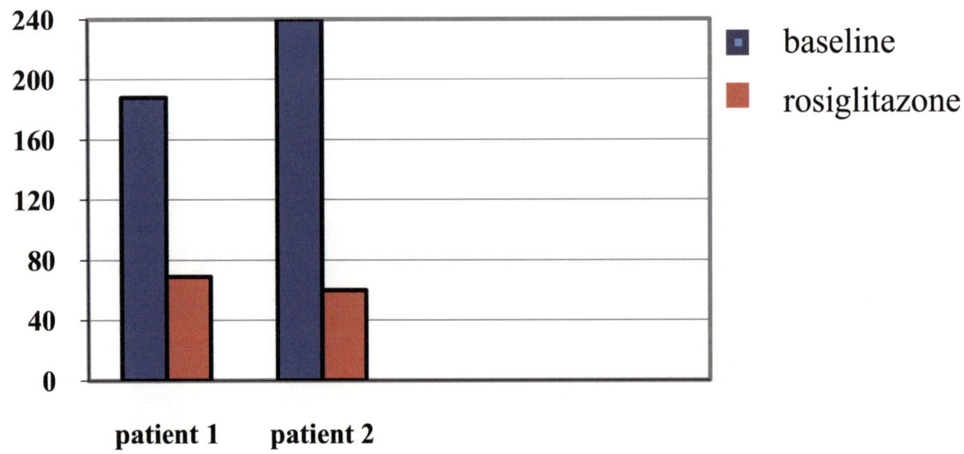

Figure 4. Effect of rosiglitazone on elevated baseline 11-Deoxycortisol level (mg/dl) in 2 patients

In 2008 we published the first report of a patient with classical, salt losing 21-hydroxylase deficiency being successfully treated with the addition of metformin to standard corticosteroid therapy (Figures 5,6) [22]. The patient was a 17 year old woman, whose CAH had been diagnosed in the nursery, where she had become profoundly dehydrated, whose current complaints were of amenorrhea, hirsutism, and acne, despite being adherent to optimal glucocorticoid/mineralocorticoid therapy. As can be seen in figure 5, her baseline serum 17-OH-progesterone on standard therapy was still very elevated, while her baseline serum total testosterone (Figure 6) was actually in the lower reference range for adult males. While maintaining this therapy, metformin 500 mg twice daily after meals was added. Co-incident with the marked reduction in both her serum 17-OH-progesterone and serum testosterone levels documented at her next visit, she noted the return of monthly menses, the absence of new acne lesions, and a reduction in hirsutism. While we would have liked to continue to titrate her metformin dose upward to 2 grams daily and, if necessary, added a second insulin-sensitizing agent in an attempt to normalize her steroid metabolite levels, and then possibly, wean her off corticosteroids altogether, the patient pronounced herself pleased with the results shown here and declined further dose titration and/or addition of other insulin sensitizers.

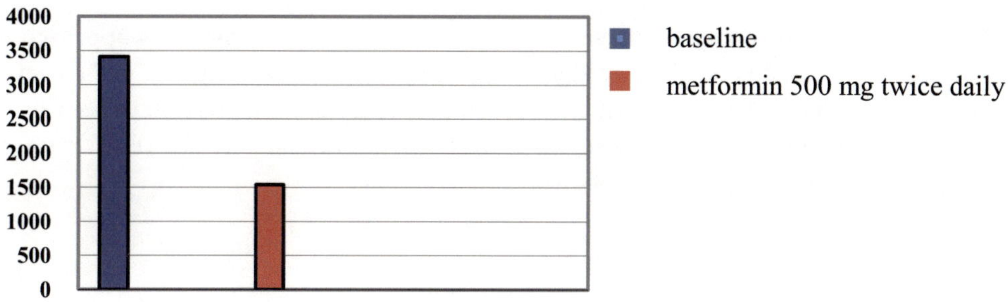

Figure 5. Effect of metformin on 17-OH-progesterone (ng/dl) in a patient with classical, salt-wasting 21-Hydroxylase deficiency

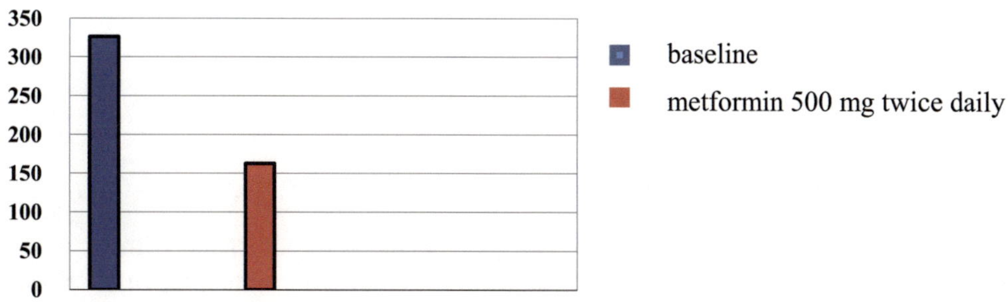

Figure 6. Effect of metformin on serum total testosterone (ng/dl) in classical, salt-wasting 21-Hydroxylase deficiency

Before proceeding to discuss other insulin-sensitizing options in the treatment of CAH and endocrine-disrupter induced/unmasked adrenal hyperplasia, it is worth discussing a few limitations to their use. Despite their demonstrated efficacy, these insulin sensitizers have still not been demonstrated to be able to totally replace corticosteroids in classical CAH nor have they been prescribed, to our knowledge, in forms of CAH such as lipoid CAH.

The main limitation of metformin use is gastrointestinal intolerance. Much of this problem may be overcome by prescribing more gastrointestinal-friendly forms of metformin such as extended release, liquid (Riomet), or matrix-embedded (Glumetza). Unfortunately, the latter two forms, which are exceptionally well-tolerated, are often not covered by prescription insurance.

Another significant limitation of metformin use is that is inappropriate to use in patients with seriously compromised renal function due to an increased risk of lactic acidosis. In the U.S. it is recommended that metformin not be used in women with serum creatinine >1.4 mg/dl or men with serum creatinine > 1.5 mg/dl. In several other countries guidelines are allowing its use at lower doses down to an eGFR > 35 ml/min.

The use of thiazolidinediones is limited because there is little experience with this class of drugs in mid-late pregnancy and there is concern about weight gain, bone loss, and bladder cancer.

Another means of improving insulin sensitivity is with diet and exercise. This approach was utilized in 2 patients with non-classic aldosterone synthase deficiency (Figure 7) [23]. Diet and exercise resulted in a 10% weight reduction accompanied by a normalization of the elevated serum deoxycorticosterone levels and normalization of the elevated LH/FSH ratio and improvement in the clinical features of virilization.

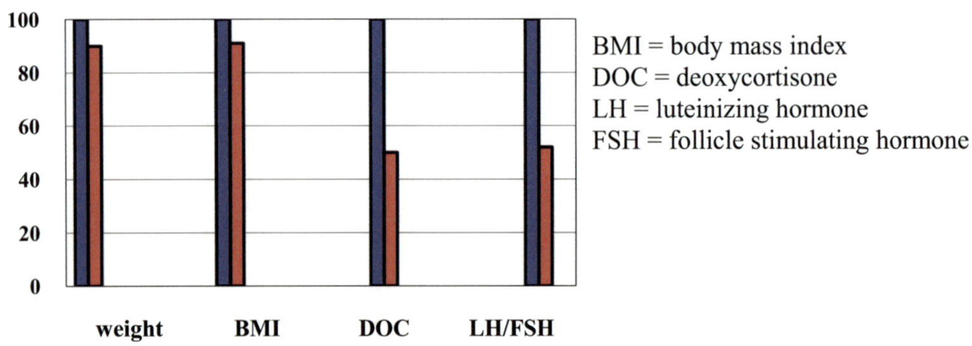

Figure 7. Changes with weight loss &exercise in 2 women with non-classic aldosterone synthase deficiency

Metabolic or bariatric surgery in obese T2DM patients has been associated with an improvement in insulin sensitivity associated with weight loss, suppression of inappropriate glucagon secretion via observed increases in GLP-1, reductions in glucose toxicity via improved glycemic control, and increased glucose utilization associated with intestinal villous hypertrophy/hyperplasia distal to the anastomotic site. It is also reported to ameliorate PCOS [24].

We reported the first patient in whom Roux-en Y gastric bypass not only caused the patient's T2DM and hypertension to remit, but also normalized the biochemical and clinical expression of her non-classical 11-hydroxylase deficiency (Figure 8) [25].

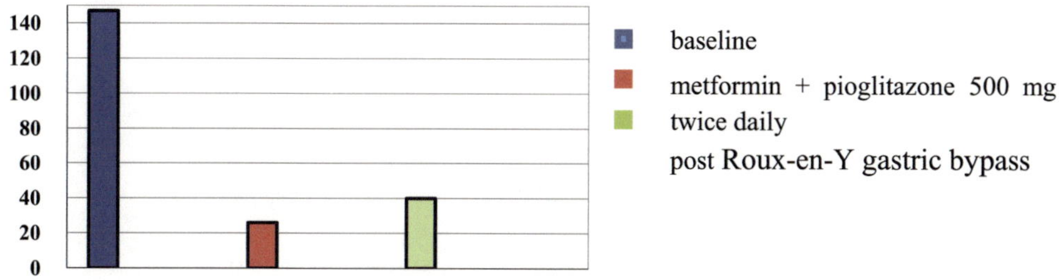

Figure 8. Response of patient's 11-Deoxycortisol (ng/dl), nl < 51 to Roux-en-Y gastric bypass

Ashwagandha root (*Withania somnifera*) has been used for millennia in Aryuvedic medicine, where it has proven effective in treating a number of specific conditions as well as being used as a general "tonic". We recently reported a patient who complained of excessive scalp hair shedding who was investigated and found to have both non-classic 3-β-ol-dehydrogenase deficiency and aldosterone synthase deficiency with elevated baseline levels of both serum 17-OH-pregnenolone and corticosterone [26]. The patient had been able to reduce her rate of scalp hair loss and normalized her serum levels of both steroid metabolites while taking pioglitazone 15 mg/day. The patient elected to, nevertheless, stop pioglitazone because of what she had read on the internet concerning osteoporosis and bladder carcinoma. She promptly started losing excessive scalp hair again. After watching the Dr. Oz television program she decided to start a standardized preparation of Ashwagandha root 400 mg twice daily as a general 'tonic" and anti-oxidant. At her next visit she reported that she was awakening in the morning with much less hair on her pillow. Repeat serum levels of 17-OH-pregnenolone and corticosterone again fell to normal while using Ashwagandha root (Figures 9,10). A report by Anwer et al. confirms that Ashwagandha, among other effects, is an insulin sensitizer [27].

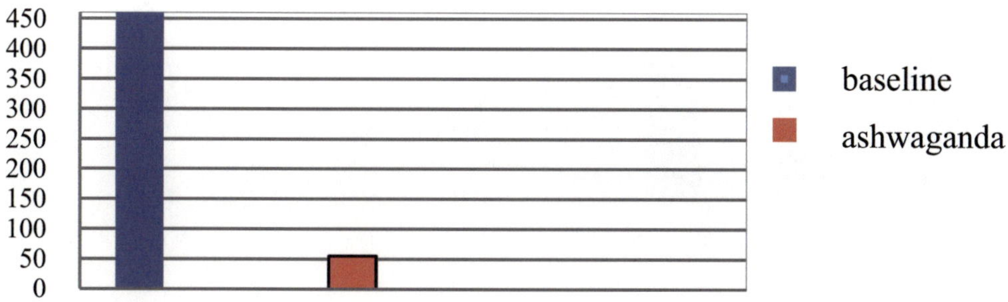

Figure 9. Response of patient's serum 17-OH-Pregnenolone (ng/dl) to Ashwagandha 400 mg twice daily

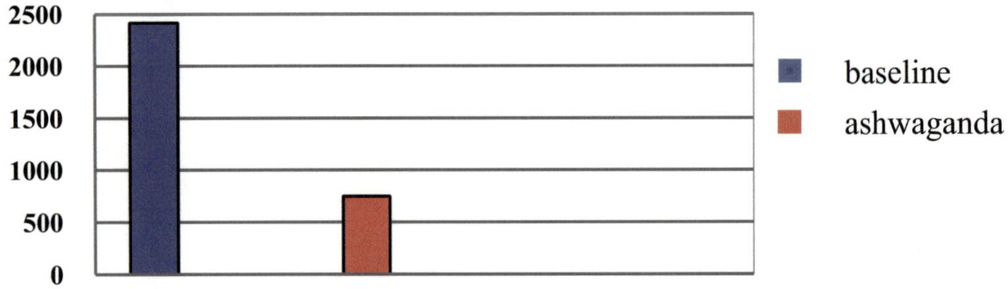

Figure 10. Response of patient's serum corticosterone (ng/dl) to Ashwagandha 400 mg Twice Daily

There is now considerable evidence that Vitamin D is an insulin sensitizer [28]. We recently reported a patient with T2DM, classical 11-hydroxylase deficiency, and severe Vitamin D deficiency [29].

Metformin treatment was not initially an option in this patient as he had a life-threatening lower extremity infection with gangrene. Metformin would have increased his risk for developing dangerous lactic acidosis. His diabetes was, therefore, treated with basal/bolus insulin. Vitamin D replacement was begun using ergocalciferol 50,000 IU once a week. His serum 11-deoxycortisol fell from a baseline value of 2024 ng/dl (nl<76) to <20 ng/dl over a period of 28 days, while his serum 25-OH-vitamin D_3 level rose concomitantly from a baseline value of 12 ng/ml (nl>30) to a level of 27 ng/dl on the 17th day of replacement (Figure 11). The 28 day Vitamin D sample was lost by the laboratory. It is known that the adrenal cortex has Vitamin D receptors (VDR's) [30]. Thus, Vitamin D may also enhance the expression of adrenal steroidogenic enzymes via cross-talk.

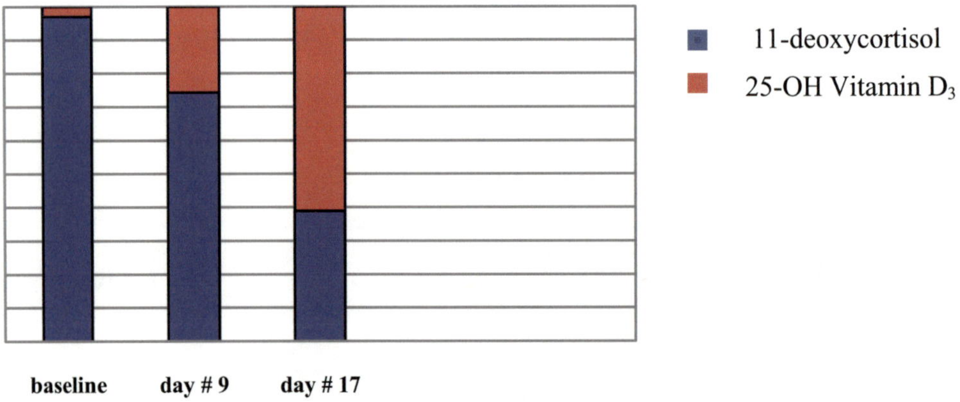

Figure 11. Changes in serum 11-deoxycortisol (left) as a function of changes in serum 25-OH-Vitamin D_3 (right) at baseline and at 9 days and 17 days after starting ergocalciferol 50,000 IU daily.

Most recently, we have reported a patient whose non-classic 11-hydroxylase deficiency was improved by taking a combination of Vitamin D and the GLP-1 receptor agonist liraglutide (Figure 12) [31]. GLP-1 receptor agonists improve insulin sensitivity by suppressing the inappropriate secretion of the counter-regulatory hormone, glucagon, decreasing glucose toxicity by lowering post-prandial and fasting glucose levels and over time by weight, (visceral fat mass) reduction.

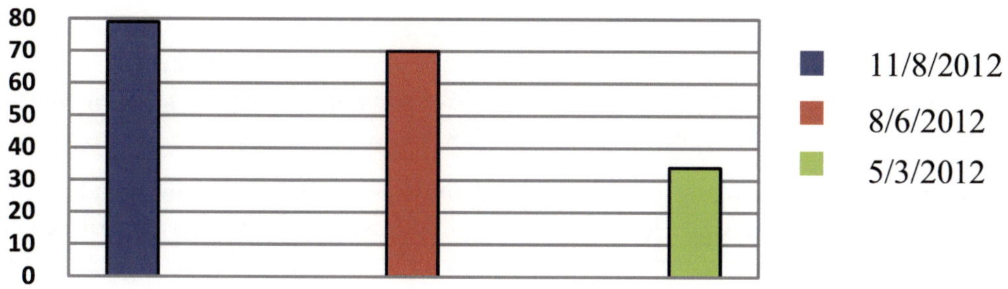

Figure 12. Response of Patient's Serum 11-Deoxycortisol (ng/dl; ref. range <42 ng/dl) to treatment with ergocalciferol & liraglutide

2.3. Possible mechanisms by which reducing insulin resistance ameliorates congenital adrenal hyperplasia

Kelly et al. studied the effects of insulin in an *in vitro* human adrenocortical cell culture [32]. They reported that steroidogenic factor-1 (SF-1) activity is up-regulated in vitro by insulin in the presence of forskolin (a functional analog of ACTH in this setting). Increased SF-1 synthesis, as well as increased binding of SF-1 to its response element, resulted in increased transcription of CYP17 causing increased adrenal androgen synthesis in both normal, human adrenocortical tissue and in cultures of the adrenocortical tumor line H-295. In these same two *in vitro* systems insulin inhibited the forskolin (ACTH) stimulated synthesis of the transcription factor *nur77*, an action that results in decreased transcription of CYP21 mRNA, further directing adrenal steroidogenesis toward androgen vs cortisol biosynthesis. Thus, hyperinsulinemia would worsen the phenotypic/biochemical expression of 21-hydroxylase deficiency as well as magnify any other deficiencies of adrenal steroidogenic enzymes.

2.4. Future directions in the treatment of congenital adrenal hyperplasia by reducing insulin resistance

A number of drugs, herbs, naturally occurring compounds, as well as other therapeutic interventions have been shown to improve insulin sensitivity. While the efficacy of metformin and the thiazolidinediones in the treatment of NCAH is now established, it is still unknown if these agents could completely replace corticosteroids in classical CAH. Similarly, while we have shown in one patient that Vitamin D replacement can obviate the need for corticosteroids in a patient with classical 11-hydroxylase deficiency, we do not know if Vitamin D would work as well in other classical forms of CAH or in CAH patients without vitamin D deficiency/insufficiency. Randomized control trials will be needed to answer these important questions.

It is now recognized that dopamine receptor agonists have an in insulin-sensitizing effect [33, 34] and a formulation of the dopamine receptor agonist, bromocriptine, is now used to treat T2DM. Both bromocriptine and cabergoline, another dopamine receptor agonist, have been used to treat PCOS [35,36]. Since most insulin sensitizing treatments that are successful in PCOS turn out to be successful in treating NCAH, a pilot study using these agents in NCAH seems reasonable.

The bile acid binding resin, colesevelam, has been reported to improve insulin sensitivity, possibly by causing an increase in endogenous GLP-1 secretion [37,38]. This finding might be a basis for a pilot study using this agent to treat CAH.

The fat absorption blocking agent orlistat is approved as a weight loss aid when combined with diet and exercise in the U.S. in both a 60 gm over the counter form and a prescription only 120 mg form. In Canada it is approved for the treatment of T2DM. Panidis et al. reported that orlistat in combination with diet produced significant weight loss and improvement in insulin sensitivity in obese women, with or without PCOS [39]. In addition, serum testosterone levels were significantly improved in women with PCOS. Based on these data pilot studies of orlistat in NCAH should be performed. Stimulation of the CB-1 cannabinoid receptor has known orexic and euphoric effects, while its blockade with rimonabant has been associated with anorexic and dysphoric effects and results in weight loss, reduced insulin resistance, and improvements in glycemia and serum lipid levels [40] and has shown efficacy in PCOS patients [41]. Rimonabant was not approved in the U.S. and its approval was withdrawn in Europe because of a higher suicide risk due, presumably, to its dysphoric effect. The risk/benefit ratio of this class of agents might be improved by better patient selection, selective co-administration of an anti-depressant, treatment of hyperhomocysteinemia (which may play a role in depression, or the development of selective cannabinoid receptor modulators, possessing the beneficial anorexic effect of the class without causing dysphoria.

The selective estrogen receptor modulators (SERM's), now in widespread clinical use, provide a model for such future development. Since CB-1 receptor blockers reduce insulin resistance, we might predict that they could ameliorate CAH.

Many, if not most, insulin resistant people have obstructive sleep apnea (OSA) [42]. Vgontzas et al. have reported that the inflammatory cytokines, TNF-α and IL-6 are elevated in patients with OSA, independently of obesity and that visceral fat was the primary parameter linked with OSA [42] and treatment with CPAP has been shown to improve insulin sensitivity in women with PCOS [43]. The fact that they found that OSA was more common in women with PCOS suggested a pathogenetic role of insulin resistance in OSA. The beneficial effect of a cytokine antagonist on excessive daytime sleepiness in obese, male apneics and on sleep disordered breathing in a general, random sample supports the hypothesis that cytokines and associated insulin resistance are mediators of excessive daytime sleepiness and OSA. Hamada et al have reported that with nasal CPAP in a CAH patient with OSA they were able to reduce the maintenance glucocorticoid dosage [44]. CAH patients, who have clinical features consistent with OSA, might benefit from undergoing a sleep study followed by a CPAP titration study if the initial sleep study is diagnostic. Alternatively, inhibitors of TNF-α and IL-6 might be useful adjuncts in the treatment of CAH.

Curcumin is a component of the popular spice, turmeric. It has been reported to decrease levels of the inflammatory cytokine, TNF-α, which, in turn, downregulates the transcription factor PPAR-γ. Administration of curcumin results in up-regulation of PPAR-γ m-RNA and protein, which we would predict would improve insulin sensitivity [45]. Pilot studies with curcumin in CAH patients, would, therefore, be of interest given the absence of any known adverse effects. Other spices, herbs, and supplements known or suspected to have insulin sensitizing effects would also be worth exploring in CAH.

Somatostatin and its analogs-octreotide, octreotide LAR, and lanreotide partially suppress insulin secretion; reduction of hyperinsulinemia by this means could result in amelioration of both PCOS and CAH. Gambineri's group reported that octreotide-LAR improved the ovulation rate and hirsutism and showed nearly significant trends toward greater reductions in serum testosterone and androstenedione compared with placebo in dieting women with abdominal obesity and PCOS [46]. Pilot studies of these drugs in these two conditions, would, therefore, be of interest; because they reduce the secretion of growth hormone they would not be suitable for use in children or adolescents.

Phenytoin and diazoxide both decrease insulin secretion and have been reported to be helpful in treating some PCOS patients [47,48]. On this basis we might predict a response in CAH patients as well. In designing pilot studies with these agents, patients with pre-diabetes or low bone density should probably be excluded due to the diabetogenic potential of both drugs and the accelerated Vitamin D clearance attributed to the latter.

2.5. Summary of treatment of CAH using insulin sensitizing approaches

- Insulin sensitizing approaches, including diet/exercise, metformin, thiazolidinediones, bariatric surgery, Ashwagandha root, Vitamin D replacement, and liraglutide can eliminate the need to use corticosteroids in the treatment of non-classical adrenal hyperplasia and valproate/anti-psychotic induced/unmasked adrenal hyperplasia due to 21-hydroxylase deficiency, 3-β-ol dehydrogenase deficiency, 11-hydroxylase deficiency, and aldosterone synthase deficiency.

- Metformin addition can improve the outcome in classical CAH due to 21-hydroxylase deficiency, exerting a corticosteroid-sparing effect.

- Vitamin D replacement in Vitamin D deficient/insufficient patients with NCAH due to the above enzyme defects can eliminate the need for corticosteroids.

- Vitamin D replacement can replace the use of corticosteroids in classical 11-hydroxylase deficiency associated with vitamin D deficiency.

- It is desirable to eliminate or minimize the use of corticosteroids in CAH in order to avoid adverse drug reactions, including hyperglycemia, bone loss, growth retardation, and affective changes.

- The amelioration of CAH by insulin-sensitizing approaches suggests that, as in PCOS, insulin resistance is an integral part of the pathogenesis of the CAH's.

3. Parasitic endocrine disruption; polycystic ovarian syndrome induced by neurocysticercosis

3.1. Background

There is growing awareness of the role of environmental endocrine disrupters in human health and reproduction as well as in the health and reproduction of other species. Most of the research in this area has dealt with the menace of manmade endocrine disrupting chemicals (EDC's), such as phthalates and hydraulic fracking chemicals. We are also rediscovering the endocrine disrupting role of parasites, which have preyed upon our species since prehistoric times. An example of this appears in statues of the pharaoh, Akhnaton which have often portrayed him as a young man with rounded hips and gynecomastia. Some historical epidemiologists have suggested that this feminized appearance might be the result of hepatic involvement by schistosomiasis, which has long been endemic in the Nile Valley.

3.2. PCOS induced by neurocysticercosis

The patient we reported was a 33 year old (at that time) Mexican woman G3P2012 with extensive neurocysticercosis, who was referred to our clinic for secondary oligomenorrhea, acne, and hirsutism [49]. She had no localizing neurologic signs and none of the cestodes directly involved the hypothalamus or the pituitary gland. There was no family history of PCOS. She had previously conceived three times without difficulty, followed by 2 normal pregnancies and 1 elective abortion. Her BMI was 28.34 kg/m^2 and was almost unchanged from 2003 to 2011. She had not become pregnant again despite having regular relations without contraception. Although her serum free and total testosterone, androstenedione, DHEA, and DHEA-S levels were normal, a diagnosis of PCOS was made by the Rotterdam criteria-the combination of oligomenorrhea plus clinical features of hyperandrogenism and the exclusion of CAH. The diagnosis was further supported by the findings of an elevated LH/FSH ratio and a low concentration of SHBG, which is evidence for both hyperandrogenism and insulin resistance. Although her baseline serum 25-OH-vitamin D_3 level was normal at 34 ng/dl, her serum 1,25-$(OH)_2$-vitamin D_3 level was elevated at 81 pg/ml. The patient refused standard treatment for cysticercosis with albendazole and dexamethasone because several of her friends had experienced adverse drug reactions with this therapy.

We initiated treatment of her PCOS with a 1200 kcal reducing diet, daily 30 minute walks, and metformin 500 mg twice daily after breakfast and supper. On this treatment monthly menses resumed, but periods lasted for only 2 days each cycle. After the metformin dosage was increased to 850 mg twice daily monthly menses continued and periods now lasted for 4 days. Hirsutism and acne noticeably diminished, however, she still did not conceive despite continuing regular relations without contraception (Table 1).

Date	LH	FSH	LH/FSH	SHBG	BMI	Insulin
June 2007	4.9	6.9	0.7		26.31	
June 2008	12.2	4.7	2.6	23	27.66	
October 2008 on metformin 500 mg twice daily pc	9.7	3.8	2.6	21	28.34	18.7
January 2009 on metformin 850 mg twice daily pc	7.6	7.9	1.0	24	27.48	9.1

Table 1. Parameters related to polycystic ovarian syndrome

Units and reference ranges for the parameters given in the table: BMI, body mass index kg/m^2 [20–25]; FSH, follicle stimulating hormone mIU/l (1.37–17.20); Insulin mIU/l (<17.0); LH, luteinising hormone IU/l (1.9–76.3); LH/FSH (≤1.0); SHBG, sex hormone binding globulin nmol/l (17–120).

In performing a literature review to ascertain if there could be an association between PCOS and cysticercosis, we learned from publications that the encysted forms of Taenia sp. are virtual steroid factories, producing such metabolites as androstenedione, testosterone, estradiol, and 17-OH-progesterone [50-56].

Morales-Montor et al., in discussing host gender preference in mammalian parasitoses, reporting that Taenia sp. exhibit a marked female host preference, and even more readily infect and reproduce in pregnant hosts. When they do infect a male host, they will feminize the host via estradiol production [55].

Given the host preference of this parasite, it would seem counterintuitive that the Taenia cestodes would produce the hyperandrogenic state of PCOS, until one remembers that PCOS is also a state of unopposed estrogen, characterized by such features as superficial cell predominance on vaginal cytology, cervical mucus ferning on low power microscopy, spinnbarkeit, and withdrawal bleeding after progesterone challenge.

3.3. Treatment of cysticercosis with selective estrogen receptor modulators (SERMs)

Vargas-Villavicencio et al. reported that treatment of mice infected with Taenia crassiceps with the SERM, tamoxifen, resulted in a rapid, dramatic 80% reduction in parasite burden in infected females and a 50% reduction in males [57]. Tamoxifen increased the Th1/Th2 ratio favoring increased expression of cellular immunity as well as being associated with a change in the cytokine pattern consistent with greater Th1 expression. They also reported that cultured Taenia crassiceps cestodes that were exposed in vitro to tamoxifen concentrations comparable with those achieved in human treatment died rapidly.

After again declining standard treatment of her neurocysticercosis with albendazole and dexamethasone, we discussed with our patient the work reported by Vargas-Villavicencio et al. and obtained her fully informed consent to initiate a course of treatment with another SERM, raloxifene 60 mg orally daily. Pregnancy and disorders predisposing to a hypercoagulable state were excluded before commencing treatment. Raloxifene, rather than tamoxifen, was chosen so as not to increase the patient's risk for endometrial cancer and because the former is known to exacerbate post-menopausal vasomotor symptoms in early post-menopausal women, suggesting that it readily crosses the blood/brain barrier, acting as an estrogen receptor antagonist within the central nervous system. Raloxifene was added to metformin 850 mg twice daily beginning on January 21, 2010. The patient was reminded of the need for reliable contraception since raloxifene is contraindicated during pregnancy.

When the patient returned to clinic on March 17, 2010 she reported apologetically that she had a positive home pregnancy test. Pregnancy was confirmed in our laboratory. She was referred to Family Planning Clinic for termination of pregnancy, because, as we re-explained to our patient, raloxifene is FDA Pregnancy Class X (should not be used in pregnancy) and therefore we could not assure her of the likelihood of a healthy baby. Raloxifene was discontinued in the event that she chose to continue the pregnancy.

A repeat brain MRI, performed on April 26, 2010 showed a diminution in the number, size, and viability of the cestodes (Figure 13).

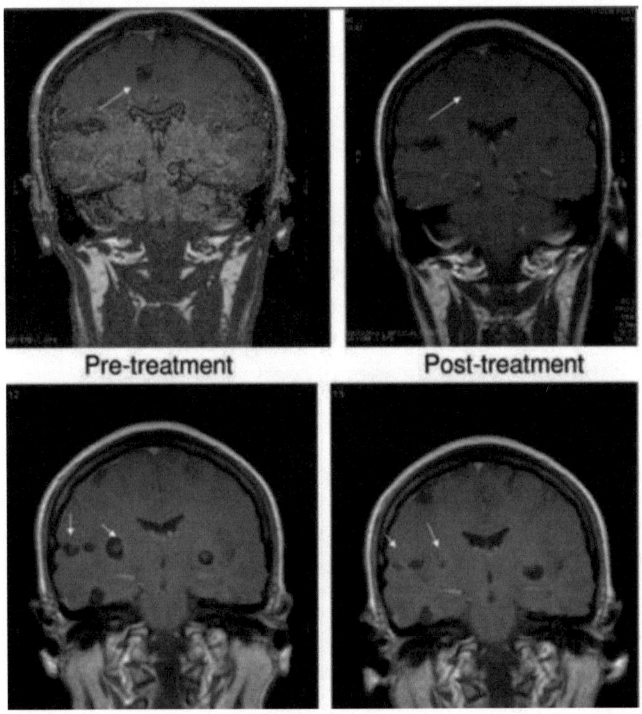

Figure 13. MRI's showing effect of raloxifene treatment 60 mg/day on a patient with extensive neurocysticercosis

The total number of lesions fell from 37 to 33. Ten lesions shrank, 5 lesions resolved, 18 lesions appeared unchanged, 4 lesions enlarged, and only 1 new lesion appeared. Concomitantly, her serum 1,25-$(OH)_2$-vitamin D_3 fell from 81 pg/ml to 41 pg/ml (Figure 14), while her serum 25-OH-vitamin D_3 only fell from 34 ng/ml to 30 ng/ml with raloxifene treatment.

Figure 14. Effect of raloxifene 60 mg/day on serum calcitriol level in a patient with neurocysticercosis

On May 5, 2010 she agreed to treatment with a 2 week standard course of albendazole and dexamethasone, which she tolerated well. Rare causes of calcitriol mediated hypercalcemia have been reported and reviewed by Kallas et al. [58] and, although our patient did not develop hypercalcemia, her apparently increased 1-α-hydroxylation of 25-OH-vitamin D_3 may be explained by the same mechanism-either the cestodes themselves or the surrounding host macrophages carrying out 1-α-hydroxylation.

Our patient thus illustrates several previously unknown features:

- Neurocysticercosis cestodes can have several endocrine disrupting effects on their human hosts including: androgenic effects, estrogenic effects, induction of insulin resistance, and enhanced 1-α-hydroxylation of 25-OH-vitamin D_3 either by the cestodes themselves or by the surrounding host macrophages in a process reminiscent of pulmonary sarcoidosis.
- Alteration of the hormonal milieu evoked by the parasites is capable of reversing the induced PCOS in a 2 step process:
  1. the use of metformin reduced the insulin resistance/hyperinsulinemia, which in turn reduced the hyperandrogenism and resulted in restoration of normal menses and resolution of acne and hirsutism, concurrently with an increase in serum SHBG and a normalization of the LH/FSH ratio, but did not, by itself result in restoration of fertility.
  2. addition of the SERM, raloxifene, by causing a less estrogenic milieu restored fertility (although this was an unintended consequence).
- Alteration of the hormonal milieu via the addition of raloxifene to metformin was effective in reducing the parasite burden in a human host. This observation suggests the possibility that alteration of the hormonal milieu may ultimately be found to be a viable primary or adjunctive treatment for various human and veterinary parasitoses.
- Given the burden of widespread cysticercosis, not only in tropical/subtropical areas, but in other area of the globe as well due to increasing migration, cysticercosis may turn out to be an important cause, not only of PCOS, but, ultimately, of the burgeoning epidemic of metabolic syndrome, pre-diabetes, and T2DM.

4. Chapter summary

- Insulin resistance/hyperinsulinemia is a constant feature of both classical and non-classic adrenal hyperplasia as well medication induced/unmasked adrenal hyperplasia.
- In vitro studies suggest that 2 mechanisms for the above observation are gain of 17-α-hydroxylase activity and decrease of 21-hydroxylase activity in the presence of hyperinsulinemia.
- Interventions which reduce insulin resistance/hyperinsulinemia dependably ameliorate the phenotypic/biochemical course of CAH and acquired/unmasked adrenal hyperplasia as they do in PCOS. In the case of NCAH insulin sensitizing interventions eliminate the need for corticosteroids and their attendant side effects, while in classical CAH insulin sensitization shows at least an ability to ameliorate the condition without resorting to supraphysiologic corticosteroid dosages.
- Other drugs and herbals with insulin sensitizing properties may ultimately prove useful in treating CAH.
- Cysticercosis is able to evoke a 4 part endocrine disrupting effect in the human host: insulin resistance, hyperandrogenism, feminization, and enhance 1-α-hydroxylation of 25-OH-vitamin D_3.
- Modifying the cysticercosis-evoked hormonal milieu with the insulin sensitizer, metformin and the SERM, raloxifene is capable of effectively treating cysticercosis induced PCOS, reducing the parasite burden, and reversing the overexpression of 1-α-hydroxylase.
- Serial measurement of vitamin D metabolites may prove to be a fairly economical way of following parasite burden and treatment response compared to serial MRI.
- Cysticercosis may ultimately prove to be a fairly common cause of insulin resistance and PCOS.

5. Nomenclature

CAH-congenital adrenal hyperplasia

NCAH-non-classic congenital adrenal hyperplasia

PCOS-polycystic ovarian (Stein-Leventhal) syndrome

17-OHP-17-hydroxyprogesterone

eGFR estimated glomerular filtration rate

http://dx.doi.org/10.5772/58953

Author details

Alan Sacerdote[1,2,3,4] and Gül Bahtiyar[1,2,3,4]

1 Division of Endocrinology, Woodhull Medical and Mental Health Center, Brooklyn, NY, USA

2 SUNY Downstate Medical Center, Brooklyn, NY, USA

3 NYU School of Medicine, New York, NY, USA

4 St. George's University, School of Medicine, St. George's, Grenada

References

[1] Speiser PW, Serrat J, New MI, Gertner JM. Insulin insensitivity in adrenal hyperplasia due to nonclassical steroid 21-hydroxylase deficiency. J Clin Endocrinol Metab 1992;75(6):1421-4.

[2] Andersson B, Marin P, Lissner L, Vermuelen A, Bjorntor P. Testosterone concentrations in women and men with NIDDM. Diab Care 1994;17(5) 405-11.

[3] Sacerdote A. Adrenal androgens and NIDDM. Diab Care 1995;18(2):278-9.

[4] Saygili F, Oge A, Yilmaz C. Hyperinsulinemia and insulin sensitivity in women with nonclassical congenital adrenal hyperplasia due to 21-hydroxylase deficiency: the relationship between serum leptin levels and chronic hyperinsulinemia. Horm Res 2005;63(6):270-4.

[5] Charmandari E, Weise M, Bornstein SR, Eisenhofer G, Keil MF, Chrousos GP, Merke DP. Children with classical congenital adrenal hyperplasia have elevated serum leptin concentrations and insulin resistance: potential clinical implications. J Ckin Endocrinol Metab 2002;87(5):2114-20.

[6] Charmandari E, Brook CG, Hindmarsh PC. Classic congenitqal adrenal hyperplasia and puberty. Eur J Endocrinol 2004;151 Suppl 3:U77-82.

[7] Charmandari E, Chrousos GP. Metabolic syndrome manifestations in classic congenital adrenal hyperplasia: do they predispose to atherosclerotic cardiovascular disease and secondary polycystic ovary syndrome? Ann NY Acad Sci 2006;1083:37-53.

[8] Sartorato P, Zuilian E, Benedini S, Marinello B, Schiavi F, Bilora F, Pozzan G, Greggio N, Pagnan A, Mantero F, Scaroni C. Cardiovascular risk factors and ultrasound evaluation of intima-media thickness of common carotids, carotid bulbs, and femoral and abdominal aorta arteries in patients with classical congenital adrenal hyperplasia due to 21-hydroxylase deficiency. J Clin Endocrinol Metab 2007;92(3):1015-8.

[9] Kim MS, Merke DP. Cardiovascular disease risk in adult women with congenital adrenal hyperplasia due to 21-hydroxylase deficiency. Semin Reprod Med 2009;27(4): 316-21.

[10] Ambroziak LI, Bednarczuk T, Ginalkska-Malinkowska M, Malanowicz EM, Grzechocinska B, Kaminski P, Bablock L, Przedlacki J, Bar-Andziak E. Congenital adrenal hyperplasia due to 21-hydroxylase deficiency—management in adults. Endokrynol Pol 2010;Suppl 1:7-21.

[11] Arlt W, Willis DS, Krone N, Doherty EJ, Hahner S, Han TS, Carroll PV, Conway GS, Rees DA, Stimson RH, Walker BR, Connell JM, Ross RJ. United Kingdom Congenital Adrenal Hyperplasia Adult Study Executive (CAHASE). J Clin Endocrinol Metab 2010;95[11]:5110-21.

[12] Zhang HJ, Yang J, Zhang MN, Liu CQ, Xu M, Li XJ, Yang SY, Li XY. Metabolic disorders in newly diagnosed young female patients with simple virilizing 21-hydroxylase deficiency, Endocrine 2010;38(2):260-5.

[13] Schneider-Rezek GS, Lemos-Marini SH, Baptista MT, Guerra-Junior G, Morcillo AM, Mello MP, Oliveira LC, D'Souza-Li L. Metabol evaluation of young women with congenital adrenal hyperplasia. Arq Bras Endocrinol Metabol 2011;55(8):646-52.

[14] Moreira RP, Gomes LC, Mendonca BB, Bachega TA. PLoS One 2012;7(9):e44893.

[15] Bahtiyar G, Sacerdote A. Management approaches to congenital adrenal hyperplasia in adolescents and adults; Latest therapeutic developments. In Chatterjee A. (ed). Amenorrhea. Rijeka: Intech 2011. P. 66-90.

[16] Osehobo E, Shaw I, Sacerdote AS. Do insulin sensitizers repair the gene defects in non-classical congenital adrenal hyperplasia. Endo 2000, 20-24 June 2000, Toronto, Canada.

[17] Sacerdote AS, Sanchez JU, Ogbeide O, Slabodkina L. Modification of expression of non-classical congenital adrenal hyperplasia by rosiglitazone. Endo 2003, 19-22 June 2003, Philadelphia, PA, USA.

[18] Sacerdote, AS. Modification of expression of non-classical congenital adrenal hyperplasia by pioglitazone. Endoc 2004, 16-19, June 2004, New Orleans, LA, USA.

[19] Arslanian SA, Levy V, Danadian K, Saad R. Metformin therapy in obese adolescents with polycystic ovary syndrome and impaired glucose tolerance: amelioration of exaggerated adrenal response to adrenocorticotropin with reduction of insulinemia/ insulin resistance. J Clin Endocrinol Metab 2002;87:1555-9.

[20] Bahtiyar G, Weiss K, Sacerdote AS. Novel endocrine disrupter effects of classic and atypical anti-psychotic agents and divalproex: induction of adrenal hyperandrogenism reversible with metformin or rosiglitazone. Endocr Pract 2007;13:601-8.

[21] Sacerdote A, Girgis E, Toosi A, Polanco H, Bahtiyar G. Additional endocrine disrupter effects of highly active anti-retroviral treatment-induction of non-classical adrenal hyperplasia. Endo 2006, 24-27, June, 2006 Boston, MA, USA.

[22] Agdere L, Bahtiyar G, Mejia J, Sacerdote A. Metformin-responsive classical, salt-losing P450c21A2B deficiency-a case report. Endocrine Practice 2008; 14(7):889-91.

[23] Sacerdote, A. Weight-dependent expression of non-classical aldosterone synthase deficiency. Endo 2002, 20-24 June 2000, Toronto, Canada.

[24] Jamal M, Gunay Y, Capper A, Eid A, Heitshusen D, Samuel I. Roux-en-Y gastric bypass ameliorates polycystic ovary syndrome and dramatically improves conception rates: a 9-year analysis. Surg Obes Relat Dis. 2012;8(4):440-4.

[25] Kalani A, Thomas N, Sacerdote A, Bahtiyar G. Roux-en-Y gastric bypass in the treatment of non-classic congenital adrenal hyperplasia due to 11-hydroxylase deficiency. BMJ Case Rep. 2013 Mar 18;2013. pii: bcr2012008416. doi: 10.1136/bcr-2012-008416

[26] Kalani A, Bahtiyar G, Sacerdote A. Ashwagandha root in the treatment of non-classical adrenal hyperplasia. BMJ Case Rep. 2012 Sep 17;2012. pii: bcr2012006989. doi: 10.1136/bcr-2012-006989.

[27] Anwer T, Sharma M, Pillai KK, Iqbal M. Effect of Withania somnifera on insulin sensitivity in non-insulin-dependent diabetes mellitus rats. Basic Clin Pharmacol Toxicol. 2008;102(6):498-503.

[28] Kramer CK, Swaminathan B, Hanley AJ, Connelly PW, Sermer M[5], Zinman B, Retnakaran R. Prospective Associations of Vitamin D Status with Beta-cell function, Insulin Sensitivity and Glycemia: The Impact of Parathyroid Hormone Status. Diabetes. 2014 May 29. pii: DB_140489. [Epub ahead of print]

[29] Thomas N, Kalani A, Vincent R, Luis Lam M, Bahtiyar G, Sacerdote A. Effect of Vitamin D in a Patient With Classical AdrenalHyperplasia due to 11-Hydroxylase Deficiency. J Med Cases 2013;4(8):569-575.

[30] Verstuyf A, Carmeliet G, Bouillon R, Mathieu C. Vitamin D: a pleiotropic hormone. Kidney Int. 2010 ;78(2):140-5.

[31] Luis Lam M, Sacerdote A, Bahtiyar G. Normalization of Serum 11- Deoxycortisol in a Patient with Non-Classic Adrenal Hyperplasia Due to 11-Hydroxylase Deficiency Treated with Vitamin D and a Glucagon-like Peptide(GLP)-1 Agonist. Endo 2014, 21-24 June, Chicago, IL, USA.

[32] Kelly SN, McKenna TJ, Young LS. Modulation of steroidogenic enzymes by orphan nuclear transcriptional regulation may control diverse production of cortisol and androgens in the human adrenal. J Endocrinol 2004; 181:355-65.

[33] .Pijl H, Ohashi S, Matsuda M. Bromocriptine: a novel approach to the treatment of Type 2 diabetes. Diab Care 2000; 23:1154-61.

[34] Scranton R, Cincotta A. Bromocriptine—unique formulation of a dopamine agonist for the treatment of type 2 diabetes. Expert Opin Pharmacother 2010; 11(2):269-79.

[35] Paoletti AM, Cagnacci A, Depau GF, Orrù M, Ajossa S, Melis GB. The chronic administration of cabergoline normalizes androgen secretion and improves menstrual cyclicity in women with polycystic ovary syndrome. Fertil Steril 1996; 66(4):527-32.

[36] Spruce BA, Kendall-Taylor P, Dunlop W, Anderson AJ, Watson MJ, Cook DB, Gray C. The effect of bromocriptine in the polycystic ovary syndrome. Clin Endocrinol (Oxf) 1984; 20(4):481-8.

[37] Shang Q, Saumoy M, Holst JJ, Salen G, Xu G. Colesevelam improves insulin resistance in a diet-induced obesity (F-DIO) rat model by increasing the release of GLP-1. Am J Physiol Gastrointest Liver Physiol 2010; 298(3):G419-24.

[38] Schwartz SL, Lai YL, Xu J, Abby SL, Misir S, Jones MR, and Nagendran S. The effect of colesevelam hydrochloride on insulin sensitivity and secretion in patients with type 2 diabetes: a pilot study. Metab Syndr Relat Disord 2010; 8(2):179-88.

[39] Panidis, D.; Farmakiotis, D.; Rousso, D.; Koutis, A.; Katsikis, I.; Krassas, G. Obesity, weight loss, and the polycystic ovary syndrome: effect of treatment with diet and orlistat for 24 weeks on insulin resistance and androgen levels. Fertil Steril 2008;.89 (4): 899-906.

[40] Migrenne S, Lacombe, A, Lefèvre AL,; Pruniaux, MP, Guillot, E. Galzin, AM. Magnan,C. Adiponectin is required to mediate rimonabant-induced improvement ofinsulin sensitivity but not body weight loss in diet-induced obese mice. Am J PhysiolRegul Integr Comp Physiol, 2009; 296, (4): 929-935.

[41] Sathyapalan T, Cho LW, Kilpatrick ES, Coady AM, Atkin SL. [2008]. A comparison between rimonabant and metformin in reducing biochemical hyperandrogenemia and insulin resistance in patients with polycystic ovary syndrome (PCOS): arandomized open-label parallel study. Clin Endocrinol 2008;69(6): 931-935.

[42] Vgontzas AN, Bixler EO, Chrousos GP. Sleep apnea is a manifestation of the metabolic syndrome. Sleep Med Rev 2005; 9, (3): 211-224.

[43] Tasali E, Van Cauter E, Hoffman L, Ehrmann DA. Impact of obstructive sleep apnea on insulin resistance and glucose tolerance in women with polycystic ovary syndrome. J Clin Endocrinol Metab 2008;93:3878-84

[44] Hamada S, Chin K, Hitomi T, Oga T, Handa, T, Tuboi T, Niimi A, Mishima M. Impact of nasal continuous positive airway pressure for congenital adrenal hyperplasia with obstructive sleep apnea and bruxism. Sleep Breath 2012; 16(1):11-15.

[45] Ghosh SS, Massey HD, Krieg R, Fazelbhoy ZA, Ghosh S, Sica DA, Fakhry I, Gehr TW. Curcumin ameliorates renal failure in 5/6 nephrectomized rats: role of inflammation. Am J Physiol Renal Physiol 2009;296,(5):1146-57.

[46] Gambineri A, Patton L, De Iasio R, Cantelli B, Cognini GE, Filicori M, Barreca A, Diamanti- Kandarakis E, Pagotto, U, Pasquali R. Efficacy of octreotide-LAR in dieting women with abdominal and polycystic ovary syndrome. J Clin Endocrinol Metab 2005:90(7):3854-62.

[47] Bercovici JM, Monguillon P, Nahoul K, Floch HH, Brettes JP. [1996]. Polycystic ovary and Diazoxide. In vivo study. Ann Endocrinol 1996;57(4):235-9.

[48] Verrotti A, D'Egidio C, Mohn A, Coppola A, Parisi P, Chiarelli F. Antiepileptic drugs, sex hormones, and PCOS. Epilepsia 2011;52(2):199-211.

[49] Sacerdote AS, Mejia JO, Bahtiyar G, Salamon O. Effect of raloxifene in human neurocysticerocosis. BMJ Case Reports 2012;doi:10.1136/bcr.06.2011.4417.

[50] Gomez Y, Valdez RA, Larralde C et al. Sex steroids and parasitism: Taenia crassiceps metabolizes exogenous androstenedione to testosterone in vitro. J Steroid Biochem Mol Biol 2000;74(3):143-7

[51] Jimenez P, Valdez RA, Romano MC. Metabolism of steroid hormones by Taenia solium and Taenia crassiceps cysticerci. J Steroid Biochem Mol Biol 2006;99(4-5):203-8.

[52] Diaz-Orea MA, DeAluja AS, Erosa M de L et al. Different effects of chorionic gonadotropin on Taenia crassiceps and Taenia solium cysticerci cultured in vitro. J Parasitol 2007;93(6):1518-20.

[53] Valdez RA, Jimenez P, Cartas AL et al. Taenia solium cysticerci synthesize androgens and estrogens in vitro. Parasitol Res 2006;98(5):472-6.

[54] Romano MC, Valdez RA, Cartas AL, et al. Steroid hormone production by parasites: the case of Taenia crassiceps and Taenia solium cysticerci. J Steroid Biochem Mol Biol 2003; 85(2-5):221-5.

[55] Morales-Montor J, Escobedo G, Vargas-Villavicencio JA et al. The neuroimmunoendocrine network in the complex host-parasite relationship during murine cysticercosis. Curr Top Med Chem 2008;8(5):400-7.

[56] Fernandez-Presas AM, Valdez RA, Wilms K et al. The key steroidogenic enzyme, 3-beta-hydroxysteroid dehydrogenase in Taenia solium and Taenia crassiceps (WFU). Parasitol Res 2008;103(4):847-52.

[57] Vargas-Villavicencio JA, Larralde C, DeLeon-Nava MA et al. Tamoxifen treatment induces protection in murine cysticercosis. J Parasitol 2007;93(6):1512-7.

[58] Kallas M, Green F, Hewison M, White C, Kline G. Rare causes of calcitriol-mediated hypercalcemia: A case report and literature review. J Clin Endocrinol Metab 2010;95(7):3111-7

Section 4

Gynecologic Oncology

Chapter 6

Screening Methods for Gynaecological Cancers

T.K. Nyengidiki

Additional information is available at the end of the chapter

http://dx.doi.org/10.5772/58947

1. Introduction

Globally life expectancy is on the increase and with this an increase in the incidence of age related gynaecological cancers and other related medical conditions. Gynaecological cancers accounted for 19% of the 5.1million estimated new cancer cases in the world with 2.9 million cancer deaths in 2002. (Sarkaranayanan et al, 2006). The essence of screening is to detect disease among healthy population without symptoms of the disease with the primary purpose of reducing the morbidity and mortality with the disease. This has been done with varying success in various countries having designed programmes aimed at reducing the scourge of gynaecological cancers.

The pattern of screening programmes can be divided into two categories namely: opportunistic and organized. The organized screening programmes are mostly observed in the developed countries like Finland, Sweden and the United states of American were specific policy decisions have been taken by the respective Government with the concentration of resources to gynaecological cancer screening with resultant of the population and improved outcome. Following the implementation of organized screening programmes especially with cervical cancer remarkable reductions in mortality in Nordic countries have been observed with largest fall in Iceland, Sweden and Finland (Laara et al, 1987) converse is the case in developing countries where most patients have poor health seeking attitude; uninformed and Disempowered population, increasing competing health needs, limited human and material needs, unaffordable treatment for gynecological cancers and lack of political will on the part of the respective governments to create policies that will focus resources on early gynaecological cancer detection(Danny L et al 2006). The economics of these countries put a lot of pressure on the limited resources in the face of multiple demand.The average per capital expenditure in many African countries is approximately USD30 compared to USD500 in the United States of `America (Denny L et al, 2005) creating an economic menu for poorly organized screening programmes. Hence screening programmes are largely opportunistic in nature relying on other channels of health care to provide a vehicle for screening like the family planning clinics and STI clinics.

Most female genital tract malignancies have identifiable precursors such as cervical intraepithelial lesions, vaginal intraepithelial, vulva intraepithelial, atypical endometrial hyperplasia for endometrial cancer while others like ovarian malignancies do not have identifiable precursors making screening modalities non specific. The potential benefits of screening includes early detection of pre invasive cancers and avenue for provision of curative services to patients identified while reassuring those that are negative and rechanneling health resources to other purposes. It must be stated that screening programme have potential limitations of false negative and positive results giving false assurances to affected patients and overtreatment of none affected patients. (Kwawukume et al, 2005)

2. Criteria for a sucessful screeening programme

Irrespective of the type of screening embarked on whether organized or opportunistic, Wilson et al (1968) stipulated certain standards to be met for a successful screening programme and these include:

- The condition should be an important health problem, have recognizable latent phase and known natural history with acceptable and available treatment options for identified patients.
- The validity and predictiveness of the screening method must be high for the identified precancerous lesion.
- Proposed screening should be a continuous process of case finding and Not "a all in one" project
- In addition to the above, policies should aim at designing programmes that will be economically balanced on medicare that will be provided for the diagnosed patients.

Judging from the above stated it is obvious why most of the screening projects designed by most governments in Sub Saharan African and Asia do not succeed as against what is obtained in the developed regions of the world. Gynaecological malignancies like cervical cancer have known life cycle and well established link with 99% of cases of cervical cancer caused by oncogenic strains of human papilloma virus of 16,18, 35 and 41 identified with a duration of 10-20 years of transformation to malignancy noted. The universality and acceptable of the screening methods and treatment options for precursors of the cancer had made it an epitome of success in the area of reducing morbidity and mortality. Ovarian malignancies do not have known precursor thus making screening a challenge without acceptable consensus on screening modalities.

http://dx.doi.org/10.5772/58947

3. Methods of gynaecological cancer screening

There are basically three broad methods of gynaecological cancer screening and a combination of method can be utilized to achieving a satisfactory result. These are:

- Biochemical: use of tumor markers such as CA125, CA 19-9,Human chorionic gonadotropin, urinary gonadotropin peptides, BRCA 1 and 2, Alpha fetoprotein.
- Physical-Radiological: The use of physical examination and ultrasound scan can be helpful in screening ovarian cancers assessing the ovarian volume and endometrial thickness screening for endometrial malignancies
- Biophysical methods: These include the PAP smears, vulva and vaginal smears, laparoscopy, colposcopy and vacuum aspiration

4. Screening for cervical cancers

The value of screening in identifying precursors of cervical cancers and reducing the cancer burden is well demonstrated in the various methods employed. Ever since the introduction of using cervical exfoliates for screening by George Papanicoloeau and coworkers in 1943, the incidence of cervical cancer related mortalities have reduced by 70% because of well organized screening programmes (Noller 2005,). The relative ease in performing screening of cervical cancer is related to the accessibility of the cervix to allow the analysis of exfoliated cells for cytology, which in turn is a fairly tolerated procedure for patients and relatively cheap to carry out. 60% of cancers of the cervix develop in the unscreened general population but despite screening 40% arise from the screened population. This is attributed to false negative results as result of sampling error or wrong interpretation of cytology reports or improper management abnormal results (Carmicheal, 1984). In addition to the traditional pap smear, other screening methods have being introduced like, liquid based cytology, computer assisted liquid based cytology, colposcopy and Human papilloma virus screening

4.1. Cervical cytology

This method uses the exfoliated cells, which are examined microscopically, and diagnosis made by recognition of well-known histopathological patterns, which identifies cellular changes of cervical intraepithelial neoplasia. These changes are graded as normal, atypical squamous cells of uncertain significance, low-grade squamous intraepithelial lesions and high grade intraepithelial lesions according to the Betheseda System of classification

The specificity of PAP smear is 98% but the sensitivity is lower and variable because of inter-observer differences in interpretation of slides and sampling error

4.2. Preparation for PAP smear

The procedure of PAP smear is usually scheduled out of menstrual flow periods but should not be deferred because of an unscheduled bleed which may as well errand a cervical pathology.It is advisable for evidence of cervicitis /vaginitis be treated if present and intercourse should be avoided with 24-48hours of the procedure in addition to avoidance of vaginal douching or application of vaginal tampons and creams which may introduce artifacts on the slides examined. Clinical information on the last menstrual period, use of hormonal contraception, intrauterine contraceptive devices, any form of immunosuppression and previous history of abnormal smears are important to the pathologist in accurate interpretation of smears.

5. Material needed

A pathologist and trained personnel in the collection of the specimen is an important ingredient in conducting the investigation. Other items needed are 95% alcohol for fixing of slides, and a jar to contain the specimen.

Over the years various sampling items have been introduced. The traditional wooden Ayrles spatula was initially used but has some limitations as the failure of accessing the endocervix, which is the point of origin of 20% of adenocarcinomas of the cervix. Specimen collections devices include the broom and the endocervical bush (cytobrush) with both having the ability to access the endocervix more than the traditional spatula. The plastic spatula is preferable to the wooden variety because the collected samples are more adherent to the wooden spatula and may be discarded with the spatula after use (Goodman, Hutchinson, 1996.)

5.1. Procedure

Following appropriate counseling of the patient and obtaining informed consent for the procedure, the patient is put in lithotomy position with the cervix exposed using a bivalve speculum. A soft cotton is used to remove any mucous material from the external cervical Os, while taking care not to contact the cervix, a tenaculum is used to grasp the anterior lip of the cervix.The collecting device which could be a spatula is introduced into the internal Os and rotated in 360^0 degree once. The samples collected are smeared on already labeled slide and fixed in 95% alcohol. A four quadrant pap smear of the vaginal walls is advised in patients with history of exposure to diethylstibesterol who are at risk of developing adenosquamous vaginal cancer (Sarina et al 2004)

5.2. Interpretation of results of PAP smear after analysis

The specimen can be categorized as satisfactory or non-satisfactory according to the Bethesda system of reporting of adequacy of smears collected. A satisfactory PAP specimen is that in which the sample collected has a adequate number of squamous epithelial cell, endocervical and representative amount of the transformation zone cell components while an unsatisfactory smear has paucity of epithelial cells poorly preserved or cellular or inflammatory cell that obscure the film.Epithelial cell abnormalities can be classified as:

Atypical squamous cells of undermined significance, low grade squamous intraepithelial lesions (CIN1) and high grade intra epithelial lesions which include carcinoma in-situ, CIN2

http://dx.doi.org/10.5772/58947

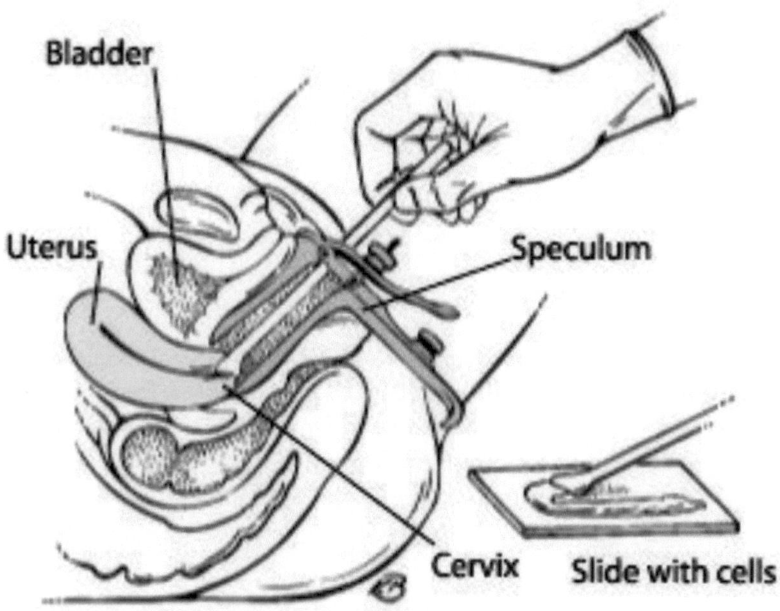

Figure 1. Taking a sample of cells

and CIN3.Other abnormalities include squamous cell abnormalities and glandular cell abnormalities. (Solomom D et al, 2001)

5.3. Limitations of PAP smear

The impact of this screening method has being felt over the years and had contributed to reducing cervical cancer related morbidities, however limitations exist which has affected its utilization. The primary need for a trained pathologist has hampered its utilization especially in the third world with scarcity of trained personnel. Even in the presence of trained personnel the interpretation of morphological alterations in the histological pattern of cervical dysplasia is highly subjective and in the presence of large pool of samples likely to be subject to observer fatigue.The sensitivity of the screening method to identify cervical intraepithelial neoplasia is 51% with a specificity of 98% with increase of sensitivity if interval of screening is made 1-3 years

6. Frequency of PAP smear screening

There are different protocols advocated by different professional bodies and country policies but latest recommended by American College of Obstetricians and Gynecologists (ACOG 2012) low and average risk patients suggest that females should start screening using PAP smear from the age of 21 years and repeating every three years until 29. From the age of 30 years PAP smear alone every three years smear screening alone every 3years with termination of screening at the age of 65 years if still negative. High-risk patients such as off springs of mothers exposed to diethylstilbestrol, immunosuppressed patients, and patients with CIN2 or higher who had been treated are however advised against following the routine screening guidelines for low risk patients.

Patients who had had hysterectomy and had never had any CIN2 or greater can have discontinuation of screening using the Pap smear or HPV testing.

6.1. Liquid based cytology

This method is an innovation to improve the sensitivity of the conventional pap smear where samples are suspended in liquid media, centrifuged to concentrate the exfoliated cells which are subjected thereafter to cytology. The Food and Drug Adminstratio in the USA approved Thinprep and BD Surepath in the years 1996/1999 for the purpose of analyzing cytology samples.

The superiority of this screening method is based on improved cell collection and the random distribution of cells collected which is more representative. This method reduced the proportion of unsatisfactory smears in a study by(Ronco et al, 2007, Arbyn et al 2008) but did not show improved sensitivity instead has a low predictive value to detect CIN 2 and above relative to the traditional Pap smear. A cost analysis also revealed increased cost relative to Pap smear (De Jager et al 2013).

7. Visual inspection using acetic acid

In areas with limited resources a resort to inspection of the cervix have assisted in the screening process without application of acetic acid (unaided). When the cervix is painted with 3-5% Acetic acid it causes reversible coagulation of nuclei proteins and prevention of the penetration of light hence abnormal tissues appearing as "aceto-white areas". This has been used with good outcome in areas like India and other less developed countries where there are absence of technical manpower such as pathologist to analyze cytology specimens. This method is simple easy to perform, cheap and acceptable by most patients and can be done by nurses, paramedics amongst others and removes the need for histological confirmation. The method enables a one stop treatment of suspected cases of premalignant lesions however there is the danger of overtreatment of postmenopausal patients when this method is applied because of non visualization of the transformation zone. This screening method has similar sensitivity to PAP but lower specificity of 64-79%. Visualization of the cervix can be aided by the use of a X4 magnification glass (Aviscope) and is said to have better sensitivity compared to VIA

7.1. Colposcopy

Following the invention of an optical device by Dr Hans Hinselmenn in 1925, the visualization of the cervix using the colposcope is now an integral part of gynaecological oncology practice.The method involves direct visualization of the cervix using a colposcopy, which a magnification of the epithelium of the cervix with the aim of identifying abnormal patterns after staining with 3-5% acetic acid under 4-40x magnification. The aim of colposcopy is to examine the transformation zone, which is the origin of cervical cancer. It should not be used as a primary screening tool but used when there is an abnormality in the smear or bleeding.

7.1.1. Colposcopy procedure

With patient in lithotomy position the cervix is exposed using a bivalve speculum allowing macroscopic examination of the cervix. The exposed cervix is subsequently painted with 3-5% acetic acid. This causes a reversible denaturing of the cellular protein the abnormal cells producing the "acetowhite reaction" of cervical intraepithelial neoplasm. The complete visualization of the squamocolumnar junction is important in this procedure because it tells the extent of anomaly of the lesion. Where there is failure of complete visualization of the SCJ the colposcopy is said to be unsatisfactory. Abnormality patterns in colposcopy include: punctuations, mosaicism and abnormal vessels

When colposcopy is used as a screening method for asymptomatic patients it is known to have a poor sensitivity of 34-43%, a specificity of 68% and a positive predictive value of 4-14% hence should not be used a primary screening method for this group of asymptomatic patients (Nidhi G et al 2009).The method of screening is relatively easy to perform with the added advantage of doing it as an office procedure but had the disadvantage of cost of equipment and the time in training a Colposcopist.

7.2. Cervicography

The absence of skilled colposcopist will hamper the use of colposcopy hence in most developing countries the use of the cervicograph have been shown to effectively identify up to 90% of lesions identified by colposcopy. The procedure involves taking two photographs using a specialized camera that develops the slides into 35mm size. Developed images can be subject to comparison from a computerized bank of pictures or reviewed by other colposcopist contacted by possible telemedicine.

7.3. HPV testing

The fact that 99% of cervical cancer is caused by identifiable onocogenic strains of human papilloma virus mainly 16,18 screening for HPV virus is a realistic modality that is currently been used. Ronco et al 2014, demonstrated that screening using HPV testing provided 60-70% greater protection against cervical cancer when compared to the conventional cytology 20% of women will have HPV infection using sensitive technologies such as hybrid capture 2 (HC2), which is a signal amplification test and polymerase chain reaction, which is a target-amplified test. It has a high sensitivity but poor specificity however has a high negative predictive value, which excludes women not likely to have cervical intraepithelial neoplasm. As part of the recommendations of the United States Preventive Service Task Force (USPSTF) screening for women above the age of 30years can be prolonged to 5years if HPV testing is added to conventional screening (Grade A recommendation)

7.4. Truscan or polarprobe

This is a portable electronic device designed by Polartechnics, Crystalaid microelectronics in Australia, which allows a non-invasive screening for cervical cancer. Its modality of operation involves emission of low voltage electrical impulses when put in contact with the cervix generate real time images of the cervix which is compared with a data base of thousands of colposcopic and cervical biopsy pictures to give a final diagnosis of the optical image generated. This is associated with less pain, removes the challenges encountered in the third world in terms of performance of the conventional Pap smear and is noted to improve compliance to screening in women(Quek et al 1998)

7.5. Ovarian carcinoma screening

Ovarian cancers are the 4th commonest cause of deaths in women in the USA and the Britain with an overall survival of 35% with about 75% of the women universally presenting in advanced stages. This is largely because of none specificity of presentations, absence of a known precursor, and the absence of specific screening test for ovarian cancers. How frequently should patients be screened for ovarian cancers is not specific the NIH in 1994 recommended that all women with a family history of hereditary cancer syndrome should have a yearly screening for ovarian cancer using the available screening methods.

7.6. Biochemical markers for ovarian cancer screening

7.6.1. CA125

CA 125 is one of the biochemical tumor markers known as cancer antigen or carbohydrate Antigen 125. This high molecular glycoprotein was identified using monoclonal antibody OC 125 was discovered by Bast et al in 1980.This modality of screening is nonspecific, which is elevated in 80% of patients with epithelial cancers and about 50% in the stage 1 cancers. It is expressed by all tissues of mullerian origin but not produced by normal ovarian epithelium This has sufficient sensitivity in post menopausal patients since other conditions that will result in a rise in the value of the CA125 such as missed miscarriages, endometriosis, pelvic inflammatory disease and benign molar pregnancy are absent in postmenopausal women with ovarian cancer.

A value of greater than 35umg/ml is considered significant for further evaluation to be done. The specificity of the screening method is about 99.9% with a poor positive predictive value of 26%. The predictive value can however be increased with serial annual CA125 as against a single value.A clinical programme by Skates et al 2003, confirmed that women with serial annual rising level of CA125 are more at risk of developing ovarian cancers than women with steady level (risk of ovarian cancer Algorithm-ROCA).If the risk is greater than 1% the patient will need evaluation using transvaginal ultrasound to determine whelter further evaluation is necessary.

7.6.2. Other tumor markers useful in the screening of ovarian malignancies

Urinary gonadotropin peptides are peptides with sequence similar to B subunit of human chorionic gonadotropin and present in 70% of women with epithelial tumours. The presence of an identifiable ovarian tumour by ultrasound, an elevated CA125 and normal urinary gonadotropin peptide are most likely a benign tumor. **Carbohydrate Antigen 19-9** is increased in patients' mucinous ovarian tumours but not in epithelial tumours

Carcinoembryonic Antigen (CEA): This is a high molecular weight glycoprotein, which is a good tumour marker for the detection of mucinous ovarian tumours and noted in 90% of mucinous tumours. **Alpha feto protein-**Albumin like protein, which is increased in patients with germ cell tumours except dysgerminonas and teratomas.

Human placentae alkaline phosphatase: This is a glycoprotein molecule which has two sub units and is useful in differentiating germ cell tumours from other ovarian tumors but has the draw back of being expressed by other mullerian structures hence is not specific

Human chorionic gonadotropin: This is elevated in non-gestational choriocarcinoma, embryonal and polyembryomas.

In order to improve the sensitivity and specificity of tumour markers use of multimarkers blood test like oviplex which has the incorporation of five tumour markers (CA125,C reactive protein, serum amyloid A(SAA), interleutin 6 and 8 have been shown to improve the sensitivity y 94% and 91% specificity especially when it concerns early ovarian cancer detection(Edgell et al, 2010).

Following diagnosis and treatment tumor markers like macrophage colony stimulating factor (MCSF) can be used in the follow up of patients which has a high predictive value for persistent disease and is raised in 68% of patients with ovarian cancer.

7.7. Genetic screening

This is based on the background information that 5-10% of women have hereditary genetic predisposition and more than 90% of inherited ovarian tumours occur as a result of genetic mutations in the BRCA1 and BRCA2 genes resulting in chromosomal structure dysfunction and increased risk of malignant transformation. The presence of BRCA 1 and 2 confers 16-90% risk of development of ovarian cancers by the age of 70years as against the 1.7% in the general population ((Brose MS et al 2002,Struewing JP et al 1997). In addition Lancaster et al 2007 also estimated that germline mutation of the above mentioned genes confers a 85% lifetime risk of breast cancer and 46% risk of ovarian cancers. Also mutations in the gene mismatch repair gene MLH, MSH or MSH6 associated with lynch /hereditary non polyposis colorectal cancer have a 9-12% of ovarian cancer and advised in favor of genetic risk assessment which will enable the physician to develop strategies prevent these genetically enabled tumour, provide counseling advice, chemoprevention and prophylactic surgeries for the benefit of the patient.

7.8. Proteomic technology

This enables analysis of cluster patterns produced based on the size and net electrical charge of serum proteins produced by the various tumours. The proteome represents all the possible gene products of the cell and the proteomic technology characterizes all protein in biological system including the complex features. This method increased the sensitivity and specificity by 100 and 95% respectively with a 94% positive predictive valve for ovarian tumours (Angela et al 2013).

7.9. Pelvic examination

It has been advocated that routine pelvic examination should be part of the screening process for ovarian cancers but non-randomized control trial has assessed the role of the bimanual pelvic examination for ovarian cancer screening. In the PLCO cancer trials no case of ovarian cancer was ovarian cancer was identified solely by bimanual examination (USPTF 2012) The American cancer society had advocated pelvic examination for asymptomatic women as one of the methods of screening for ovarian cancer in combination with other screening methods like CA 125 and transvaginal ultrasound scan (ACS 2012).

7.10. Use of ultrasonography

The measurement of the volume of the ovaries has being used in screening of ovarian cancer. Transvaginal ultrasound scan can detect changes in the ovarian size and morphology. The upper limit of ovarian size for premenopausal women was $20cm^3$ and $10cm^3$ for postmenopausal women (Parlik EJ et al). Adding the parameters of cyst wall, characteristics and septation increases the sensitivity to 86% and a specificity of 99% for differentiating benign from malignant lesions(Depriest et al). It is however not recommended for population screening because of its low predictive value and lack of specificity. The combination of colour flow Doppler with transvaginal scan may assist in distinguishing malignant from benign lesions by measurement of the vascular resistance pattern of blood vessels supplying the ovaries

A combination of ultrasound scan, CA125 and menopausal status can be used in calculating the risk of malignancy index for patients and may buttress the need for more vigilance. The risk of malignancy index of greater than 200 connotes a higher risk of malignancy.

RMI=M x C x U (RCOG guideline,2003) where

M: Score of 1=premenopausal, 3=postmenopausal

C: value of the CA125

U: 1=normal scan

1 for each of the following presence of multilocular, bilateral,solid components ascities and metastatic disease with a maximum score of 3

7.11. Laparoscopy

The presence of the following features at laparoscopy may be suggestive of an ovarian malignancy size of the ovaries, bilaterally, surface excrescence dense adhesions, ascites and peritoneal lesions noted on laparoscopy. A combination of laparoscopy with transvaginal can improve the specificity of these methods but has the risk of tumor spill. This method of screening is expensive in terms of equipment, training of manpower and the surgical risk associated with the procedure for it to be advocated as a screening tool globally.

7.12. Screening for endometrial cancer

There is no known standard recommendation for screening of endometrial cancers and the ACOG consider the process not cost effective and not warranted (ACOG 1997).Despite that there is need for appropriate medical history of menstrual abnormalities and occurrence of postmenopausal bleeding should initiate the need for further evaluation of the patient.The history of tamoxifen use in a patient on hormonal therapy for breast cancer should increase the suspicion of possible endometrial malignancy. Physical examination and subsequent finding of bulky uterus in a postmenopausal patient should arouse the need for additional evaluation. Routine screening using transvaginal or biopsy is not recommended for low risk or average risk patients however in patients with hereditary nonpolyposis colon cancer it is advised that screening be done as a routine from the age of 35 years annually (Birke 1997, Smith 2011)

7.13. Endometrial biopsy/PAP smear

There are different methods of assessment of the endometrial cavity amongst these are fractional curettage of the endometrium where samples are obtained from the uterus in four quadrants and sample send for histology looking out for premalignant lesions of the uterus such as atypical endometrial hyperplasia which is a possible precursor to endometrial cancer

However fractional curettage has the disadvantage of the samples collected not representative of the endometrial tissues. Other methods of collection of samples include vacuum aspiration and hysterscopically directed biopsy of suspicious lesions can also be done

Conventional PAP smear as a screening method for endometrial cancer is not advised since 50% of patients with endometrial cancer will have normal results (Gu, 2001) but improved specificity can be achieved if liquid based cytology is used in detecting glandular lesions

7.14. Ultrasound scan

This assesses the endometrial thickness using transvaginal ultrasound scan can be helpful in screening of patients with endometrial pathology. An endometrial thickness of 5mm has a high sensitivity and specificity for detecting endometrial pathology and a higher negative predictive value of about 100%(Smith –Bindman et at 1998)

8. Screening for vaginal/vulva cancers

Vulva and vaginal cancers account for 7% and 2% of all gynaecological cancers in the United Kingdom in with 80% of them been squamous cell carcinoma and 60% of vulva and 68% of vaginal cancers occur in developing countries (WHO 2009). In Nigeria cancers of the vulva and vagina constitute 1.3% and 1.4% of all gynaecological cancers (Clement et al 2013). It is worthy of note that 40 % of all vulva and vagina cancers are attributed to Human Papilloma virus in the United States of America with HPV 16 the main aetiological agent (Wu X et al 2008,Saraiya et al 2008). In developing countries like Nigeria HPV 16 and 36 have been identified in most cases of vaginal /vulva cancer (Thomas et al). This identification of this etiological agents makes one of the modalities of screening HPV genotype screening a possibility in addition visual inspection with acetic acid for vulva lesions. However there is no consensus on the modality of screening of vaginal and vulva lesions but it is advised that careful examination of vulva/perineal lesions must be undertaken and a biopsy of suspicious lesions taken. Despite the absence of supporting data e expert opinion recommend that annual visual inspection for vulva/vaginal lesions can be undertaken as part of the screening(Crum CP, 1992)

9. Geographical variations in screening programmes in gynaecological cancer

Screening of gynaecological cancers is largely dependent on the cancer burden in the respective country with each country strategizing to reduce the burden. Before the 1940s there was a notable rise in the incidence and mortality associated with cancer such as cervical cancer necessitating the organization of organized screening programmes especially in the `Nordic countries which were largely nationwide and population based resulting in a near nation wide coverage. This was largely achieved by the direction of national resources aided by well-formulated policies by the respective Governments with resounding achievements.

Converse is the case in developing countries with limited resources competing for numerous challenges. The screening programmes of countries are largely opportunistic, poorly organized and not entered on national coverage of the population. The obvious lack of political will on the part of the various Governments has also compounded this problem. Most times screening programmes in these countries are cost driven With governments relying on methods that are relatively less expensive though not necessarily ideal screening methods. The absence of suitable manpower to handle more complex screening methods make such methods unavailable for generality of the population. Thus screening for cervical cancer in developing are usually based on the traditional cytology using the spatula with its drawbacks already highlighted as opposed to liquid based cytology. Less expensive methods for screening such as VIA and cervicography are also used to meet up with the challenges of the draught of the challenges of the draught of histopathologist to analyse samples collected. The absence of histopathologists puts a lot on pressure on already burdened histopathologists resulting in delays of screening results with a back lash on the patients zeal for further follow up in subsequent appointments. The lack of information on credible treatment plans for those diagnosed is also as rate limiting step in achieving national coverage in most of these countries.

10. Conclusion

Gynaecological cancer screening have been shown over the years to be life saving as exemplified by the have shown over the years to be life saving as exemplified by the experience of the Nordic countries as regard cervical cancer where the traditional PAP smears had been used with resounding success reducing incidence and mortality. Same can not be said of other gynaecological cancers were there is currently no consensus on the ideal screening tool. The use of tumour markers like CA 125 solely had not been shown to be good screening tool hence the need for multimodal approach in dealing with ovarian tumours with some still in clinical trials hence the need for the multimodal means for screening for ovarian cancer with some still in the clinical trial phase.

Author details

T.K. Nyengidiki

Department of Obstetrics and Gynecology, College of Health Sciences, University of Port Harcourt, Rivers State, Nigeria

References

[1] Sankaranayanan R, Ferley J. World wide burden of Gynaecological cancer, the size of the burden.Bailliere's Best Practice. Res.2006; 20:207-225

[2] Laara E,Day NE, Hakama M : Trends in morttality from cervical cancer in the Nordic countries: association with organized screening programmes. Lancet : 1987.30;1(8544)1247-9

[3] Kwawukume EY, Srofenyoh EK. Premalignant lesions of the female Genital tract. In EY Kwawukume Ejiro EE edn Comprehensive Gynaecology in the Tropics. Graphic Packaging limited publishers, 2005. 395-411

[4] Denny L, Micheal Q, Sankaranarayanan R. Screening for cervical cancers in developing countries. Vaccine 2453.(2006):S3/71-S3/77

[5] Denny L. Prevention of cervical cancer in developing countries .Br J Obstet Gynaecol, 2005; 112:1204-12.

[6] Wison JM, Junngner. Principle and Practice of screening of disease. Geneva: WHO. 1968.Available from http//www.who.int/bulletin/volume/86/4/07-050112BP.pdf

[7] Noller KL. Cervical cancer screening and evaluation. Obste Gynaecol.vol 106(2) 2005:391-397.

[8] Goodman A, Hutchinson ML. Cell surplus on sampling devices after routine cervical cytologic smears. A study of residual cell populations. *J Reprod Med* 1996; 41: 239-241.

[9] Sarina S, Beth EP.Diethylstilbesterol Exposure. Am. Fam Physician 2004.15; 69(10): 2395-2400

[10] Solomon D,Davey D ,Kurman R et al. The 2001 Bethesda System. Terminology for Reporting Results of Cervical Cytology. JAMA 2002;287(16):2114-2119(doi 10.1001/ Jama.287.26.2114

[11] The American Congress of Obstetricians and Gynecologists. ACOG Practice Bulletin. Clinical Management Guidelines for Obstetrician-Gynecologists: Screening for Cervical Cancer. November, 2012

[12] Ronco G, Cuzick J , Confortini M. Accuracy of liquid based cytology vs conventional cytology: overall result of new technology for cervical cancer screening randomized controlled trials.BMJ.2007.335(7609):28

[13] Arbyn M, Christine B, Paul K, et al. Liquid compared to conventional cervical cytology.A systematic Review and Meta Analysis.ACOG.2008.111.(1).167-177

[14] De Jager P, Singh E, Kistnasamy B, Bertram,MY et al .Cost and cost effectiveness of conventional and liquid based cytology in South Africa- A laboratory service providers perspective SAJOG.2013.19(2).44-48.Doi: 10.7196.SAJOG.619

[15] Nidhi G, Mukesh C : Colposcopy made easy. A handbook on Manual for practicing Doctors and Postgraduates. Jaypee brothers' medical publishers. 72

[16] Ronco G,Dillner J, Elfstrom MK, Sara Tunesi et al. Efficacy of HPV-based screening for prevention of invasive cervical cancer: follow-up of four European randomized controlled trials. The Lancet 2014.383.8.9916.524-532.doi.10.1016/S0140-6736(13) 62218-7

[17] USPSTFrecommendations.2012.Http//www.uspreventiveservicetaskforce.org/uspstf/ uspscerv.htm.

[18] Quek SC, Mould T, Canfell T et al. The polar probe-emerging technology for cervical cancer screening. Ann Acad Med. Singapore. 1998.27:717-21

[19] Bast RC, Fenney M, Lazarus H, Nadler LM, Colvin RB et al. Reactivity of a monoclonal antibody with human ovarian carcinoma. J Clin Invest; 1981.68:1331-1337.

[20] Skates SJ, Menon U, Macdonald N et al. Calculation of the risk of ovarian cancer from serial CA125 values for preclinical detection of postmenopausal women. J Clinc Oncol.2003; 21:206S-210S

[21] Edgell T, Martin R, Barker G, et al. Phase 11 biomarkers trial of multimarker diagnostic for ovarian tumors. J Cancer Res Oncol.2010; 136 (7): 1079-1088.

[22] Brose MS, Rebbeck TR, Calzone KA et al. Cancer risk estimates for BRCA 1 mutation carriers identified in a risk evaluation programme. J Natl Cancer Inst 2002; 94:1365-72.

[23] Struewing JP, Hartge P, Wacholder S et al. The risk of cancer associated with specific mutations of BRCA 1 and BRCA 2 among Ashkenazi Jews .N Engl J Med . 1997:336:1401-8

[24] Lancester MJ, Powell BC, Kauff ND et al. Society of Gynaecologic Oncologist education committee statement in risk assessment for inherited gynaecological cancers predisposition. Gyn Onc.2007.107: 159-162.

[25] Angela Toss, Elisabetta D, Elena R, Lara D et al .Ovarian cancer: can proteomics give new insight for therapy and diagnosis. Int J.Mol.Sci.2013.14.8271-8290;doi 10.3390/ IJMS 14048271.

[26] American Cancer Society. Cancer Facts & Figures 2012. Atlanta: American CancerSociety.www.cancer.org/Research/cancerfactsFigures/cancerfactsFigures/cancrfacts. 2012

[27] US preventive service Taskforce reaffirmation Recommendation statement. Accessed at www.us preventiveservicetaskforce.org/uspstf 12/ovarian/ovariancancers.htm

[28] Pavlik EJ, DePriest PD, Gallion HH, Ueland FR, Reedy MB, Kryscio RJ, et al. Ovarian volume related to age. Gynecol Oncol 2000;77: 410–2.

[29] DePriest PD, Gallion HH, Pavlik EJ, Kryscio RJ, van Nagell JR Jr. Transvaginal sonography as a screening method for the detection of early ovarian cancer. Gynecol Oncol 1997;65: 408–14.

[30] The Royal College of Obstetricians and Gynecologist Guideline No 34.Ovarian cyst in Postmenopausal women. Oct 20013

[31] American college of Obstetricians and Gynaecologist. Routine cancer screening. ACOG opinion no 185.Washington DC.1997

[32] Gu M, Shi W, Barakat RR, Thaler HT et al. Pap smear in women with endometrial carcinoma. Acta Cytol.2001.45 (4) 555-60

[33] Nigeria. Human Papilloma virus and related cancers.Summary report update. WHO/ILO HPV information centreWHO and institute catala .2010. http:// app.who.int/hpvcentre/statisitics/dynamic/ico/country. Pdf/NGA .pdf

[34] Clement Okolo, Olatokunboh MO, Olulosin AA, Effiong EU .A review of vulva and vaginal cancers in Ibadan. Nigeria. NAJ Med Sci.2013;6(2):76-81

[35] Crum CP. Carcinoma of the Vulva: Epidemiological and pathogenesis. Obstet Gynaecol.1992;79: 448-54

[36] W u X, Matanoski G, Chen VW et al. Descriptive epidemiology of the vaginal cancer incidence survival by race, ethnicity and age in the United States. Cancer supplement. 2008; 113(S10):2873-2882

[37] Saraiya M, Watsom M, Wu X et al. Incidence of insitu and invasive vulva cancer in the United States. 1998-2003. Cancer supplement .2008.113(S10):2865-2872

[38] Thomas JO,Herrero R, Omigbodum AA et al .Prevalence of Papilloma virus infection in women in Ibadan. A population based study.Br J cancer.2004;90(3):638-645.

Chapter 7

From the Ovary to the Fallopian Tube: A History of Ovarian Carcinogenesis

G. Chene, G. Lamblin, K. Le Bail-Carval, P. Chabert,
J.D. Tigaud and G. Mellier

Additional information is available at the end of the chapter

http://dx.doi.org/10.5772/58945

1. Introduction

Because of the poor prognosis for ovarian cancer due to the fact it is most often diagnosed late at an advanced stage, screening and early detection could likely reduce the mortality rate. Epithelial ovarian cancer represents 90% of all ovarian cancers [1, 2]. Initialy divided into a double-pathway, epithelial subtypes are in fact distinct diseases with specific characteristics and molecular signatures (see tables 1 and 2) [3, 4]. Recent persuasive data support the idea that high grade serous carcinoma (HGSC) may arise from the Fallopian tube epithelium whereas endometrioid and clear cell cancers could arise from atypical endometriosis through the Fallopian tube. Opportunistic salpingectomy could reduce both HGSC, and endometriosis-associated ovarian cancers (EAOC) (i.e. endometrioid and clear cell cancers).

	Type 1	Type 2
Molecular signatures	BRAF, KRAS, PTEN, b catenin	TP53
Genomic instability	low	high
Frequency	20%	80%
Precursors	adenoma/ borderline tumors, endometriosis	de novo
Prognosis	stage 1, slow evolution	> stage 1, fast evolution
Histological sub-types	low grade serous, endometrioid, mucinous, clear cell carcinoma	high-grade serous, non-differentiated carcinoma, carcinosarcoma

Table 1. Diagram of double-pathway oncogenesis [2]

	Low grade serous	Clear cell	Endometrioid	Mucinous	High grade serous
Molecular signatures	BRAF KRAS HER2	ARID1A HNF 1B PI3KCA PTEN	ARID1A PTEN B-catenine KRAS	KRAS HER2	TP53 BRCA
Genomic instability	low	low	low	low	high
Frequency	5%	10%	10%	3%	70%
Precursors	Borderline serous	Endometriosis Adenofibroma	Endometriosis Adenofibroma	Sequence: Adenoma/ Borderline	-Fallopian tube (STIC) -Ovary (dysplasia)
Prognosis	Favourable	Intermediate	Favourable	Favourable	Poor
Initial response to platinum salt chemotherapy	Intermediate (20-30%)	Chemoresistance (15%)	Good	Chemoresistance (15-20%)	Good (80%)
Potential therapeutic targets	BRAF inhibitors MEK inhibitors	PI3K inhibitors	mTOR inhibitors	MEK inhibitors	PARP inhibitors Cell cycle inhibitors

Table 2. Diagram of quintuple-pathway oncogenesis [3, 4]. This classification shows the clinico-pathological differences along with potential therapeutic targets for each histological sub-type. An advantage of this new classification is that it describes the heterogeneous nature of ovarian cancer.

We propose to discuss the origin of HGSC and EAOC cancers and the potential clinical implications.

2. High-grade serous ovarian cancer (see figure 1)

At this point it seems appropriate to recall the anatomy and embryology involved in order to clarify the close relationship and interaction between Fallopian tube and ovary. During embryonic development, the coelomic epithelium gives rise to the peritoneum and ovarian surface epithelium (OSE). The Mullerian duct develops as an invagination of the coelomic epithelium in direct continuity of the OSE. So the OSE and Fallopian tube share the same origin. Moreover, there is a direct histological connection between the epithelium of the fimbria and the OSE [6] (see figure 1). As we will show below, all these various elements suggest that we should no longer use the term ovarian cancer, but rather tubo-ovarian cancer.

http://dx.doi.org/10.5772/58945

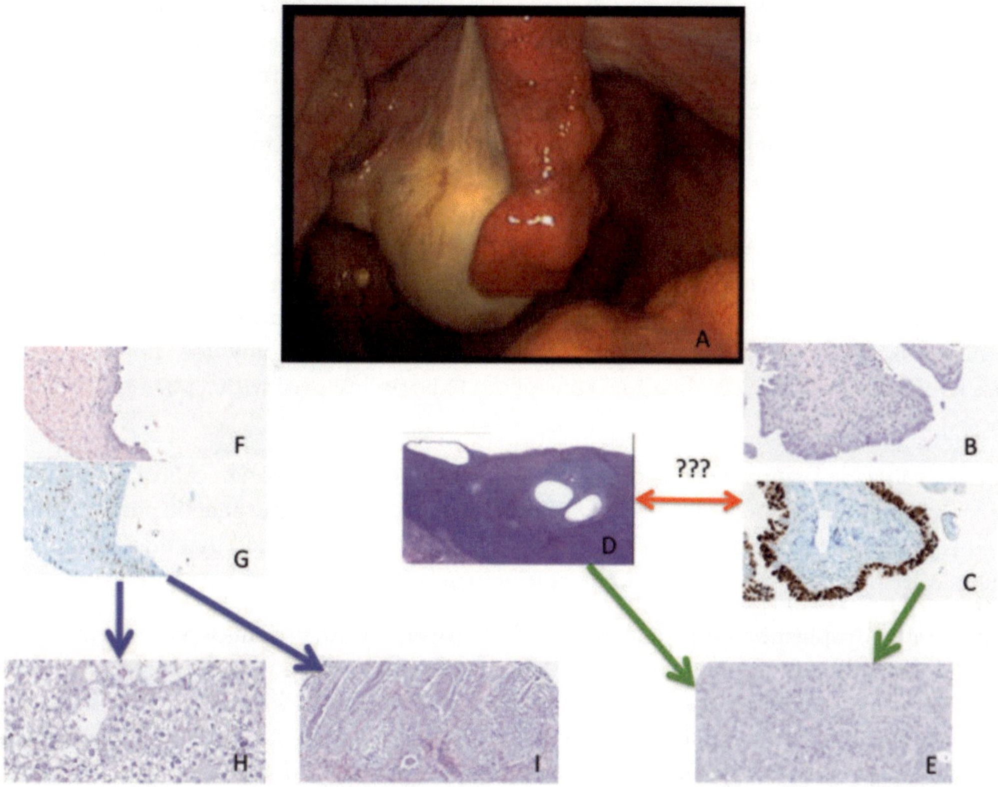

Figure 1. A-In this laparoscopic view, we can see the close anatomical interaction between the fallopian tube and the ovary; In the high-grade serous ovarian carcinogenesis, serous tubal intraepithelial carcinoma (STIC in photo B) may be the non-invasive precursor of high-grade ovarian cancer (E). STIC is characterized by a p53 immunohistochemical signature (C); On the other hand, ovarian epithelial dysplasia (see the inclusion cysts in D) may be also a preinvasive lesion in the high-grade serous ovarian carcinogenesis. This raises the question of the temporal relationships and chronology of events: what is the exact relationship between ovarian dysplasia and STIC ? In the clear cell (H) and endometrioid (I) ovarian carcinogenesis, endometriosis (F) may be a non-invasive precursor when there is loss of ARID1A expression (G). The fallopian tube may be considered as both as a source in the high-grade serous ovarian carcinogenesis and as a conduit for endometriosis in the clear cell and endometrioid ovarian carcinogenesis [60].

a. Once upon a time the ovarian hypothesis:

In 1971, Fathalla [7] developed the theory of incessant ovulation after noting the high frequency of ovarian cancer in nulliparous women and the high prevalence of peritoneal carcinosis of ovarian origin in battery hens (ovulation every 28 hours, rate of spontaneous ovarian cancer between 30 and 40% at 4 years of age). Inversely, the protective role of oral contraception, pregnancy and breastfeeding thanks to their inhibition of ovulation has been well-established [8-10]: repeated ovulations are pro-inflammatory events and could result in the formation of ovarian epithelium inclusion cysts in the OSE. These inclusion cysts, exposed as they are to cellular, paracrine and hormonal growth factors in the pro-inflamatory stromal microenvironment, could thus be the origin of a neoplastic process.

While 90% of cases of ovarian cancer are sporadic, 10% are hereditary in nature with a high proportion linked with BRCA mutations. There is a 35 to 60% cumulative risk at age 70 in case of BRCA 1 mutation. The risk is a little lower in case of BRCA2 mutations, lying between 10 and 27% [11]. These patients, their ovaries and tubes provide an excellent model for studies aiming at a better understanding of ovarian carcinogenesis. Due to the fact that bilateral adnexectomy is recommended in this group at risk, after the age of 35 and after completion of childbearing, these ovaries (and then the tubes, see below) have received particular attention in histopathological and molecular level studies. As a consequence histopathological anomalies called ovarian epithelial dysplasia (by analogy with other preinvasive lesions of the genital tract) were initially described in ovaries with a genetic risk (BRCA mutation) [12]. In view of the high risk of ovarian cancer in these patients if bilateral ovariectomy does not take place, these dysplastic lesions were therefore considered to be preinvasive with a potential towards cancer.

Similar dysplastic lesions were also revealed in areas adjacent to ovarian cancer, and also in the contralateral ovary in case of unilateral ovarian cancer without any genetic predisposition [13-18]. The molecular and histopathological similarities thus suggested that these dysplastic lesions were the initial phases of ovarian carcinogenesis.

More recently dysplastic anomalies were revealed in ovaries from patients who had undergone an ovulation stimulation process in a context of infertility [19, 20]. However since the histopathological, immunohistochemical and molecular characteristics differed from those of dysplastic lesions found in patients with a BRCA genetic mutation, it would appear that there may be several types of dysplasia that evolve differently (towards cancer in case of BRCA mutation, unlike the case after an *in vitro* fertilisation protocol) [21, 22].

b. ...and all of a sudden the tubal hypothesis:

In 2001, Piek *et al* [23] revealed for the first time 6 cases of tubal dysplasia including one case of severe dysplasia in a cohort of 12 patients with a genetic predisposition for ovarian cancer. Other studies have corroborated these results with nearly 10% Serous Tubal Intraepithelial Carcinoma (or STIC), 57% to 100% of which were located in the fimbriated end of the Fallopian tube [24-27]. These lesions consist of nonciliated cells exhibiting 3 or more of the following features: abnormal chromatin pattern, nuclear enlargement, marked nuclear pleomorphism, epithelial stratification and/or loss of polarity, and nuclear moulding. They are also characterised by high immunohistochemical expression of TP53 (expression level between 80% and 92%) and highly positive levels for proliferation marker Ki67 and DNA double-strand break marker γ-H2AX [24-27].

Other even earlier tubal lesions have also been described and it was possible to propose a serous carcinogenic sequence with a tubal origin: after a genotoxic stress and subsequent to various mutations (such as TP 53 mutation and BRCA mutation or epigenetic loss which play an important role in the maintenance of genomic integrity), very early histopathological anomalies of the tube would appear: these SCOUT lesions (Secretory Cell Outgrowths), characterised by a succession of at least 30 pseudostratified secretory epithelial cells with a low expression of PAX2, PTEN and Ki67, and no p53 mutation, would then evolve towards

http://dx.doi.org/10.5772/58945

p53 signatures [28, 29]. These p53 signatures, defined by a succession of at least 12 secretory cells with intense nuclear p53 staining and a low proliferative index, could evolve towards STIC (same TP53 molecular mutation suggesting a clonal relationship and a genetic identity). However, these p53 signatures are found in around 50% of normal control Fallopian tubes and it is not possible at the time of writing to tell which signature(s) might evolve towards STIC and which would not undergo this unfavourable evolution [30].

Finally, STIC lesions may metastase in the ovary and adjacent peritoneum [31].

Several series of sporadic high-grade serous ovarian and serous peritoneal cancers (without BRCA mutation) were re-analysed and revealed the presence of the same serous carcinogenic sequence in almost 50% of cases [31].

c. Tubal or ovarian origin?

STIC lesions present preinvasive characteristics, as shown by the following elements:

- identical TP 53 mutations in STIC lesions and invasive cancer [32]
- up-regulation of other genes (RSF1, Cyclin E, p16, FAS, Stathmin 1, Lamnin 1) as it is the case in invasive ovarian cancer [33-35]
- genomic instability: telomeric shortening and chromosomic rearrangements [36-38]
- animal experiments: development of peritoneal carcinosis with a tubal origin

But, other arguments plead in favour of an ovarian origin. Notably, the fact that STIC lesions are not found in all genetic or sporadic series of ovarian cancer. If there are no STIC lesions or at the very least histological scarring due to STIC of the tube, what would the origin of the cancer be? So this raises the question of the temporal relationships and chronology of events: like for the chicken and the egg, do STIC lesions precede invasive cancer, or the contrary?

To conclude, although during the last century the postulate was raised that ovarian cancer originates in the ovary itself (which seemed logical and is the case for other organs), it would today appear that ovarian cancer has a dual origin, both tubal (predominating in case of genetic risk with BRCA mutation) and ovarian. It remains to be seen how and why one patient will have a cancer of tubal origin while another will have one of ovarian origin [31]. Furthermore, what triggers the transformation of normal secretory Fallopian tube epithelium into HGSC?

The solution is likely in in the interaction between the tube and the ovary. Some authors have described the chronic inflamatory therory [39, 40]. They stated that there is less retrograde flow of inflamatory mediators from the genital tract and through the tube with tubal ligature, hysterectomy, oral contraception or pregnancy (closed cervix). For other authors, the release of inflamatory follicular fluid during ovulation may cause damage on the ovarian and fallopian tube epithelial cells [41, 42]. All these arguments point to the concept of tubo-ovarian cancer, i.e. a disease both in tube and ovary.

The potential clinical implications are discussed in the following paragraphs.

3. Endometrioid and clear cell cancers (see figure 1)

Women with CC and EC frequently present with endometriosis. In a review of 29 studies, Van Gorp *et al* [43] found a statistical association between endometriosis and endometriosis-associated ovarian cancers (EAOC): 36% of clear cell carcinoma were associated with endometriosis (11-70%), and 10% in case of endometrioid carcinoma (5-43%). A precursor lesion called atypical endometriosis was proposed. Atypical endometriosis (AE) is defined by the presence of hyperplasia or cytological atypia, increased nuclear/cytoplasmic ratio, mild hyperchromosomia, mild to moderate pleomorphism, crowded and occasionally stratified epithelial cells. AE has been identified adjacent to concomitant EAOC, with a demonstrated transition from benign endometriosis through AE to EAOC. At the molecular level, AE and EAOC share common molecular abnormalities such as PTEN and PIK3CA mutations, HNF 1b up-regulation, MET amplification and loss of ARID1A [44].

ARID1A (loss or mutation) and PIK3CA are early events and likely occur in precursor lesions as well as in EAOC: mutation of ARID1A gene (AT rich interactive domain 1A) was found in 41 to 57% of clear cell cancers and 30 to 48% of endometrioid cancers [31, 45-47]. ARID1A is a tumour suppressor gene and encodes BAF 250a protein that is involved in the multi-protein SWI/SNF chromatin-remodelling complex.

It has been well established that the SWI/SNF complex is involved in DNA repair through cell cycle arrest and apoptosis, cell survival after DNA damage (particularly by promoting γH2AX induction) and genomic stability. ARID1A has recently been demonstrated to act as a negative regulator of the cell cycle through interaction with TP53 and its mutation may lead to cellular dysfunction as dysregulation of chromatin remodelling [48]. Moreover, loss of expression of this gene was recently found in benign endometriosis (20%) and AE (38.5%) adjacent to malignant lesions (57.7%), suggesting a chronological association from benign through atypical endometriosis to AEOC [44]. Samartzis et al [49] found also loss of ARID1A/ BAF 250a expression in presumably benign ovarian endometriomas (n=3/20, 15%) particularly in the form of cell clusters that could suggest a clonal loss of BAF 250a and a risk of carcinogenic transformation [31].

Finally tubal ligation is protective against AEOC suggesting passage of endometriosis through the tube as a key oncogenic step with potential clinical implications (see below).

4. Clinical implications

The challenge is to detect a microscopic lesion during the occult period. We know also the preclinical natural history of HGSC which lasts on average 4 years as *in situ*, stage 1 and 2 cancers and approximately 1 year as stage 3 /4 cancers before they become clinically apparent [50].

To date, there is no screening test for ovarian cancer. ROCA screening (Risk of Ovarian Cancer) may be promising. It is based on a computerised Bayesian algorithm comparing each individual's CA125 profile to the pattern in ovarian cancer and healthy women. If the CA125 rate is closer to known cases of ovarian cancer, the risk may be greater and a specific clinical assessment with ultrasonography is performed. UKCTOCS will report on the impact on mortality in January 2015 [51, 52].

In the other non invasive methods, evaluation of DNA obtained by Papanicolaou test to detect ovarian cancers is probably encouraging: 41% (9/22) of ovarian cancers were identified using a panel of mutated genes from liquid Papanicolaou smear specimens [53].

However, none of these methods can currently be considered as a safe alternative to risk-reducing surgery. It has been thoroughly demonstrated that carrying out preventive bilateral adnexectomy significantly reduces the risk of ovarian cancer (by over 98%) in at-risk groups (BRCA mutations, Lynch syndrome, family history of breast/ovarian cancer). Nevertheless, while operative morbidity can remain limited thanks to minimally invasive laparoscopic surgery, the complications of surgically induced menopause should not be minimised in women who are still young [54].

The new tubal theories in which the Fallopian tube is considered to be a conduit for EAOC (endometriosis as a precursor lesion) and as an origin for HGSC could result in a preference for exclusive bilateral salpingectomy instead of adnexectomy.

The current Canadian recommendations in British Columbia in gynaecological clinical and surgical practice are in line with this [55]:

- removal of Fallopian tube along with fimbriated end at the time of hysterectomy
- perform salpingectomy instead of tubal ligation
- genetic counseling and BRCA mutation screening in women at high genetic risk of HGSC, with risk-reducing surgery in patients with BRCA mutations

However, we believe a distinction should be drawn between HGSC and EAOC:

- in HGSC risk groups carrying out salpingectomy could be an attractive alternative in that it avoids inducing menopause [56], but this preventive attitude appears to be premature as yet since the origin of this cancer does not seem to be the tube in absolutely all cases, and also because the impact of salpingectomy on ovarian reserves is still the subject of debate. Kwon *et al* [58] have developed a simulation model comparing three strategies in the BRCA population: bilateral salpingo-oophorectomy, bilateral salpingectomy, bilateral salpingectomy with delayed oophorectomy. The authors conclude that prophylactic adnexectomy is best in terms of reducing the risk of ovarian and breast cancer. However, bilateral salpingectomy with delayed oophorectomy could be an interesting option in terms of cost-effective strategy and higher quality of life.
- in groups at risk of EAOC, the problem is not so much the Fallopian tube but rather that of endometriosis. Endometriosis very often developes early (sometimes during adolescence) and removal of the Fallopian tube could only be carried out far later and consequently would be of no interest. Only by drawing the distinction between (atypical) endometriosis with a risk of degeneration and benign endometriosis could efficient screening become possible. The use of specific markers such as ARID1A could be promising [54].

Finally, *ex vivo* optical imaging using reflectance and fluorescence may detect preinvasive lesions. McAlpine *et al* [58] were able to view STIC tubal lesions with 73% sensitivity, 83% specificity, 57% positive predictive value and 91% negative predictive value.

In the future, the development of real time *in vivo* high resolution imaging for STIC through falloposcopy (transcervical route) or salpingoscopy (confocal microlaparoscopy) could certainly be useful in patients with a genetic risk of ovarian cancer and who want to remain fertile, by allowing a precise histopathological diagnosis for the ovaries and tubes in real time and *in vivo* [59].

5. Conclusions

We have moved from one paradigm to another: instead of an exclusively ovarian origin, it appears that ovarian cancer may also have a tubal origin (probably in the majority of genetic risk cases) with the consequent questions concerning clinical implications and exclusively preventive salpingectomy.

We consider that more studies are still needed in order to validate these new concepts. It is clear now that, just as for breast cancer, ovarian cancer is a heterogeneous disease involving specific molecular signatures. Molecular characteristics may likely define personalized treatment specific to subtypes as is the case in breast cancer [31].

Author details

G. Chene*, G. Lamblin, K. Le Bail-Carval, P. Chabert, J.D. Tigaud and G. Mellier

*Address all correspondence to: chenegautier@yahoo.fr

Department of Gynecology, Hôpital Femme Mère Enfant, HFME, Lyon CHU, Lyon, France

References

[1] Chene G, Dauplat J, Bignon Y J, Cayre A, Raoelfils I, Pomel C, Penault-Llorca F. Ovarian carcinogenesis: recent and old hypothesis. Gynecol Obstet Fertil. 2011; 39: 216-23

[2] Ming-Shih I, Kurman RJ. Ovarian tumorigenesis. A proposed model based on morphological and molecular genetic analysis. Am J Pathol 2004; 164: 1511-18

[3] Prat J. Ovarian carcinomas : five distinct diseases with different origins, genetic alterations, and clinicopathological features. Virchows Arch. 2012 ; 460 : 237-49

[4] Chene G, Dauplat J, Cayre A, Robin N, Penault-Llorca F. The fallopian tube odyssey: from the ovary to the tube. About high-grade serous ovarian carcinoma. Bull Cancer 2013; 100: 757-64

[5] Crum CP. Intercepting pelvic cancer in the distal fallopian tube : Theories and realities. Mol Oncol 2009 ; 3 : 165-70

[6] Auersperg N. The origin of ovarian cancers--hypotheses and controversies. Front Biosci (Schol Ed). 2013; 5: 709-19.

[7] Fathalla M. Incessant ovulation : a factor in ovarian neoplasia ? Lancet 1971; 2: 163.

[8] Riman T, Nilsson S, Persson IR. Review of epidemiological evidence for reproductive and hormonal factors in relation to the risk of epithelial ovarian malignancies. Acta Obstet Gynecol Scand 2004; 83: 783-95.

[9] Schuetz AW, Lessman C. Evidence for follicle wall involvement in ovulation and progesterone production by frog follicles in vitro. Differentiation, 1982; 22: 79-84.

[10] Colgin DC, Murdoch WJ. Evidence for a role of the ovarian surface epithelium in the ovulatory mechanism of the sheep: secretion of urokinase-type plasminogen activator. Animal Reproduction Science, 1997; 47: 197-204.

[11] Chene G, Dauplat J, Robin N, Caure A, Penault-Llorca F. Tu-be or tu-be: that is the question… About serous ovarian carcinogenesis. Critical Reviews in Oncol/Hematol 2013; 88: 134-43

[12] Deligdisch L. Ovarian dysplasia: a review. Int J Gynecol Cancer 1997; 7: 89-94.

[13] Salazar H, Godwin AK, Daly MB, Laub PB, Hogan M, Rosenblum N, Boente MP, Lynch HT, Hamilton TC. Microscopic benign and invasive malignant neoplasms and a cancer-prone phenotype in prophylactic oophorectomies. J Natl Cancer Inst 1996: 88: 1810/20.

[14] Werness BA, Afify AM, Bielat KL, Eltabbakh GH, Piver MS, Paterson JM. Altered surface and cyst epithelium of ovaries removed prophylactically from women with a family history of ovarian cancer. Hum Pathol 1999, 30: 151-157.

[15] Plaxe S, Deligdish L, Dottino P, Cohen C. Ovarian intraepithelial neoplasia demonstrated in patients with stage I ovarian carcinoma. Gynecol Oncol 1990; 38: 367-72.

[16] Mittal KR, Jacquotte AZ, Cooper JL, Demopoulos R. Controlateral ovary in unilateral ovarian carcinoma: a search for preneoplastic lesions. Int J Gynecol Patho 1993; 12: 59-63.

[17] Tressera F, Grases PJ, Labastida R, Ubeda A. Histological features of the controlateral ovary in patients with unilateral ovarian cancer : a case control study. Gynecol Oncol 1998; 71: 437-441.

[18] Chene G, Penault-Llorca F, Le Bouedec G, Dauplat MM, Mishellany F, Jaffeux P, Aublet-Cuvelier B, Pouly JL, Dechelotte P, Dauplat J. Ovarian epithelial dysplasia

and prophylactic oophorectomy for genetic risk. Int J Gynecol Cancer. 2009 ; 19: 65-72

[19] Nieto JJ, Crow J, Sundaresan M, Constantinovici N, Perret CW, Mc Lean AN, et al. Ovarian epithelial dysplasia in relation to ovulation induction and nulliparity. Gynecol Oncol 2001; 82: 344-349.

[20] Chene G, Penault-Llorca F, Le Bouedec G, Mishellany F, Dauplat MM, Jaffeux P, et al. Ovarian epithelial dysplasia after ovulation induction: time and dose effect. Human Reprod 2009; 24: 132-138.

[21] Dauplat J, Chene G, Pomel C, Dauplat MM, Le Bouedec G, Mishellany F, et al. Comparison of dysplasia profiles in stimulated ovaries and in those with a genetic risk for ovarian cancer. Eur J Cancer 2009; 45 (17): 2977-83.

[22] Chene G, Penault-Llorca F, Tardieu A, Cayre A, Lagarde N, Jaffeux P, et al. Is there a relationship between ovarian epithelial dysplasia and infertility? Obstet Gynecol Int. 2012; 2012: 429085.

[23] Piek JM, van Diest PJ, Zweemer RP. Dysplastic changes in prophylactic removed fallopian tubes of women predisposed to developping ovarian cancer. J Pathol 2001; 195 : 451-6.

[24] Finch A, Shaw P, Rosen B, Murphy J, Narod SA, Colgan TJ. Clinical and pathologic findings of prophylactic salpingo-oophorectomies in 159 BRCA1 and BRCA2 carriers. Gynecol Oncol 2006; 100: 58-64

[25] Callahan MJ, Crum CP, Medeiros F, Kindelberger DW, Elvin JA, Garber JE, Feltmate CM, Berkowitz RS, Muto MG. Primary fallopian tube malignancies in BRCA-positive women undergoing surgery for ovarian cancer risk reduction. J Clin oncol. 2007; 25: 3985-90

[26] Leeper K, Garcia R, Swisher E, Goff B, Greer B, Paley P. Pathologic findings in prophylactic oophorectomy specimens in high-risk women. Gynecol oncol 2002; 87: 52-6

[27] Medeiros F, Muto MG, Lee Y, Elvin JA, Callahan MJ, Feltmate C, Garber JE, Cramer DW, Crum CP. The tubal fimbria is a preferred site for early adenocarcinoma in women with familial ovarian cancer syndrome. Am J Surg Pathol 2006; 30: 230-6

[28] Chen YE, Mehra K, Mehrad M, Ning G, Miron A, Mutter GL, Monte N, Quade BJ, McKeon FD, Yassin Y, Xian W, Crum CP. Secretory cell outgrowth, PAX2 and serous carcinogenesis

[29] Tung CS, Mok SC Tsang YT et al. PAX2 expression in low malignant potential ovarian tumors and low grade ovarian serous carcinomas. Mod Pathol 2009; 22: 1243-50.

[30] Mehra KK, Chang MC, Folkins AK, Raho CJ, Lima JF, Yuan L, Mehrad M, Tworoger SS, Crum CP, Saleemuddin A. The impact of tissue block sampling on the detection

of p53 signatures in fallopian tubes from women with BRCA 1 or 2 mutations (BRCA +) and controls. Mod Pathol 2011; 24: 152-6

[31] Chene G, Lamblin G, Le Bail-Carval K, Chabert P, Bakrin N, Mellier G. Early preinvasive lesions in ovarian cancer. Biomed Research International 2014; 1-12: ID 639252

[32] Kuhn E, Kurman RJ, Vang R, Sehdev AS, Han G, Soslow R, Wang TL, Shih IE; TP53 mutations in serous tubal intraepithelial carcinoma and concurrent pelvic high-grade serous carcinoma-evidence supporting the clonal relationship of the two lesions. J Pathol 2012; 226: 421-26

[33] Sehdev AS, Kurman RJ, Kuhn E, et al. Serous tubal intraepithelial carcinoma upregulates markers associated with high-grade serous carcinomas including RSF-1 (HBXAP), Cyclin E and fatty acid synthase. Mod Pathol 2010 ; 23 : 844-55.

[34] Karst AM, Levanon K, Duraisamy S, et al. Stathmin 1, a marker of PI3K pathway activation and regulator of microtubule dynamics, is expressed in early pelvic serous carcinomas. Gynecol Oncol 2011; 123 : 5-12

[35] Roland IH, Yang WL, Yang DH, Daly MB, Ozols RF, Hamilton TC. Loss of surface and cyst epithelial basement membranes and preneoplastic morphologic changes in prophylactic oophorectomies. Cancer 2003; 98: 2607-23

[36] Kuhn E, Meeker A, Wang TL, et al. Shortened telomeres in serous tubal intraepithelial carcinoma : an early event in ovarian high-grade serous carcinogenesis. Am J Surg Pathol 2010 ; 34 : 829-36

[37] Chene G, Tchirkov A, Eymard-Pierre E, Dauplat J, Raoelfils I, Cayre A, Watkin E, Vago P, Penault-Llorca F. Early telomere shortening and genomic instability in tubo-ovarian preneoplastic lesions. Clin Cancer Res 2013; 19: 2873-82

[38] Chene G, Ouellet V, Rahimi K, Barres V, Caceres K, Meunier L, Cyr L, De Ladurantaye M, Provencher D, Mes Masson AM. DNA damage signalling and apoptosis in preinvasive tubal lesions of ovarian carcinoma. Int J Gynecol Cancer; 2014: in press

[39] Bosetti C, Negri E, Trichopoulos D, Franceschi S, Beral V, Tzonou A, Parazzini F, Greggi S, La Vecchia C. Long-term effects of oral contraceptives on ovarian cancer risk.

[40] Fleming JS, Beaufie CR, Haviv I, Chenevix-Trench G, Tan OL. Incessant ovulation, inflammation and epithelial ovarian carcinogenesis: revisiting old hypotheses. Molecular and cellular endocrinology, 2006; 247: 4-21.

[41] Emori MM, Drapkin R. The hormonal composition of follicular fluid and its implications for ovarian cancer pathogenesis. Reprod Biol Endoccrinol 2014; 12: 60.

[42] Lau A, Kollara A, St John E, Tone AA, Virtanen C, Greenblatt EM, King WA, Brown TJ. Altered expression of inflammation-associated genes in oviductal cells following

fluid exposure: implications for ovarian carcinogenesis. Exp Biol Med 2014; 239: 24-32

[43] Van Gorp T, Amant F, Neven P, Vergore I, Moerman P. Endometriosis and the de velopment of malignant tumours of the pelvis. A review of literature. Best Pract Res Clin Obstet Gynaecol 2004; 18: 349-71.

[44] Xiao W, Awadallah A, Xin W. Loss of ARID1A/BAF 250a expression in ovarian endometriosis and clear cell carcinoma. Int J Clin Exp Pathol 2012; 5: 642-50

[45] Wiegand KC, Shah SP, Al-Agha OM, et al. ARID 1A mutations in endometriosis-associated ovarian carcinomas. N Eng J Med 2010; 363: 1532-43

[46] Jones S, Wang TL, Shih Ie M, et al. Frequent mutations of chromatin remodeling gene ARID 1A in ovarian cell carcinoma. Science 2010; 330: 228-31

[47] Lowery WJ, Schildkraut JM, Akushevich L, Bentley R, Marks JR, Huntsman D, Berchuck A. Loss of ARID 1A-associated protein expression is a frequent event in clear cell and endometrioid ovarian cancers

[48] Lee HS, Park JH, Kim SJ, Kwon SJ, Kwon J. A cooperative activation loop among SWI/SNF, H2AX, and H3 acetylation for DNA double-strand break repair. EMBO J 2010; 29: 1434-45

[49] Samartzis EP, Samartzis N, Noske A, Fedier A, Caduff R, Dedes KJ, Fink D, Imesch P. Loss od ARID1A / BAF 250a-expression in endometriosis: a biomarker for risk of carcinogenic transformation? Modern Pathol 2012; 1-8

[50] Brown PO, Palmer C. The preclinical natural history of serous ovarian cancer: defining the target for early detection. PLoS Med 2009; 6: e1000114.

[51] Menon U, Skates SJ, Lewis S, Rosenthal AN, McDonald N, Jacobs IJ. Prospective study using the risk of ovarian cancer algorithm to screen for ovarian cancer. J Clin Oncol 2005; 23: 7919-26.

[52] Menon U, Griffin M, Gentry-Maharaj A. Ovarian cancer screening-current status, future directions. Gynecol oncol 2014; 132: 490-5

[53] Kinde L, Bettegowda C, Wang Y, Wu J, Agrawal N, Shih IeM, Kurman R, Dao F, Levine DA, Giuntoli R, Roden R, Eshleman JR, Carvalho JP, Marie SK, Papadopoulos N, Kinzler KW, Vogelstein B, Diaz LA Jr. Evaluation of DNA from the Papanicolaou test to detect ovarian and endometrial cancers. Sci Transl Med 2013; 5: 167ra4.

[54] Chene G, Rahimi K, Mes Masson AM, Provencher D. Surgical implications of the potential new tubal pathway for the ovarian carcinogenesis. J Minim Invasive Gynecol, 2013; 20: 153-9

[55] McAlpine JN, Hanley GE, Woo MM, Tone AA, Rozenberg N, Swenerton KD, Gilks CB, Finlayson SJ, Huntsman DG, Miller DM; ovarian cancer research program of British Columbia. Opportunistic salpingectomy: uptakes, risks and complications of

http://dx.doi.org/10.5772/58945

a reguinal initiative for ovarian cancer prevention. Am J Obstet Gynecol 2014; 210: 471.e1-11

[56] Dietl J, Wischhusen J, Hausler SFM. The post-reproductive fallopian tube: better removed? Human reprod 2011; 26: 2918-24

[57] Kwon JS, Tinker A, Pansegrau G, McAlpine J, Housty M, McCullum M, Gilks CB. Prophylactic salpingectomy and delayed oophorectomy as an alternative for BRCA mutation carriers. Obstet Gynecol 2013; 121: 14-24

[58] McAlpine JN, El Hallani S, Lam SF, Kalloger SE, Luk M, Huntsman DG, McAulay C, Gilks CB, Miller DM, Lane PM. Autofluorescence imaging can identify preinvasive or clinically occult lesions in fallopian tube epithelium: a promising step towards screening and early detection. Gynecol oncol 2011; 120: 385-92

[59] Chene G, Penault-Llorca F, Cayre A, Robin N, Dauplat J. Early detection of ovarian cancer : tomorrow ? J Gynecol Obstet Biol Reprod. 2013; 42: 5-11

[60] Tone AA, Salvador S, Finlayson SJ, Tinker AV, Kwon JS, Lee CH, Cohen T, Ehlen T, Lee M, Carey MS, Heywood M, Pike J, Hoskins PJ, Stuart GC, Swenerton KD, Huntsman DG, Gilks CB, Miller DM, McAlpin JN. The role of the fallopian tube in ovarian cancer. Clin Adv Hematol Oncol 2012; 10: 296-306

Chapter 8

Past, Present and Future Perspectives on the Management of Endometrial Cancer— A Comprehensive Review

Ahmed Abu-Zaid and Ismail A. Al-Badawi

Additional information is available at the end of the chapter

http://dx.doi.org/10.5772/58946

1. Introduction

Endometrial cancer is the most frequent gynecologic malignancy in the United States and the sixth most frequent malignancy worldwide. The highest incidence of endometrial cancer is reported in North America, followed by Central and Eastern Europe. Conversely, the lowest incidence of endometrial cancer is reported in developing countries such as Central and Western Africa [1]. In the United States, roughly 47,000 new cases of endometrial cancer and 8,000 related deaths are recorded yearly [2]. The incidence of endometrial cancer has dramatically increased by 21% since 2008, and unfortunately, the mortality rate per 100,000 cases has increased by more than 100% over the last two decades, and by 8% since 2008 [3].

At the time of clinical diagnosis, it has been estimated that approximately 75% of endometrial cancer patients have early stage disease (FIGO stage I and II) with a 5-year overall survival of 80% to 90% [4, 5]. However, nearly 10% to 15% of patients with early-stage disease develop recurrences after the primary surgical treatment [6, 7]. Conversely, a very small group of patients are unlucky and present with advanced stage disease with unfortunate prognoses. The 5-year survival rates for regional disease (FIGO stage III) and distant disease (FIGO stage IV) are 57% and 19%, respectively [8].

Management of endometrial cancer can be very challenging, even for early-stage disease. The objective of the chapter is to comprehensively shed light on the past, present and future perspectives on the different treatment modalities employed in the management of endometrial cancer.

2. The role of surgery in management of endometrial cancer:

Despite the vast majority of patients diagnosed with endometrial cancer present to clinical attention with early stage disease limited to uterus, metastatic disease is recognized in a substantial proportion when comprehensive surgical staging is carried out [9]. In 1988, the International Federation of Gynecologists and Obstetricians (FIGO) officially suggested surgical staging as part of the primary management plan for endometrial cancer. Despite the recent amendments of the staging system in 2009, comprehensive staging (total hysterectomy, bilateral salpingooophorectomy, peritoneal cytology, intraoperative bilateral pelvic and para-aortic lymph node dissection) continue to be recommended [10-12].

The major advantages of comprehensive surgical staging are directly related to the diagnosis, prognosis, and proper categorization of patients who may benefit from adjuvant therapy. FIGO endometrial cancer staging is chiefly based on surgical pathology and comprehensive surgery permits accurate delineation of disease extent.

2.1. The role of laparotomy, conventional laparoscopy and robotic-assisted laparoscopy in management of endometrial cancer

Conventionally, laparotomy has been the primary mode for surgical staging in patients with endometrial cancer [10-12].

However, several studies examined the practicality of minimally invasive approaches such as laparoscopy for surgical staging of endometrial cancer [13,14].

Afterwards, randomized controlled trials endeavored to compare laparotomy versus conventional laparoscopic approaches. In Gynecologic Oncology Group Study (GOG) LAP2, more than 2000 patients with endometrial cancer were randomized to receive comprehensive surgical staging via conventional laparoscopy or laparotomy [15]. Conventional laparoscopic arm experienced fewer post-surgery complications (14% vs 21%, respectively; p=0.0001), shorter hospitalization rates over 2 days (52% vs 94%, respectively; p=0.0001), however, longer operating periods (204 minutes vs 130 minutes, respectively; p=0.001). The incidence of intraoperative adverse events was similar. Operative conversion from conventional laparoscopy to laparotomy happened in roughly 17.5% of patients with body mass index (BMI) of 25, and 26.5% of patients with BMI of 35 and above, mainly due to poor surgical exploration. Over the 6-week recovery period, the conventional laparoscopic arm patients articulated much higher scores on multiple quality-of-life aspects (less pain, more cosmetics, faster resumption of daily and social activities) [16].

A recently published meta-analysis of survival data compiling 3 randomized controlled clinical trials did identify survival differences between the surgical approaches in patients receiving the conventional laparoscopy and laparotomy for surgical staging of endometrial cancer [17]. A secondary survival analysis showed largely comparable 5-year overall survival rate (around 90% in both groups) and 3-year recurrence rate (around 11% vs 10% in conventional laparoscopy and laparotomy groups, respectively). Based on these findings, it was concluded that conventional laparoscopic approach was not inferior to laparotomy for surgical staging of endometrial cancer [15,18]. Rather, it was concluded that conventional laparoscopic surgical management of endometrial cancer is superior to laparotomy in terms of hospital stay and short-term safety with comparable overall survival and free-recurrence rates. Hence, conventional laparoscopy —whenever technically possible— should be considered as the recommended (primary) approach for comprehensive surgical staging in management of patients with endometrial cancer.

The daVinci Surgical System (Intuitive Surgical, Sunnyvale, CA) is widely used by many gynecologic oncologists and designed to facilitate robotic-assisted laparoscopy. Despite the many benefits (seated and long-distance operating setting, three-dimensional image of surgical field, tremor omission, etc), one of the major disadvantages is lack of haptic feedback [2].

There are multiple published retrospective case series studies that journeyed to explore the use of robotic-assisted laparoscopy for comprehensive surgical staging of endometrial cancer [19,20]. Primary results showed that robotic-assisted laparoscopy was feasible and safe (highly governed by hands-on surgical expertise). Unfortunately, robotic-assisted laparoscopy has not been prospectively compared in randomized controlled trials to conventional laparoscopy for evaluating the efficacy of endometrial cancer surgical staging, and hence data about survival, safety, and performance differences are lacking. Nevertheless, current literature data point out that robotic-assisted laparoscopy has advantages closely comparable to conventional laparoscopy. Moreover, over time, technical expertise can be simply acquired with robotic assistance as compared to conventional laparoscopy, and thus enabling the achievement of complete comprehensive staging of endometrial cancer in the obese and morbidly obese patients, as laparotomy possesses high potential adverse events in such populations [21]. For communities concerned about financial matters, cost differences between surgical approaches for staging endometrial cancer has been reported [22]. Laparotomy was the most expensive, followed by robotic-assisted laparoscopy, and followed by conventional laparoscopy.

Port-site tumor implantation taking place in patients undergoing minimally invasive laparoscopic techniques for gynecologic cancers is always a major concern for many patients and surgeons [10]. Generally speaking, the incidence of port-site tumor metastatic deposits following laparoscopic procedures in patients with malignant cancer is very minimal, and mostly takes place in the setting of already locally widely spread intra-abdominal disease or distant metastatic disease [23]. Precisely, the risks of port-site tumor implantation in patients with early-stage endometrial cancer following laparoscopic procedures (conventional or robotic-assisted approaches) are very low (less than 1%) [24]. Therefore, minimally invasive laparoscopic techniques can be used safely, to a greater degree, in patient with early-stage disease.

2.2. The role of lymphadenectomy in management of endometrial cancer

The issue of bilateral pelvic and para-aortic lymphadenectomy for surgical staging of endometrial cancer remains a topic of argument [10, 25-27]. Although lymphadenectomy is required for accurate staging, lymphadenectomy should generally be considered in patients with high risk for lymph nodal involvement [28-31]. Such risk factors include: tumor grade 3 (poorly differentiated), more than 50% of myometrial invasion, lymphovascular space invasion, non-endometrioid histology (serous, clear cell, undifferentiated, small cell, anaplastic, etc), cervical stromal involvement, advanced FIGO stage (III and IV), and older age (above 60 years) [28].

Several randomized controlled clinical trials demonstrated no survival benefits from systematic lymphadenectomy in patients with early-stage and low-risk endometrial cancer. Benedetti Panici and colleagues [25] explored the effect of systematic lymphadenectomy in patients with stage I endometrial cancer and documented no difference in overall survival (90% vs. 86%) and disease-free survival (80% vs. 82%) rates between lymphadenectomy and no lymphadenectomy arms. Moreover, the ASTEC trial from United Kingdom [26] studied approximately 1400 patients with endometrial cancer limited to uterus, and showed no recurrence-free or overall survival benefits from pelvic lymphadenectomy in patients with early-stage endometrial cancer. Another randomized clinical trial from Italy [25] reported no difference in rates of survival or recurrence between patients who underwent lymphadenectomy versus who did not undergo lymphadenectomy for early-stage endometrial cancer. Furthermore, 2 cohort studies showed that patients with low-risk endometrial cancer disease (neoplasm size ≤2 cm, less than 50% myometrial invasion, grade 1 and 2 endometrioid neoplasms) had no lymphadenopathy at time of surgical staging and did not gain advantage from systematic lymphadenectomy [30, 31]. Collectively, these data suggest no therapeutic benefit of lymphadenectomy in patients with early-stage and low-risk endometrial cancer.

Bristow and associates [32] conducted a retrospective cohort study examining 41 patients with advanced stage IIIC endometrial cancer, and found statistically significant disease-specific survival benefit of 37.5 months versus 8.8 months (p=0.006) between patients who received optimal (completely debulked) lymphadenectomy and patients who received suboptimal lymphadenectomy groups. They concluded that patients with stage IIIC endometrial carcinoma, complete debulking of gross nodal disease and subsequent administration of combined adjuvant radiation therapy and chemotherapy are correlated with improved disease-specific survival.

There are continuing disputes regarding whether to perform complete bilateral para-aortic lymphadenectomy in all patients. Positive para-aortic lymph nodes can occur in the absence of pelvic lymphadenopathy [30, 33]. Abu-Rustum and colleagues [33] identified 1.6% rate of para-aortic lymphadenopathy in 734 patients with negative pelvic lymphadenopathy and low- and high-grade endometrial cancer. As such, the current practice is to perform pelvic lymphadenectomy, in addition to para-aortic lymphadenectomy, or to propose sentinel lymph node mapping [34, 35]. Khoury-Collado and partners [34] evaluated a sum of 266 patients with endometrial cancer for lymph node mapping. Sentinel lymph node recognition was positive in 223 patients (84%). The utility of sentinel lymph node mapping may surface as a plausible suggestion to decide whether patients with early stage endometrial cancer will get advantage from pelvic and/or para-aortic lymph node evaluation.

Other studies recommend that para-aortic lymphadenectomy should be offered to patients with advanced stage and high-risk histopathological endometrial cancer [29-32]. Mariani and colleagues [30] explored 281 patients who had lymphadenectomy at the time of endometrial cancer staging and identified that approximately 22% of high-risk patients had lymph node invasion. Of these, roughly 33% had isolated pelvic lymphadenopathy, 16% had isolated para-aortic lymphadenopathy and 51% had both pelvic and para-aortic lymphadenopathy.

Although straightforward disease-free survival and overall survival benefits of pelvic and para-aortic lymphadenectomy have not been solidly reported, the procedure of lymphadenectomy offers accurate staging of endometrial cancer, and recognizes node-positive patients who may benefit from adjuvant treatment.

2.3. The role of "Cytoreduction" in management of recurrent endometrial cancer

Around 25% of endometrial cancer related mortality is primarily due to recurrent disease [6, 36, 37]. More than half of patients with endometrial cancer experience recurrence following the initial surgical treatment [38]. Recurrence rates can be as low as 15% in early-stage disease and benign pathology, and as high as 50% in late-stage disease and aggressive pathology [39-41]. Prognosis of patients with recurrent disease and peritoneal metastasis is very graving (median survival less than 12 months) [42, 43]. Optimal Surgical debulking (whenever feasible), even with multiple recurrences, is the standard of care followed with adjuvant radiotherapy, chemotherapy or hormonal therapy [43].

Bristow and associates [44] reported a cohort of 61 patients undergoing cytoreduction for recurrent endometrial cancer. Optimal cytoreduction (no gross residual disease) was achieved in 66% of patients and yielded longer median recurrence-free survival rates of 39 months as opposed to patients with suboptimal cytoreduction of only 13 months ($p=0.0005$).

Awtrey and partners [45] reported a cohort of 27 patients undergoing cytoreduction for recurrent endometrial cancer. Optimal cytoreduction (no gross residual disease) and suboptimal cytoreduction (less than 2 cm residual disease) was achieved in roughly 56% and 67% of patients, respectively, and, yielded longer median survival rates (43 months vs. 10 months, respectively; $p< 0.05$).

In the above-mentioned two studies, the absence of residual disease was correlated with improved disease-free survival and overall survival rates [44, 45]. Collectively, Barlin and colleagues [46] conducted a meta-analysis and showed that optimal cytoreduction to no macroscopic disease was correlated with overall survival benefits ranging from 9 to 25 months in patients with recurrent endometrial cancer.

2.4. The role of Hyperthermic Intraperitoneal Chemotherapy (HIPEC) in management of recurrent endometrial cancer

The utilization of hyperthermic intraperitoneal chemotherapy (HIPEC) has yielded significantly substantial improvements in disease-free survival and overall survival rates in patients with peritoneal recurrence from pseudomyxoma peritonei [47], colon cancers [48], gastric cancers [49] and ovarian cancers [50]. Its use in management of recurrent endometrial cancer is minimal and has not gained much popularity.

Bakrin and colleagues [43] studied the combination of cytoreduction and HIPEC in 5 patients with recurrent endometrial cancer. Optimal cytoreduction was achieved in all patients. HIPEC was carried out with mitomycin C and cisplatin. Intraoperative and postoperative adverse events were uneventful. Two patients developed early recurrences at 2 and 10 months and both died afterwards. The remaining three patients were alive and disease-free at 7, 23 and 39 months with fair performance status.

Abu-Zaid and colleagues [51] studied the combination of cytoreduction and HIPEC in 2 and 4 patients with primary advanced and recurrent endometrial cancer, respectively. Optimal cytoreduction was achieved in 5 patients. HIPEC was carried out with doxorubicin and cisplatin. Intraoperative and postoperative adverse events were uneventful. All patients received adjuvant chemotherapy (carboplatin and paclitaxel). Despite optimal debulking, one patient with an aggressive histology (clear cell carcinoma) relapsed within 6 months and died 5 months later because of metastatic spread to liver and pelvis. One patient with suboptimal cytoreduction (more than 2 cm residual disease) developed liver recurrence within 3 months and was still alive with disease at a follow-up of 6 months. The remaining patients were alive and disease-free without recurrence at follow-up at 35, 34, 19, and 7 months.

Another study done in France [52] included 13 patients treated with cytoreduction and HIPEC for management of endometrial cancer with peritoneal metastases. One patient was lost to follow-up. Following HIPEC, three patients died before the first year, and two patients approximately died at first year and first year and half, respectively. Three patients were alive with disease, and 4 patients were alive without disease, between approximately 2 and 125 months period.

In the above-mentioned studies, disease-free survival and overall survival rates were largely affected by degree of peritoneal cancer index, cytoreduction completeness and tumor pathology [43, 51, 52].

Despite promising results, almost all the existing studies are limited by their retrospective study designs, lack of randomized controlled trials, short follow-up periods and small sample sizes. This is an interesting arena for research and further studies are needed.

The logic for using HIPEC is chiefly attributed to the straightforward temperature-improved cytotoxicity of the intraperitoneal chemotherapeutic agents [53, 54]. Moreover, HIPEC aims to deeply penetrate the residual microscopic deposits [53, 54]— the primary source of surgical failure and early recurrence rates [43, 51, 52, 55, 56] in recurrent endometrial cancer. Moreover, HIPEC avoids the needless chemotherapy-related systemic toxicities while maximizing the local concentrations [57]. The most frequently used HIPEC agents include cisplatin [58] doxorubicin [59] and mitomycin C [60].

Generally, morbidity and mortality of cytoreduction and HIPEC are greatly influenced by the surgeons' expertise and learning curve [61]. A recent systematic review by Chua and colleagues [62] demonstrated that the morbidity rate associated with cytoreduction and HIPEC range from approximately 12% to 52%, whereas mortality rate range from 1% to 6%.

http://dx.doi.org/10.5772/58946

3. The role of adjuvant radiation therapy in management of endometrial cancer

The role of radiation therapy in management of endometrial cancer is still under investigation with inconsistent findings and there are no solid conclusions. Improvement in disease-free survival rates is noted only.

3.1. Pelvic external beam radiation therapy (EBRT)

The efficacy of adjuvant external beam radiotherapy (EBRT) was studied in five randomized clinical trials [40, 41, 63-69]. Only ASTEC/EN.5 clinical trial included a substantial percentage of patients with aggressive serous or clear cell histology (6.5%) [64]. Conversely, in all the other remaining trials, endometrioid adenocarcinoma was the most predominant histology. All trials demonstrated advantages of EBRT in terms of loco-regional control (disease-free survival) only, but failed to yield any survival benefits. Furthermore, at a median follow-up of 21 years, an update of Oslo trial demonstrated that patients under 60 years of age who were administered adjuvant EBRT experienced lower overall survival rates and higher risks of harboring secondary malignancies, as high as 30% [69]. Moreover, in the PORTEC trial, patients who received EBRT had worse quality of life as opposed to the observation patients [68]. The EBRT toxicities commonly involved the urogenital and gastro-intestinal tract systems and included urinary leakage and urgency, in addition to frequent diarrheal attacks and stool incontinence. These findings were endorsed in two recently published meta-analyses [70, 71]. Subgroups analyses were completed and demonstrated that EBRT had improved disease-free survival in patients with high risk of recurrence (p=0.03), however, EBRT had harmful outcomes on overall survival in patients with low or intermediate risk of recurrence (p=0.03) [70]. Therefore, it can be concluded that adjuvant EBRT should be largely employed for management of high-risk patients with primary advanced or recurrent endometrial cancer. Moreover, long-term related toxicities of EBRT should be considered wisely when adjuvant EBRT is selected for younger patients. EBRT should be selected in patients with high-risk histological features, positive lymph nodes or primary advanced stage disease (III/IV) [28]. The suggested histopathological features for determining high-risk disease include: tumor grade 3 (poorly differentiated), more than 50% of myometrial invasion, lymphovascular space invasion, non-endometrioid histology (serous, clear cell, undifferentiated, small cell, anaplastic, etc), cervical stromal involvement, advanced stage disease (FIGO stage III and IV) and older age (more than 60 years) [28].

3.2. Vaginal brachytherapy

The efficacy of adjuvant vaginal brachytherapy (VB) was evaluated in two randomized clinical trials [72, 73]. Patients with serous or clear cell histology were exempted from the studies and only patients with endometrioid adenocarcinomas were included. In low-risk patients with endometrial cancer (stage IA–B, grades 1–2), vaginal brachytherapy did not add benefit over observation [72]. However, in PORTEC-2 clinical trial, in high-intermediate risk patients, vaginal brachytherapy was demonstrated to be non-inferior to EBRT and provided comparable loco-regional control (less than 2% at 5-year period for both arms), disease-free survival and overall survival [63, 73]. Vaginal brachytherapy is associated with considerably fewer gastrointestinal tract toxicities (less diarrheal attacks and stool incontinence) and a better functioning social quality of life [72-74]. Sorbe and colleagues [63] compared combination of EBRT and brachytherapy versus brachytherapy alone: there was no 5-year overall survival benefit (89% and 90%, respectively; p=0.548). However, the 5-year pelvic and loco-regional recurrences were much more common in the vaginal brachytherapy alone group (1.5% and 5%, respectively; p=0.013). It was concluded that combined radiation therapy (EBRT and vaginal brachytherapy) should possibly be reserved for high-risk patients, whereas vaginal brachytherapy alone should be reserved for purely medium-risk patients.

In conclusion, vaginal brachytherapy, to a certain degree, effectively decreases the risk of vaginal recurrence in patients with risk factors while minimizing the radiation-related toxicities. In patients with early-stage endometrial cancer, vaginal brachytherapy should the adjuvant treatment of choice over EBRT.

4. The role of adjuvant chemotherapy in management of endometrial cancer

The role of adjuvant chemotherapy has been studied in patients with early-stage intermediate-to-high risk endometrial cancer, as well as patients with primary advanced, inoperable or recurrent late-stage endometrial cancer [39, 75-81]. The efficacy of postoperative chemotherapy was studied in a total of nine randomized clinical trials [39, 75-81]. The following trials included a substantial percentage of patients with the aggressive serous or clear cell histology: NSGO-EORTC (37%), GOG122 (25%), GOG184 (18%) [39, 78, 81]; the vast majority of patients had endometrioid adenocarcinoma histology.

Three clinical trials compared chemotherapy schedules with radiotherapy [39, 75, 76]. Two randomized clinical trials compared between one group of patients receiving cyclophosphamide–doxorubicin–cisplatin, and one group of patients receiving pelvic EBRT. There were no benefits between both groups with respect to 5-year progression-free survival and overall survival rates [75, 76]. Conversely, GOG122 trial demonstrated statistically significant 5-year progression-free survival (50% and 38%, respectively; p=0.007) and overall survival (55% and 42%, respectively; p=0.004) rates between one group of patients receiving doxorubicin–cisplatin, and one group of patients receiving EBRT. All patients studied in COG122 study had advanced stage disease (III/IV) with less than 2 cm residual disease post-surgery [39].

Four clinical trials explored the advantage of adding a chemotherapy regimen to EBRT [77-79]. Three clinical trials (MaNGO ILIADE-III, Kuoppala and GOG34) demonstrated no progression-free survival or overall survival benefits of combined treatment (chemotherapy plus radiotherapy) versus EBRT alone. However, the NSGO-EORTC trial showed that postoperative chemotherapy was correlated with an improved 5-year progression-free survival rate (79% and 72%; p=0.004), but not overall survival benefits [77]. There are discrepancies for the reported results among studies and these can be attributed to the variances of treatment methods such as: percentage of patients with advanced stage disease (stage III–IV) and choice of chemotherapy regimens. Therefore, such studies must be interpreted with caution.

However, overall, a recently published meta-analysis covering a total of nine clinical trials showed that adjuvant chemotherapy was correlated with a statistically significant overall survival benefit (HR=0.74 [95% CI: 0.62–0.89]; p=0.0009), associating with an absolute difference of 3% in 5-year survival rate [80].

Two clinical trials endeavored to compare chemotherapy regimens and the superiority of either of them in terms of progression-free survival or overall survival rates failed to take place [81, 82]. Fujimura and colleagues [81] considered one group of patients with cyclophosphamide–doxorubicin–cisplatin, and one group of patients with etoposide–cisplatin. Homesley and colleagues (the GOG184 trial) [82] considered one group of patients for doxorubicin–cisplatin–placitaxel, and one group of patients for doxorubicin–cisplatin. In this study, the addition of paclitaxel to a cisplatin–doxorubicin regimen was accompanied with substantial chemotherapy-related side effects, mainly neurologic and hematologic [82].

There is an ongoing randomized clinical trial GOG209 phase III (paclitaxel–carboplatin versus paclitaxel–doxorubicin–cisplatin for management of recurrent/advanced endometrial cancer) [83]. Preliminary findings demonstrated that carboplatin–placitaxel combination was not inferior to doxorubicin–cisplatin–placitaxel with respect to progression-free survival (comparable median of 13-14 months; $p > 0.05$) and overall survival (32 versus 38 months, respectively; no statistical significant difference: $p > 0.05$) and was associated with reduced toxicity: peripheral neuropathic toxicity grade 2 or higher (19% versus 26%), thrombocytopenia (12% versus 23%), metabolic imbalances (8% versus 14%), vomiting (4% versus 7%) and diarrhea (2% versus 6%) [10]. However, in consideration of the paclitaxel–doxorubicin–cisplatin associated toxicity, the combination of paclitaxel–carboplatin probably stands as the most preferred utilized chemotherapy regimen, and its administration is supported by the GOG209 trial above [83] and many other retrospective studies [51]. More studies are needed.

Previous studies have demonstrated that neoadjuvant chemotherapy with subsequent optimal cytoreduction for patients presenting with primary advanced endometrial cancer yielded no residual disease in 79% to 100% of all patients treated [84, 85]. Additional studies are needed.

5. The role of hormonal therapy in management of endometrial cancer

Many endometrial cancers express estrogen (ER) and progesterone (PR) receptors, and hence hormonal therapy can be applied as reasonable therapeutic choice in patients with hormone receptor-positive endometrial cancers. The presence of ER and PR receptors largely provides a powerfully predictive value in evaluating therapeutic response to hormonal therapy.

Primary hormonal therapy (without surgical intervention) to preserve fertility in child-bearing women with endometrial cancer has shown some degree of success, although the vast majority of patients ended up receiving the definitive therapy (that is, total abdominal hysterectomy) [86, 87]. As opposed to adjuvant radiotherapy, chemotherapy or combined radio-chemotherapy, hormonal therapy is hardly ever considered as one of the "primary" adjuvant treatment regimens in management of patients with endometrial cancer [86, 87]. Currently, hormonal therapy is largely employed for management of patients with poor performance status or recurrent/advanced/metastatic endometrial cancers, with the advantages of low morbidity, few drug-related side effects and relatively suboptimal therapeutic response [86, 87].

The most frequently employed hormonal agents for management of endometrial cancer include: progesterone/progestin, selective estrogen receptor modulators (SERMs), gonadotropin-releasing hormone (GnRH) agonists, and aromatase inhibitors [86-90].

5.1. Progesterone/progestin

Progesterone/progestin has been proven to be an effective inhibitor (suppressor) of endometrial carcinogenesis mediated through estrogen exposure [91, 92].

Many retrospective studies and clinical trials have been conducted to evaluate the role of multiple progestin-based hormonal therapy regimens in management of patients with recurrent endometrial cancer. The most commonly used regimens are megestrol acetate (MA) and medroxyprogesterone acetate (MPA).

In 1996, a meta-analysis of 6 randomized trials comprising a sum of 3339 patients with endometrial cancer failed to produce any survival benefits when adjuvant progesterone/progestin therapy was administered [93]. Moreover, a successively reported randomized clinical trial recruiting more than 1000 patients with endometrial cancer also failed to produce any survival benefits when adjuvant progesterone/progestin therapy was administered [94]. Furthermore, in 2011, a recently published Cochrane meta-analysis demonstrated no survival benefits of adjuvant progesterone/progestin in 4556 patients with endometrial cancer [95]

5.2. Selective estrogen receptor modulators (SERMs)

The expression of ER in endometrial cancer justifies the use of selective estrogen receptor modulators (SERMS), such as tamoxifen and raloxifene [96]. The tamoxifen-induced increased risk of developing endometrial cancer is a well-known adverse effect and must always be considered in mind [97], as opposed to raloxifene that is not associated with any endometrial cancer risk.

Thigpen and partners [98] used adjuvant tamoxifen (2 doses of 20 mg/day) in management of patients with recurrent and advanced endometrial cancer. The response rate was 10%. The median progression-free survival and overall survival rates were roughly 2 and 9 months, respectively. Raloxifene produced equally unsatisfactory results.

Arzoxifene is a modified drug of raloxifene. Two phase II clinical trials by McMeekin et al. [99] and Burke et al. [100] explored the role of adjuvant arzoxifene (20 mg/day) for management of patients with recurrent, metastatic and advanced endometrial cancer. The response rates were 25% and 31%, respectively. The median response periods were approximately 19.3 and 12.9 months, respectively.

Rendina and associates [101] compared the efficacy of adjuvant tamoxifen versus MPA in patients with recurrent endometrial cancer, and response rates were roughly 53% and 56%, respectively.

Pandya et al. [102] randomized 20 patients and 42 patients with endometrial cancer to receive MA (standard progestin) and combination of MA plus tamoxifen, respectively. The response rates were 20% (1 complete and 3 partial responses) and 19% (1 complete and 7 partial responses), respectively. It was decided that the combination of MA plus tamoxifen did not yield clinical benefits over MA alone in management of patients with advanced endometrial cancer.

Whitney et al. [103] in a phase II trial of MPA (200 mg/week) plus tamoxifen (40 mg/day) in patients with advanced and recurrent endometrial cancer demonstrated a 33% response rate (13 partial and 6 complete responses among a total of 58 patients). The median progression-free survival and overall survival were 3 month and 13 months, respectively. It was concluded that daily tamoxifen (40 mg/day) and alternating weekly MPA (200 mg/week) constitutes an effective therapeutic regimen in management of patients with recurrent and advanced endometrial cancer.

5.3. Gonadotropin-releasing hormone (GnRH) agonists

Gonadotropin-releasing hormone (GnRH) agonists can effectively suppress estrogen production levels by ovarian cells — a process mediated by down-regulation of GnRH receptors [87]. Multiple studies in the United Kingdom explored the usefulness of GnRH agonists in the management of patients with recurrent endometrial cancer [104, 105]. In a phase II clinical trial, 6 out of 17 patients (35%) experienced a response rate at a median of 20 months without drug-related toxicities [104]. A long-term follow-up study, five years afterwards, the same research team documented that the response rate was 28% in 32 patients with recurrent endometrial cancer [105]. The response rate was higher in the previously irradiated regions (35%) versus non-irradiated regions (28%) of relapse. The study concluded that utilization of GnRH agonists greatly exhibit beneficial anti-cancer outcomes in patients with recurrent and advanced endometrial cancer, particularly in those patients who received previous radiation therapy.

Another GOG clinical trial explored the influence of Goserelin acetate (GnRH agonist) in 42 patients with advanced and recurrent endometrial cancer. A total of 5 patients (11%) experienced a response rate. The median progression-free survival and overall survival rates were roughly 2 and 7.3 months, respectively [106].

5.4. Aromatase inhibitors (AIs)

Aromatase inhibitors (AIs), such as anastrozole and letrozole, directly block the aromatase enzyme, and subsequently decrease the estrogen production and suppress its estrogen-driven neoplastic endometrial proliferation [87].

A phase II clinical trial by Rose and colleagues [107] studied the efficacy of anastrozole (1 mg a day for 28 days) in 23 patients with advanced or recurrent endometrial cancer. The response rate was 9% and progression-free interval ranged from 1 to 6 months. Despite the drug-related adverse events were well-tolerated, it was concluded that anastrozole does not offer any survival advantages.

Another multi-center phase II clinical trial by Ma and colleagues [108] studied the effect of letrozole in 28 patients with metastatic or recurrent endometrial cancer who previously received progestin-based and/or chemotherapy regimens. One patient (3.6%), two patients (7.1%) and eleven patients (39%) experienced a complete response, a partial response and a median 6.7-month stable disease, respectively. The median time to progression and overall survival were approximately 4 and 9 months, respectively. The most frequently encountered drug-related adverse events in a descending order were: hot flashes, grade I and II (28%), followed by fatigue and anemia

In short, it can be concluded that AIs greatly failed to offer survival benefits in management of patients with endometrial cancer

6. The role of molecular-target therapy in management of endometrial

As opposed to conventional cytotoxic drugs, molecular-targeted cytotoxic drugs are able to differentiate between normal cells and cancerous cells, and therefore specifically damage only the cancerous cells by inhibiting the cellular molecules/pathways associated with neoplastic proliferation and metastasis [109].

6.1. Mammalian target of rapamycin (mTOR) inhibitors

PTEN genetic mutations are associated with reduced apoptosis and are implicated in more than 80% of endometrioid cancer of the uterus [109]. The effects of PTEN genetic mutations can be decreased by utilizing mammalian target of rapamycin (mTOR) inhibitors (for example, temsirolimus, ridaforolimus, everolimus, and AP2357) by interrupting phosphoinositide 3-kinase◎AKT◎mTOR pathway [109, 110]. In a phase II clinical trial of temsirolimus in previously chemotherapy-untreated patients with recurrent endometrial cancer, 26% and 63% of patients experienced partial response and stable disease, respectively [111]. In a phase II clinical trial of temsirolimus in previously chemotherapy-treated patients with recurrent endometrial cancer, 7% and 44% of patients experienced partial response and stable disease, respectively [112].

In a phase II clinical trial of ridaforolimus as a single agent in patients with advanced endometrial cancer, a total 29% of patients experienced clinical beneficial response in the form of complete response, partial response or prolonged stable disease for more than 16 weeks [113].

In a phase II clinical trial of everolimus as a single agent in patients with recurrent endometrial cancer, 21% of patients experienced confirmed clinical beneficial response in the form of complete response, partial response or prolonged stable disease at 20 weeks after therapy [114].

There is an ongoing randomized controlled trial single-agent temsirolimus versus a combination of temsirolimus and hormonal therapy [109]

6.2. Human Epidermal Growth Factor Receptor (EGFR) Inhibitors

Epidermal Growth Factor Receptor (EGFR) is frequently expressed in normal endometrial tissues; however, its overexpression is correlated with advanced endometrial cancer and poor prognosis [110]. Examples of EGFR inhibtors include erlotinib and gefitinib, both of which are low-molecular weight tyrosine kinase inhibitors.

In a phase II clinical trial of erlotinib in 23 patients with recurrent endometrial cancer, only one patient (4.3%) experienced partial response [115]. In a phase II clinical trial of gefitinib in 29 patients with recurrent endometrial cancer, only one patient (3.4%) experienced complete response [116].

Cetuximab is a monoclonal antibody targeted against EGFR. A phase II clinical trial of cetuximab in management of recurrent endometrial cancer is still ongoing [110].

Trastuzumab belongs to human EGFR type 2 (HER-2)-related inhibitors [110]. HER-2 overexpression is implicated in the development of advanced endometrial cancer and poor prognosis [117, 118], and specifically found in up to 20-30% of patients with serous endometrial cancer [119]. A phase II clinical trial of trastuzumab in 33 patients with HER-2 amplified recurrent/ advanced endometrial cancer did not result in any clinical beneficial response [120]

Lapatinib is an inhibitor targeting EGFR and HER-2 receptors. A phase II clinical trial of lapatinib in management of recurrent endometrial cancer is still ongoing [110].

6.3. Angiogenesis Inhibitors

Vascular Endothelial Growth Factor (VEGF) plays central roles in angiogenesis and overexpression is a feature in advanced endometrial cancer and correlated with poor prognosis [110, 121].

In a phase II clinical trial of single agent bevacizumab (a recombinant humanized immunoglobulin monoclonal antibody targeted against VEGF) in 52 patients with recurrent endometrial cancer, only 7 patients (around 14%) showed complete/partial response at 6 months following treatment. The median progression-free survival and overall survival were roughly 4 and 11 months, respectively. The adverse side effects were tolerated [122]. Wright and colleagues [123] studied the role of bevacizumab in 10 patients with recurrent endometrial cancer. Only two (20%) and three (30%) patients responded to treatment and experienced stable disease, respectively. A GOG 229-E phase II clinical trial of single-agent bevacizumab, and GOG 229-G phase II clinical trial of a combination of bevacizumab and temsirolimus in management of patients with metastatic endometrial cancer are still ongoing [109, 110].

Aflibercept is a fusion protein with high-affinity against VEGF receptors [110]. In a phase II clinical trial of single agent Aflibercept in 44 patients with recurrent endometrial cancer, only 3 patients (around 8%) experienced partial response. Moreover, 18 patients (41%) experienced progression-free survival of 6 months; however, of these, 8 patients had to withdraw aflibercept secondary to drug-related adverse events. The median progression-free survival and overall survival were roughly 3 and 15 months, respectively [124].

Thalidomide possesses anti-angiogenetic action [110]. In a phase II clinical trial in 24 patients with chemotherapy-unresponsive recurrent endometrial cancer, 3 patients (12.5%) experienced partial response and 2 patients (8.3%) had a progression-free survival of more than 6 months. The median progression-free survival and overall survival were roughly 1.7 and 6.3 months, respectively [125].

Sunitinib is a multi-kinase inhibitor with an anti-angiogenetic action. It is currently under investigation in clinical trials to assess its effectiveness in management of patients with recurrent endometrial cancer [109, 110].

The existing response rates to molecular-targeted regimen as single-agent treatment are largely insignificant and additional randomized clinical trials are necessary, probably with a combination of currently available treatments and an exploration for elements influencing molecular targeted drug sensitivity.

7. Conclusion

- Management of endometrial cancer is challenging.
- Endometrial cancer is primarily treated with surgical staging.
- Comprehensive surgical staging for endometrial cancer is recommended (total hysterectomy, bilateral salpingooophorectomy, peritoneal cytology, intraoperative bilateral pelvic and para-aortic lymph node dissection). It allows accurate delineation of the extent of the disease and subsequently allows identifying patients who may benefit from adjuvant therapy.
- The extent of lymph node dissection (bilateral pelvic and/or para-aortic) in surgical staging of patients with endometrial cancer, regardless of FIGO staging, remains controversial.
- As opposed to laparotomy, conventional laparoscopy —whenever technically possible— should be considered as the recommended (primary) approach for comprehensive surgical staging in patients with endometrial cancer
- For patients with recurrent endometrial cancer, optimal cytoreduction (even if multiple) is associated with increased disease-progression survival.
- For patients with recurrent endometrial cancer and peritoneal metastasis, the role of hyperthemic intraperitoneal chemotherapy is still experimental. Despite initial promising results, additional studies are needed.
- For high-risk patients with endometrial cancer, adjuvant treatment (radiation therapy, chemotherapy, or both) is recommended, and appropriate selection of patients for adjuvant therapy is critical.
- For high-risk patients with endometrial cancer, adjuvant pelvic external beam radiation therapy is recommended over vaginal brachytherapy. Conversely, in low-risk patients with

endometrial cancer, adjuvant vaginal brachytherapy, and not external beam radiation therapy, should be primarily used (if deem necessary by treating physicans). Radiation therapy can improve disease-free survival.

- For high-risk patients with endometrial cancer, carboplatin—placitaxel adjuvant chemotherapeutic regimen is recommend over the standard doxorubicin—cisplatin (with or without placitaxel) chemotherapeutic regimen, due to its well-tolerated drug-related adverse effects and non-inferiority to the standard chemotherapeutic regimen. It is associated with improved disease-free survival.
- For high-risk patients with endometrial cancer, a combination therapy of radiation therapy and chemotherapy could probably decrease the disease progression and overall death.
- Hormonal therapy is not recommended, and its use should be restricted to clinical trials.
- Molecular-targeted therapy is not recommended, and its use should be restricted to clinical trials.
- Long-term follow-up of patients is necessary.
- Further randomized controlled clinical trials are needed.

Author details

Ahmed Abu-Zaid [1,2*] and Ismail A. Al-Badawi[1,2]

*Address all correspondence to: i_albadawi@yahoo.com

1 Department of Obstetrics and Gynecology, King Faisal Specialist Hospital and Research Center, Riyadh, Saudi Arabia

2 College of Medicine, Alfaisal University, Riyadh, Saudi Arabia

References

[1] International Agency for Research on Cancer. GLOBALCAN 2008: cancer incidence and mortality worldwide. Lyon, France: IARC Press; 2010.

[2] American Cancer Society. Cancer facts & figures 2012. Atlanta, GA: American Cancer Society; 2012.

[3] Sorosky JI. Endometrial cancer. Obstet Gynecol 2012;120:383–397.

[4] Lewin SN, Herzog TJ, Barrena Medel NI, et al. Comparative performance of the 2009 international Federation of gynecology and obstetrics' staging system for uterine corpus cancer. Obstet Gynecol 2010;116(5):1141–1149.

[5] Kao MS. Management of recurrent endometrial carcinoma. Chang Gung Med J 2004;27(9):639-645.

[6] Morrow CP, Bundy BN, Kurman RJ, et al. Relationship between surgical-pathological risk factors and outcome in clinical stage I and II carcinoma of the endometrium: a Gynecologic Oncology Group study. Gynecol Oncol 1991;40(1):55-65.

[7] Hirahatake K, Hareyama H, Sakuragi N, et al. A clinical and pathologic study on para-aortic lymph node metastasis in endometrial carcinoma. J Surg Oncol 1997;65(2):82-87.

[8] Siegel R, Naishadham D, Jemal A. Cancer statistics, 2013. CA Cancer J Clin 2013;63(1):11–30.

[9] Creasman WT, Morrow CP, Bundy BN et al. Surgical pathologic spread patterns of endometrial cancer. A Gynecologic Oncology Group Study. Cancer 1987;60 (8 Suppl.): 2035–2041.

[10] SGO Clinical Practice Endometrial Cancer Working Group, Burke WM, Orr J, et al. Endometrial cancer: A review and current management strategies: Part I. Gynecol Oncol 2014;134(2):385-392.

[11] Morneau M, Foster W, Lalancette M, et al. Adjuvant treatment for endometrial cancer: literature review and recommendations by the Comité de l'évolution des pratiques en oncologie (CEPO). Gynecol Oncol 2013;131(1):231-240.

[12] Dinkelspiel HE, Wright JD, Lewin SN, et al. Contemporary clinical management of endometrial cancer. Obstet Gynecol Int 2013;2013:583891.

[13] Childers JM, Brzechffa PR, Hatch KD, et al. Laparoscopically assisted surgical staging (LASS) of endometrial cancer. Gynecol Oncol 1993;51(1):33–38.

[14] Spirtos NM, Schlaerth JB, Spirtos TW, et al. Laparoscopic bilateral pelvic and paraaortic lymph node sampling: an evolving technique. Am J Obstet Gynecol 1995;173(1):105–111.

[15] Walker JL, Piedmonte MR, Spirtos NM, et al. Laparoscopy compared with laparotomy for comprehensive surgical staging of uterine cancer: Gynecologic Oncology Group Study LAP2. J Clin Oncol 2009;27(32):5331–5336.

[16] Kornblith AB, Huang HQ, Walker JL, et al. Quality of life of patients with endometrial cancer undergoing laparoscopic international federation of gynecology and obstetrics staging compared with laparotomy: a Gynecologic Oncology Group study. J Clin Oncol 2009;27(32):5337–5342.

[17] Palomba S, Falbo A, Russo T, et al. Updating of a recent meta-analysis of randomized controlled trials to assess the safety and the efficacy of the laparoscopic surgery for treating early stage endometrial cancer. Gynecol Oncol 2009;114(1):135–136.

[18] Walker JL, Piedmonte MR, Spirtos NM, et al. Recurrence and survival after random assignment to laparoscopy versus laparotomy for comprehensive surgical staging of uterine cancer: Gynecologic Oncology Group LAP2 Study. J Clin Oncol 2012;30(7): 695–700.

[19] Boggess JF, Gehrig PA, Cantrell L, et al. A comparative study of 3 surgical methods for hysterectomy with staging for endometrial cancer: robotic assistance, laparoscopy, laparotomy. Am J Obstet Gynecol 2008;199(4):360 [e1-9].

[20] Seamon LG, Cohn DE, Richardson DLet al. Robotic hysterectomy and pelvic-aortic lymphadenectomy for endometrial cancer. Obstet Gynecol 2008;112(6):1207–1213.

[21] Gehrig PA, Cantrell LA, Shafer A, et al. What is the optimal minimally invasive surgical procedure for endometrial cancer staging in the obese and morbidly obese woman? Gynecol Oncol 2008;111(1):41–45.

[22] Bell MC, Torgerson J, Seshadri-Kreaden U, et al. Comparison of outcomes and cost for endometrial cancer staging via traditional laparotomy, standard laparoscopy and robotic techniques. Gynecol Oncol 2008;111(3):407–411.

[23] Zivanovic O, Sonoda Y, Diaz JP, et al. The rate of port-sitemetastases after 2251 laparoscopic procedures in women with underlying malignant disease. Gynecol Oncol 2008;111(3):431–437.

[24] Martinez A, Querleu D, Leblanc E, et al. Low incidence of port-site metastases after laparoscopic staging of uterine cancer. Gynecol Oncol 2010;118(2):145–150.

[25] Benedetti Panici P, Basile S, Maneschi F, et al. Systematic pelvic lymphadenectomy vs. no lymphadenectomy in early-stage endometrial carcinoma: randomized clinical trial. J Natl Cancer Inst 2008;100(23):1707–1716.

[26] ASTEC study group, Kitchener H, Swart AM, et al. Efficacy of systematic pelvic lymphadenectomy in endometrial cancer (MRC ASTEC trial): a randomised study. Lancet 2009;373(9658):125–136.

[27] May K, Bryant A, Dickinson HO, et al. Lymphadenectomy for the management of endometrial cancer. Cochrane Database Syst Rev 2010;1:CD007585.

[28] Amant F, Mirza MR, Creutzberg CL. Cancer of the corpus uteri. Int J Gynaecol Obstet. 2012;119 Suppl 2:S110-117.

[29] Aalders JG, Thomas G. Endometrial cancer – revisiting the importance of pelvic and para aortic lymph nodes. Gynecol Oncol 2007;104(1):222–231.

[30] Mariani A, Dowdy SC, Cliby WA, et al. Prospective assessment of lymphatic dissemination in endometrial cancer: a paradigm shift in surgical staging. Gynecol Oncol 2008;109(1):11–18.

[31] Dowdy SC, Aletti G, Cliby WA, et al. Extra-peritoneal laparoscopic para-aortic lymphadenectomy—a prospective cohort study of 293 patients with endometrial cancer. Gynecol Oncol 2008;111(3):418–424.

[32] Bristow RE, Zahurak ML, Alexander CJ, Zellars RC, Montz FJ. FIGO stage IIIC endometrial carcinoma: resection of macroscopic nodal disease and other determinants of survival. Int J Gynecol Cancer 2003;13(5):664–672.

[33] Abu-Rustum NR, Gomez JD, Alektiar KM, et al. The incidence of isolated paraaortic nodalmetastasis in surgically staged endometrial cancer patients with negative pelvic lymph nodes. Gynecol Oncol 2009;115(2):236–238.

[34] Khoury-Collado F, Murray MP, Hensley ML, et al. Sentinel lymph node mapping for endometrial cancer improves the detection of metastatic disease to regional lymph nodes. Gynecol Oncol 2011;122(2):251–254.

[35] Abu-Rustum NR, Khoury-Collado F, Pandit-Taskar N, et al. Sentinel lymph node-mapping for grade 1 endometrial cancer: is it the answer to the surgical staging dilemma? Gynecol Oncol 2009;113(2):163–169.

[36] Aalders JG, Abeler V, Kolstad P. Recurrent adenocarcinoma of the endometrium: a clinical and histopathological study of 379 patients. Gynecol Oncol. 1984;17(1):85–103.

[37] Di Saia PJ, Creasman WT, Boronow RC, et al. Risk factors and recurrent patterns in Stage I endometrial cancer. Am J Obstet Gynecol. 1985;151(8):1009–1015.

[38] Sohaib SA, Houghton SL, Meroni R, et al. Recurrent endometrial cancer: patterns of recurrent disease and assessment of prognosis. Clin Radiol. 2007;62(1):28–34.

[39] Randall ME, Filliaci VL, Muss H, et al. Randomized phase III trial of whole abdominal irradiation versus doxorubicin and cisplatin chemotherapy in advanced endometrial carcinoma: a Gynecologic Oncology Group Study. J Clin Oncol 2006;24(1):36–44.

[40] Keys HM, Roberts JA, Bruneto VL, et al. A phase III trial of surgery with or without adjunctive external pelvic radiation therapy in intermediate risk endometrial adenocarcinoma: a Gynecologic Oncology Group Study. Gynecol Oncol 2004;92(3):744–751.

[41] Creutzberg CL, van Putten WL, Koper PC, et al. PORTEC Study Group. Survival after relapse in patients with endometrial cancer: results from a randomized trial. Gynecol Oncol 2003;89(2):201–209.

[42] Obel JC, Friberg G, Fleming GF. Chemotherapy in endometrial cancer. Clin Adv Hematol Oncol 2006;4(6):459-468.

[43] Bakrin N, Cotte E, Sayag-Beaujard A, et al. Cytoreductive surgery with hyperthermic intraperitoneal chemotherapy for the treatment of recurrent endometrial carcinoma confined to the peritoneal cavity. Int J Gynecol Cancer 2010;20(5):809-814.

[44] Bristow RE, Santillan A, Zahurak ML, et al. Salvage cytoreductive surgery for recurrent endometrial cancer. Gynecol Oncol 2006;103(1):281-287.

[45] Awtrey CS, Cadungog MG, Leitao MM, et al. Surgical resection of recurrent endometrial carcinoma. Gynecol Oncol 2006;102(3):480-488.

[46] Barlin JN, Puri I, Bristow RE. Cytoreductive surgery for advanced or recurrent endometrial cancer: a meta-analysis. Gynecol Oncol 2010;118(1):14-18.

[47] Elias D, Gilly F, Quenet F, et al. Pseudomyxoma peritonei: a French multicentric study of 301 patients treated with cytoreductive surgery and intraperitoneal chemotherapy. Eur J Surg Oncol 2010;36(5):456–462.

[48] Sugarbaker PH. Peritoneal surface oncology: review of a personal experience with colorectal and appendiceal malignancy. Tech Coloproctol 2005;9(2):95–103.

[49] Yonemura Y, Endou Y, Shinbo M, et al. Safety and efficacy of bidirectional chemotherapy for treatment of patients with peritoneal dissemination from gastric cancer: selection for cytoreductive surgery. J Surg Oncol 2009;100(4):311–316.

[50] Cotte E, Glehen O, Mohamed F, et al. Cytoreductive surgery and intraperitoneal chemo-hyperthermia for chemo-resistant and recurrent advanced epithelial ovarian cancer: prospective study of 81 patients. World J Surg 2007;31(9):1813-1820.

[51] Abu-Zaid A, Azzam AZ, AlOmar O, et al. Cytoreductive surgery and hyperthermic intraperitoneal chemotherapy for managing peritoneal carcinomatosis from endometrial carcinoma: a single-center experience of 6 cases. Ann Saudi Med 2014;34(2): 159-166.

[52] Jérôme D, Mariangela D, Mélanie F, et al. Cytoreductive surgery with hyperthermic intraperitoneal chemotherapy for the treatment of endometrial cancerwith peritoneal carcinomatosis. Eur J Obstet Gynecol Reprod Biol 2014;172:111-114.

[53] Witkamp AJ, de Bree E, Van Goethem R, et al. Rationale and techniques of intra-operative hyperthermic intraperitoneal chemotherapy. Cancer Treat Rev. 2001;27(6): 365-374.

[54] Mohamed F, Marchettini P, Stuart OA, et al. Thermal enhancement of new chemotherapeutic agents at moderate hyperthermia. Ann Surg Oncol 2003;10(4):463-468.

[55] Scarabelli C, Campagnutta E, Giorda G, et al. Maximal cytoreductive surgery as a reasonable therapeutic alternative for recurrent endometrial carcinoma. Gynecol Oncol 1998 Jul;70(1):90-93.

[56] Glehen O, Mithieux F, Osinsky D, et al. Surgery combined with peritonectomy procedures and intraperitoneal chemohyperthermia in abdominal cancers with peritoneal carcinomatosis: a phase II study. J Clin Oncol 2003;21(5):799-806.

[57] Glehen O, Beaujard AC, Arvieux C, et al. Peritoneal carcinomatosis. Surgical treatment, peritonectomy and intraperitoneal chemohyperthermia (In French). Gastroenterol Clin Biol 2002;26(3):210-215.

[58] Rietbroek RC, van de Vaart PJ, Haveman J, et al. Hyperthermia enhances the cytotoxicity and platinum-DNA adduct formation of lobaplatin and oxaliplatin in cultured SW 1573 cells. J Cancer Res Clin Oncol 1997;123(1):6-12.

[59] Herman TS, Henle KJ, Nagle WA, et al. Effect of step-down heating on the cytotoxicity of adriamycin, bleomycin, and cis-diamminedichloroplatinum. Cancer Res 1984;44(5):1823-1826.

[60] Teicher BA, Kowal CD, Kennedy KA, et al. Enhancement by hyperthermia of the in vitro cytotoxicity of mitomycin C toward hypoxic tumor cells. Cancer Res 1981;41(3): 1096-1099.

[61] Glehen O, Gilly FN, Boutitie F, et al. Toward curative treatment of peritoneal carcinomatosis from nonovarian origin by cytoreductive surgery combined with perioperative intraperitoneal chemotherapy: a multi-institutional study of 1290 patients. Cancer 2010;116(24):5608–5618.

[62] Chua TC, Yan TD, Saxena A, et al. Should the treatment of peritoneal carcinomatosis by cytoreductive surgery and hyperthermic intraperitoneal chemotherapy still be regarded as a highly morbid procedure?: a systematic review of morbidity and mortality. Ann Surg 2009;249(6):900–907.

[63] Sorbe B, Horvath G, Andersson H, et al. External pelvic and vaginal irradiation versus vaginal irradiation alone as postoperative therapy in medium-risk endometrial carcinoma — a prospective randomized study. Int J Radiat Oncol Biol Phys 2012;82(3):1249–1255.

[64] Blake P, Swart AM, Orton J, et al. Adjuvant external beam radiotherapy in the treatment of endometrial cancer (MRC ASTEC and NCIC CTG EN.5 randomised trials): pooled trial results, systematic review, and metaanalysis. Lancet 2009;373(9658):137–146.

[65] Creutzberg CL, van Putten WL, Koper PC, et al. Surgery and postoperative radiotherapy versus surgery alone for patients with stage-1 endometrial carcinoma: multicentre randomised trial. PORTEC Study Group. Post Operative Radiation Therapy in Endometrial Carcinoma. Lancet 2000;355(9213):1404–1411.

[66] Creutzberg CL, van Putten WL, Koper PC, et al. The morbidity of treatment for patients with Stage I endometrial cancer: results from a randomized trial. Int J Radiat Oncol Biol Phys 2001;51(5):1246–1255.

[67] Scholten AN, van PuttenWL, Beerman H, et al. Postoperative radiotherapy for Stage 1 endometrial carcinoma: long-term outcome of the randomized PORTEC trial with central pathology review. Int J Radiat Oncol Biol Phys 2005;63(3):834–838.

[68] Nout RA, van de Poll-Franse LV, Lybeert ML, et al. Long-term outcome and quality of life of patients with endometrial carcinoma treatedwith orwithout pelvic radiotherapy in the post operative radiation therapy in endometrial carcinoma 1 (PORTEC-1) trial. J Clin Oncol 2011;29(13):1692–1700.

[69] Lindemann K, Onsrud M, Kristensen G, et al. Survival after radiation therapy for early-stage endometrial carcinoma: the Oslo study revisited after up to 43 years of follow-up. J Clin Oncol 2012;30 (Suppl.): abstr 5008.

[70] Johnson N, Cornes P. Survival and recurrent disease after postoperative radiotherapy for early endometrial cancer: systematic review and meta-analysis. BJOG 2007;114(11):1313–1320.

[71] Kong A, Johnson N, Kitchener HC, et al. Adjuvant radiotherapy for stage I endometrial cancer. Cochrane Database Syst Rev 2012;3:CD003916.

[72] Sorbe B, Nordstrom B, Maenpaa J, et al. Intravaginal brachytherapy in FIGO stage I low-risk endometrial cancer: a controlled randomized study. Int J Gynecol Cancer 2009;19(5):873–878.

[73] Nout RA, Smit VT, Putter H, et al. Vaginal brachytherapy versus pelvic external beam radiotherapy for patients with endometrial cancer of high-intermediate risk (PORTEC-2): an open-label, non-inferiority, randomised trial. Lancet 2010;375(9717): 816–823.

[74] Nout RA, Putter H, Jurgenliemk-Schulz IM, et al. Quality of life after pelvic radiotherapy or vaginal brachytherapy for endometrial cancer: first results of the randomized PORTEC-2 trial. J Clin Oncol 2009;27(21):3547–3556.

[75] Susumu N, Sagae S, Udagawa Y, et al. Randomized phase III trial of pelvic radiotherapy versus cisplatin-based combined chemotherapy in patients with intermediate- and high-risk endometrial cancer: a Japanese Gynecologic Oncology Group study. Gynecol Oncol 2008;108(1):226–233.

[76] Maggi R, Lissoni A, Spina F, et al. Adjuvant chemotherapy vs radiotherapy in high-risk endometrial carcinoma: results of a randomised trial. Br J Cancer 2006;95(3):266–271.

[77] Hogberg T, SignorelliM, de Oliveira CF, et al. Sequential adjuvant chemotherapy and radiotherapy in endometrial cancer–results from two randomised studies. Eur J Cancer 2010;46(13):2422–2431.

[78] Kuoppala T, Maenpaa J, Tomas E, et al. Surgically staged high-risk endometrial cancer: randomized study of adjuvant radiotherapy alone vs. sequential chemo-radiotherapy. Gynecol Oncol 2008;110(2):190–195.

[79] Morrow CP, Bundy BN, Homesley HD, et al. Doxorubicin as an adjuvant following surgery and radiation therapy in patients with high-risk endometrial carcinoma, stage I and occult stage II: a Gynecologic Oncology Group Study. Gynecol Oncol 1990;36(2):166–171.

[80] Johnson N, Bryant A, Miles T, et al. Adjuvant chemotherapy for endometrial cancer after hysterectomy. Cochrane Database Syst Rev 2011;10:CD003175.

[81] Fujimura H, Kikkawa F, Oguchi Het al. Adjuvant chemotherapy including cisplatin in endometrial carcinoma. Gynecol Obstet Invest 2000;50(2): 127–132.

[82] Homesley HD, Filiaci V, Gibbons SK, et al. A randomized phase III trial in advanced endometrial carcinoma of surgery and volume directed radiation followed by cisplatin and doxorubicin with or without paclitaxel: a Gynecologic Oncology Group study. Gynecol Oncol 2009;112(3):543–552.

[83] Miller D, Filiaci V, Fleming G, et al. Late-breaking abstract 1: randomized phase III noninferiority trial of first line chemotherapy for metastatic or recurrent endometrial carcinoma: a Gynecologic Oncology Group Study. Gynecol Oncol 2012;125(3):771.

[84] Despierre E, Moerman P, Vergote I, et al. Is there a role for neoadjuvant chemotherapy in the treatment of stage IV serous endometrial carcinoma? Int J Gynecol Cancer 2006;16(Suppl 1):273–277.

[85] Vandenput I, Moerman Ph, Leunen K, et al. Neoadjuvant chemotherapy followed by interval debulking surgery for stage IV uterine papillary serous carcinoma: an interim analysis. 2009 Oral Abstract IGCS Bangkok.

[86] Lee WL, Lee FK, Su WH, et al. Hormone therapy for younger patients with endometrial cancer. Taiwan J Obstet Gynecol 2012;51:495-505.

[87] Lee WL, Yen MS, Chao KC, et al. Hormone therapy for patients with advanced or recurrent endometrial cancer. J Chin Med Assoc 2014;77(5):221-226.

[88] Tsikouras P, Bouchlariotou S, Vrachnis N, et al. Endometrial cancer: molecular and therapeutic aspects. Eur J Obstet Gynecol Reprod Biol 2013;169(1):1-9.

[89] Decruze SB, Green JA. Hormone therapy in advanced and recurrent endometrial cancer: a systematic review. Int J Gynecol Cancer 2007;17:964–978.

[90] Carlson MJ, Thiel KW, Leslie KK. Past, present, and future of hormonal therapy in recurrent endometrial cancer. Int J Womens Health. 2014;6:429-435.

[91] Lee WL, Tsui KH, Seow KM, et al. Hormone therapy for postmenopausal women-dAn unanswered issue. Gynecol Minim Invasive Ther 2013;2:13-17.

[92] Cheng MH, Wang PH. Uterine myoma: a condition amenable to medical therapy? Expert Opin Emerg Drugs 2008;13:119-133.

[93] Martin-Hirsch PL, Lilford RJ, Jarvis GJ. Adjuvant progestagen therapy for the treatment of endometrial cancer: review and meta-analyses of published randomised controlled trials. Eur J Obstet Gynecol Reprod Biol 1996;65(2):201–207.

[94] COSA-NZ-UK Endometrial Cancer Study Groups. Adjuvant medroxyprogesterone acetate in high-risk endometrial cancer. Int J Gynecol Cancer 1998;8(5):387–391.

[95] Martin-Hirsch PP, Bryant A, Keep SL, et al. Adjuvant progestagens for endometrial cancer. Cochrane Database Syst Rev 2011;6:CD001040.

[96] Mountzios G, Pectasides D, Bournakis E, et al. Developments in the systemic treatment of endometrial cancer. Crit Rev Oncol Hematol 2011;79:278-292.

[97] Tsui KH, Wang PH, Chen CK, et al. Nonclassical estrogen receptors action on human dermal fibroblasts. Taiwan J Obstet Gynecol 2011;50:474-478.

[98] Thigpen T, Brady MF, Homesley HD, et al. Tamoxifen in the treatment of advanced or recurrent endometrial carcinoma: a Gynecologic Oncology Group Study. J Clin Oncol 2001;19:364-367.

[99] McMeekin DS, Gordon A, Fowler J, et al. A phase II trial of arzoxifene, a selective estrogen response modulator, in patients with recurrent or advanced endometrial cancer. Gynecol Oncol 2003;90:64-69.

[100] Burke TW, Walker CL. Arzoxifene as therapy for endometrial cancer. Gynecol Oncol 2003;90(2 Pt 2):S40–S46.

[101] Rendina GM, Donadio C, Fabri M, et al. Tamoxifen and medroxyprogesterone therapy for advanced endometrial carcinoma. Eur J Obstet Gynecol Reprod Biol 1984;17:285-291.

[102] Pandya KJ, Yeap BY, Weiner LM, et al. Megestrol and tamoxifen in patients with advanced endometrial cancer: an Eastern Cooperative Oncology Group Study (E4882). Am J Clin Oncol 2001;24:43-46.

[103] Whitney CW, Brunetto VL, Zaino RJ, et al. Phase II study of medroxyprogesterone acetate plus tamoxifen in advanced endometrial carcinoma: a Gynecologic Oncology Group study. Gynecol Oncol 2004;92:4-9.

[104] Gallagher CJ, Oliver RT, Oram DH, et al. A new treatment for endometrial cancer with gonadotropin releasing-hormone analogue. Br J Obstet Gynaecol 1991;98:1037-1041.

[105] Jeyarajah AR, Gallagher CJ, Blake PR, et al. Long-term follow-up of gonadotrophin-releasing hormone analog treatment for recurrent endometrial cancer. Gynecol Oncol 1996;63:47-52.

[106] Asbury RF, Brunetto VL, Lee RB, et al. Gynecologic Oncology Group. Goserelin acetate as treatment for recurrent endometrial carcinoma: a Gynecologic Oncology Group study. Am J Clin Oncol 2002;25:557-560.

[107] Rose PG, Brunetto VL, VanLe L, et al. A phase II trial of anastrozole in advanced recurrent or persistent endometrial carcinoma: a Gynecologic Oncology Group study. Gynecol Oncol 2000;78:212-216.

[108] Ma BB, Oza A, Eisenhauer E, et al. The activity of letrozole in patients with advanced or recurrent endometrial cancer and correlation with biological markersda study of the National Cancer Institute of Canada Clinical Trials Group. Int J Gynecol Cancer 2004;14:650-658.

[109] Nogami Y, Banno K, Kisu I, et al. Current status of molecular-targeted drugs for endometrial cancer (Review). Mol Clin Oncol 2013; 1(5):799-804.

[110] Zagouri F, Bozas G, Kafantari E, et al. Endometrial cancer: what is new in adjuvant and molecularly targeted therapy? Obstet Gynecol Int 2010;2010:749579

[111] Oza AM, Elit L, Biagi J, et al. Molecular correlates associated with a phase II study of temsirolimus (CCI-779) in patients with metastatic or recurrent endometrial cancer-NCIC IND 160. J Clin Oncol 2006;24:e3003.

[112] Oza AM, Elit L, Provencher D, et al. A phase II study of temsirolimus (CCI-779) in patients with metastatic and/or locally advanced recurrent endometrial cancer previously treated with chemotherapy: NCIC CTG IND 160 b. J Clin Oncol 2008;26:e5516

[113] Colombo N, McMeekin S, Schwartz P, et al. A phase II trial of the mTOR inhibitor AP23573 as a single agent in advanced endometrial cancer. J Clin Oncol 2007;25: e5516.

[114] Slomovitz BM, Lu KH, Johnston T, et al. A phase 2 study of the oral mammalian target of rapamycin inhibitor, everolimus, in patients with recurrent endometrial carcinoma. Cancer 2010;116(23):5415-5419.

[115] Jasas KV, Fyles A, Elit L, et al. Phase II study of erlotinib (OSI 774) in women with recurrent or metastatic endometrial cancer: NCIC CTG IND 1. J Clin Oncol 2004; 22:e5019.

[116] Leslie KK, Sill MW, Darcy KM, et al. Efficacy and safety of gefitinib and potential prognostic value of soluble EGFR, EGFR mutations, and tumor markers in a Gynecologic Oncology Group phase II trial of persistent or recurrent endometrial cancer. J Clin Oncol 2009;27:e16542.

[117] Konecny GE, Santos L, Winterhoff B, et al. HER2 gene amplification and EGFR expression in a large cohort of surgically staged patients with nonendometrioid (type II) endometrial cancer. Br J Cancer 2009;100(1):89–95.

[118] Grushko TA, Filiaci VL, Mundt AJ, et al. An exploratory analysis of HER-2 amplification and overexpression in advanced endometrial carcinoma: a gynecologic oncology group study. Gynecol Oncol. 2008;108(1):3–9.

[119] Hye SC, Hu W, Kavanagh JJ. Targeted therapies in gynecologic cancers. Curr Cancer Drug Targets 2006;6(4):333–363.

[120] Fleming GF, Sill MW, Darcy KM, et al. Phase II trial of trastuzumab in women with advanced or recurrent, HER2-positive trastuzumab in women with advanced or recurrent, HER2-positive endometrial carcinoma: a Gynecologic Oncology Group study. Gynecol Oncol 2010;116:15-20.

[121] Kamat AA, Merritt WM, Coffey D, et al. Clinical and biological significance of vascular endothelial growth factor in endometrial cancer. Clin Cancer Res 2007;13: 7487-7495.

[122] Aghajanian C, Sill MW, Darcy KM, et al. Phase II trial of bevacizumab in recurrent or persistent endometrial cancer: a Gynecologic Oncology Group study. J Clin Oncol 2011;9: 2259-2265.

[123] Wright JD, Powell MA, Rader JS, Mutch DG, Gibb RK. Bevacizumab therapy in patients with recurrent uterine neoplasms. Anticancer Res 2007;27(5):3525–3528.

[124] Coleman RL, Sill MW, Lankes HA, et al. A phase II evaluation of aflibercept in the treatment of recurrent or persistent endometrial cancer: a Gynecologic Oncology Group study. Gynecol Oncol 2012; 127: 538-543.

[125] McMeekin DS, Sill MW, Benbrook D, et al. A phase II trial of thalidomide in patients with refractory endometrial cancer and correlation with angiogenesis biomarkers: a Gynecologic Oncology Group study. Gynecol Oncol 2007;105: 508-516.

Chapter 9

Endometrial Cancer Prevention with Levonorgestrel-Releasing Intrauterine System

Dirk Wildemeersch, Maciej Jóźwik and Marcin Jóźwik

Additional information is available at the end of the chapter

http://dx.doi.org/10.5772/59211

1. Introduction

Endometrial cancer is a potentially preventable disease but still many new cases occur each year. In the USA, the incidence of endometrial cancer has increased by more than 30% over the past 20 years. [1] Globally, about 4% of all cancers in women are endometrial cancers that occur predominantly in postmenopausal women, although many are now also diagnosed in younger women. [2] It is the leading gynecological malignancy with approximately 47,130 women diagnosed in 2012 in the USA. [3] Endometrial cancer is often diagnosed at an early stage due to abnormal vaginal bleeding which occurs as a prominent clinical feature in most women. Two types of endometrial cancer can be distinguished. Type 1, occurring in approximately 80% of women, carries a better prognosis, has predominantly endometrioid histology and is well or moderately differentiated (grading G1-G2), and Type 2 includes worse prognosis, poorly differentiated (grade G3) carcinomas, like serous and clear cell carcinomas. [4] The epidemiology of Type 1 endometrial cancer is fairly well understood: 1) prolonged unopposed estrogen exposure is the endocrine background of this hormonally regulated neoplasm; 2) hereditary factors are associated with an increased risk and high parity and later age at last birth are protective [5, 6]; 3) the role of obesity as an important risk factor is well established; 4) combined oral contraceptives are protective, whereas 5) hormone replacement therapy (HRT) in the menopause is an important risk factor and the risk increases markedly with the use of estrogen only and sequential HRT. Understanding the causative role of these conditions constitutes the basis for prevention strategies. The rising obesity epidemic and decreased fertility are likely to result in a higher incidence of endometrial cancer and may become an important public health problem globally in the coming years. This communication will focus on the risk groups and will formulate some strategies for the prevention of cancer of the endometrium in women at increased risk.

2. Risk factors for endometrial cancer

2.1. Hormone replacement therapy

The primary role of progestin in postmenopausal estrogen therapy is endometrial protection to prevent hyperplasia. [7] Prior to the widespread use of combined estrogen-progestin therapy (EPT), the risk of developing hyperplasia due to unopposed estrogen stimulation was substantial. Endometrial hyperplasia in postmenopausal women with an intact uterus, treated with unopposed oral estrogen, was found in 20% of women during the first year and in 62% after 3 years of estrogen therapy (ET). [8] In support of this finding, in the Postmenoapausal Estrogen/Progestin Intervention Trial, 62% of women who received only estrogen (0.625 mg of conjugated equine estrogen orally daily) developed endometrial hyperplasia. One third of these women had complex hyperplasia with or without atypia. [9] Hyperplasia is characterized by a proliferation of the endometrial glands. In non-atypical hyperplasia, the glands are outgrown yet normal, but in atypical hyperplasia glandular abnormality is already present both structurally and at cellular level. [10] Non-atypical hyperplasia rarely progresses to more severe conditions. Atypical adenomatous hyperplasia, on the other hand, has been observed to progress to adenocarcinoma of the uterus in 29% of cases. [11]

Progestins should, therefore, be added to ET in all postmenopausal women with an intact uterus. Since the mid-1980s, EPT has increasingly been prescribed. The North American Menopause Society reviewed the types of EPT regimen used in the USA and concluded that standard regimens provide adequate endometrial protection. [7] A Cochrane review devoted to this subject also came to the conclusion that the addition of an oral progestin to ET, administered either continuous cyclic or continuous combined, is associated with reduced rates of hyperplasia. [12] An important drawback of postmenopausal EPT is the occurrence of withdrawal or breakthrough bleedings. Withdrawal uterine bleedings occur in 80% of women using cyclic EPT. Continuous combined regimens avoid withdrawal bleeding, but breakthrough bleeding has been observed in up to 40% of women during the first 6 months. Most postmenopausal women dislike breakthrough bleedings and this is the most common reason for discontinuation and non-adherence to the treatment regimen. With EPT, therefore, irregular bleeding should be kept to a minimum. Depending on the EPT type, dose and route of administration, progestins may have adverse effects on the cardiovascular system, coagulation and breast tissue. The Women's Health Initiative (WHI) reported an increased risk for heart disease, stroke and breast cancer. [13] Since these adverse effects were not observed with ET alone, it is speculated that adding progestins may diminish the beneficial effects on atherosclerosis, vasodilatation and plasma lipids and may contribute to the increased risk of breast cancer. Indeed, the WHI study suggests that EPT may stimulate breast cancer growth and hinder breast cancer diagnosis due to increased mammographic density when a progestin is added to ET. [14, 15] This was confirmed in the Million Women Study and other studies, in particular a Swedish cohort study. [16, 17, 18]

Intrauterine-administered progestin, such as levonorgestrel (LNG), delivered directly to the target cells of the endometrium, has a profound suppressive effect on endometrial growth rendering the endometrium inactive and simultaneously eliminating uterine bleeding. [19,

http://dx.doi.org/10.5772/59211

20] Pharmacokinetic studies with an intrauterine system (IUS) releasing 20 μg of LNG/day (Mirena®; Bayer AG, Germany) have shown substantially lower plasma LNG concentrations than those seen with a subdermal LNG implant (Norplant®; Pfizer Pharmaceuticals Inc, USA), the combined oral contraceptive pill and the mini-pill; moreover, unlike with oral contraceptives, LNG levels with the Mirena LNG-IUS do not display peaks and troughs. [21] This is important because the low plasma levels may have a significantly lower impact on organs and tissues, such as the breast, coagulation system, and cardiovascular system.

Studies conducted by us and by others using continuous combined estrogen plus low-dose LNG-IUS after 5 years of use in postmenopausal women, provided data on the endometrial morphology to verify endometrial safety. The main objective of these studies was to evaluate an alternative route of progestin administration in postmenopausal women using ET. They suggest that continuous combined ET with intrauterine delivery of a progestin was highly accepted by the participating women. The rationale of the development of LNG-IUSs specifically for postmenopausal women is to minimize the potential adverse systemic effects. As progestins are required only to oppose the stimulating effects of estrogens on the endometrium, locally acting progestins, by definition, could avoid these unwanted metabolic effects. Intrauterine LNG delivery with low-dose systems, even though minimal absorption may occur, should be regarded as essentially locally acting. This regimen also offers important additional benefits that could be exploited, such as high adherence to treatment and a low discontinuation rate because of bleeding problems and progestin-like side effects. In addition, a LNG-IUS that adapts to the decreasing dimensions of the uterus gradually reduced in size due to the suppressive effect of LNG and the decreasing levels of endogenous estrogen, will be optimally tolerated by the women. [22, 23]

2.2. Polycystic ovary syndrome

Women with polycystic ovary syndrome (PCOS) are about three times more likely to develop endometrial cancer compared with women without this condition. [24] PCOS affects approximately 5 to 10% of women of reproductive age. The disorder is characterized by a disruption of normal reproductive physiology and should be diagnosed in women with oligomenorrhea or amenoorrhea, hyperandrogenemia and polycystic ovaries defined by ultrasonography after exclusion of medical conditions that cause irregular menstrual cycles and androgen excess. [25] Women with PCOS have a higher prevalence of obesity, impaired glucose tolerance and type 2 diabetes. They are at risk of cardiovascular disease and often have features of metabolic syndrome, including hypertension, dyslipidemia, visceral obesity and insulin resistence. [26] Women with PCOS should, therefore, be screened for type 2 diabetes and for cardiovascular risk by fasting glucose followed by a glucose tolerance test, BMI, fasting lipid and lipoprotein levels, and other metabolic syndrome risk factors. The condition that makes PCOS patients vulnerable to endometrial cancer is chronic anovulation as prolonged exposure to unopposed estrogen can lead to endometrial hyperplasia and cancer. It is important to identify individuals at risk at an early stage.

From 2 to 14% of patients diagnosed with endometrial cancer are women younger than 40 and the diagnosis is typically associated with the detection of an accompanying hyperestrogenic state. [25] According to studies in the United States, an estimated prevalence in very young women is 0.8%. [27, 28] A comprehensive review of PCOS was published by the American College of Obstetricians and Gynecologists. [29] Of note, PCOS can occur both in normal weight and overweight women. Yet classically, the young woman with endometrial hyperplasia or cancer is obese and nulliparous but, recently, several studies found up to 50% of women with endometrial cancer to be slender and with regular menstrual cycles. The proportion of estrogen and progesterone receptor positivity is similar in both obese and slim patients. Such women should be evaluated for concurrent ovarian malignancy (see Lynch syndrome below) which occurs in some studies in approximately 10% of cases. Therefore, 3-D ultrasound and magnetic resonance imaging (MRI) can be valuable additions in the diagnosis and staging of these patients.

2.3. Excessive body mass: Overweight and obesity

Obesity has become a major public health problem on a global scale. Overweight and obesity are not only an established risk factor for cardiovascular disease and type 2 diabetes; they are also an important risk factor for the development of endometrial cancer. [30] Renehan at al. found that each increase in BMI of 5 kg/m^2 significantly increased a woman's risk for the development of endometrial cancer. [31] Estrogen is a known endometrial growth factor in these women. The excess estrogens originate mostly from the conversion of androstenedione to estrone and testosterone to estradiol by peripheral adipose tissue. [32] Consequently, in obese postmenopausal women, adipose tissue becomes the primary source of circulating estrogen. Concentrations of estrogens in the adipose tissue have been measured at levels several-fold above that observed in plasma. Also, higher levels of insulin in obese women contribute to the increased risk for endometrial cancer as insulin demonstrates mitotic and antiapoptotic activity. Furthermore, serum sex hormone-binding globulin (SHBG) levels decrease with increasing adiposity, thus rising the fraction of circulating unbound estrogen.

The relationship between obesity and endometrial cancer has been well studied and has been acknowledged as a risk factor in women over 30 years of age. A strong association between early age at diagnosis and Type 1 endometrial cancer was found. The relationship was linear, suggesting that as obesity becomes more severe, the underlying carcinogenic mechanisms are more vividly activated. [4] There is limited public knowledge of the relationship between obesity and cancer risk. Making the data available to overweight and obese women could be useful to inform them about the risks which could affect their lives at an early age, and about the steps they could undertake to reduce or eliminate this risk, since prevention and other risk reduction strategies in the obese/overweight female population are possible with a high degree of success.

2.4. Lynch syndrome

Lynch syndrome is one of the most common cancer predisposition syndromes estimated to affect as many as 1 in 370 individuals. [33, 34] Often called hereditary nonpolyposis colorectal cancer it is an inherited disorder that increases the risk of many types of cancer, particularly

http://dx.doi.org/10.5772/59211

cancers of the colon and rectum, which are collectively referred to as colorectal cancer. Individuals with Lynch syndrome also have an increased risk for cancers of the stomach, small intestine, liver, gallbladder ducts, upper urinary tract, brain, and skin. Additionally, women with this disorder have a high risk for cancer of the ovaries and endometrium. Patients with Lynch syndrome may occasionally have noncancerous polyps in the colon. For many women with Lynch syndrome, the risk for endometrial cancer is comparable or even exceeds their risk for colorectal cancer. In the United States, about 140,000 new cases of colorectal cancer are diagnosed each year. Approximately 3 to 5 percent of these cancers are caused by Lynch syndrome. Estimates suggest that as many as 1 in 10 young age (< 50) endometrial cancers are associated with Lynch syndrome. Broader knowledge of population carrier frequency for DNA mismatch repair gene mutations could contribute to the understanding of the burden of cancer due to genetic susceptibility, but robust prevalence estimates are lacking. The lifetime endometrial cancer risk is between 27% and 71% which exceeds that of colorectal cancer. Mean age of occurrence is approximately 50 years (62 years in non-Lynch) and 18% are diagnosed under the age of 40 years. Practical guidelines for Lynch syndrome and early detection can be found via website: http://ghr.nlm.nih.gov/condition/lynch-syndrome. We are of opinion that women diagnosed with Lynch syndrome should be counseled on and consider the prophylactic long-term use of a LNG-IUS in relation to their increased endometrial cancer risk.

2.5. Tamoxifen adjuvant treatment for breast cancer

The long-term recurrence and mortality rates of breast cancer have been substantially reduced due to adjuvant treatment with tamoxifen. Tamoxifen is a selective estrogen receptor modulator (see Table 1) which exerts an anti-estrogenic effect on mammary tissue. [35] However, it also induces endometrial proliferation and women using tamoxifen harbor significantly more endometrial polyps than other women of which up to 36% could have hyperplasia or cancer. [36] The prophylactic use of LNG-IUS in women with breast cancer treated with tamoxifen is still controversial as the effect of the progestin released from the device on breast cancer recurrence remains uncertain notwithstanding the significantly reduced incidence of endometrial polyps. [37] Nonetheless, in the future, this situation could be clarified by the advent of an intrauterine system impregnated with a selective progesterone receptor modulator (SPRM; see Table 2) that would demonstrate powerful progestin action on the endometrium without any stimulatory, if not purely inhibitory, properties with regards to hormonally sensitive breast glandular tissue.

Compound	Commercial name(s)	Principal indication(s)
Clomiphene	Clomid, Clomifen	Ovulation induction
Tamoxifen	Tamoxiphene, Nolvadex	Breast cancer
Raloxifene	Evista	Breast cancer, osteoporosis
DT56a	Femarelle, Tofupill	Menopause, osteoporosis

Table 1. Examples of selective estrogen receptor modulators, or SERMs, for the use in the clinical setting.

Compound	Commercial names	Principal indications
Ulipristal	Ella, ellaOne, Esmya	Emergency contraception, uterine leiomyomas
Asoprisnil (J867)	Investigational - no commercial name given	Uterine leiomyomas, endometriosis
Telapristone (CDB-4124)	Investigational - bears names: Progenta, Proellex	Uterine leiomyomas, endometriosis

Table 2. Examples of selective progesterone receptor modulators, or SPRMs, for the use in the clinical setting.

3. Biology of progesterone and progestins

The endometrium is highly sensitive to sex steroid hormones. Estrogens cause endometrial proliferation and progesterone inhibits this growth by converting the endometrium to its secretory stage to prepare the uterus for implantation. In relation to endometrial protection, progesterone is the key inhibitor of carcinogenesis. The balance between the estrogen and progesterone activity during the menstrual cycle must be precisely maintained as an increase in the estrogen activity and/or a reduction in the antagonistic activity by progesterone will stimulate carcinogenesis. Estrogens act upon the endometrium through estrogen receptors (ERs), resulting in the induction of growth factors such as the epidermal growth factor, insulin-like growth factor-1 and growth-enhancing protooncogenes c-fos and c-myc. Besides these genomic effects of estrogens in the endometrium, estrogens exert nongenomic effects via activation of the PI3K/Akt prosurvival signaling pathway. Progesterone acts by binding to progesterone receptors (PRs), thus regulating multiple signaling pathways through PR-dependent transcriptional activity. In addition to ligand-mediated regulation, PR activity is also modulated by a variety of factors including microRNAs and epigenetic factors. [38] Despite their high degree of sequence identity, the PR isoforms maintain a number of unique biological functions, including: differences in transcriptional activity, ligand response, gene regulation, and tissue-specific physiological effects. [39] Unbeneficial role of some progestins is highlighted by the finding that medroxyprogesterone acetate, a widely used and quite powerful progestin, stimulates vascular thrombin receptor *in vitro,* thus being capable of triggering thromboembolic events. [40, 41]

4. Biology of progesterone receptor antagonists — Potentially stronger acting compounds?

Following the discovery of the antiprogestin mifepristone, hundreds of similar compounds have been synthesized, which can be grouped in a large family of PR ligands. This family includes pure agonists, such as progesterone itself and progestins, and, at the other end of the biological spectrum, pure progesterone antagonists (PAs). An intermediate position of the spectrum is occupied by SPRMs which demonstrate mixed agonist–antagonist properties. These compounds have numerous applications in healthcare of women.

Most PAs and SPRMs display direct antiproliferative effects in the endometrium when given orally, although with variable strength being compound- and dose-dependent. PAs can also be released using an IUS and induce endometrial atrophy in nonhuman primates. PAs and SPRMs have two important effects in primates: 1) they suppress endometrial growth by blocking the action of progesterone on endometrial progestational development and consequently induce amenorrhea; and 2) they suppress the proliferative effects of estrogen on endometrial proliferation and prevent unopposed action on this tissue. [42] These properties indicate the potential for clinical applications of these compounds which cover a broad field and are very promising in major public health areas. These include emergency contraception, long-term estrogen-free contraception (administered alone, or in association with a progestin-only pill to improve bleeding patterns), uterine leiomyomas (where they induce a marked reduction in tumor volume and produce amenorrhea) and endometriosis. Further developments might also include the treatment of hormone-dependent tumors. [43, 44]

5. Rationale for prevention using levonorgestrel-releasing intrauterine system

The first beneficial results with frameless FibroPlant® (Contrel Research, Ghent, Belgium) LNG-IUS in women with non-atypical and atypical endometrial hyperplasia were published in 2003. [45] Later, several reports followed using the framed Femilis® (Contrel Research) LNG-IUS and included two cases of endometrial carcinoma, all successfully managed. [46, 47] No failures occurred during follow-up for many years. The numbers were small but indicative of the extraordinary impact of LNG to suppress the hyperplastic and atypical endometrium.

The risk of developing cancer in women with atypical endometrial hyperplasia untreated for 20 years is between 8.6 and 42.5%. [48] In contrast, less than 5% of women with nonatypical endometrial hyperplasia will experience progression to carcinoma. The lower risk for women with nonatypical than atypical hyperplasia can assist in decision making for nonsurgical management of endometrial hyperplasia. The higher risks with atypical hyperplasia progressing to carcinoma warrant consideration of appropriate approaches as concurrent carcinoma among patients with atypical endometrial hyperplasia can range from 17 to 52% across studies. [49]

The standard treatment for endometrial hyperplasia with atypia or early stage (pT1a) adenocarcinoma of the endometrium is staging hysterectomy with bilateral oophorectomy. It is rather clear that for many young women who wish to preserve their fertility, such a decision is unacceptable. Studies using LNG-IUS releasing 20 μg of LNG/day indicate that successful treatment is possible especially when such potent progestins as LNG are administered. Intrauterine route of delivery appears much more effective than oral administration. [50, 51, 52] Successful treatment of early endometrial carcinoma has been reported with a 65 μg/day progesterone-releasing IUS, followed up to 36 months, yet, results of biopsies were negative only in 7 of 11 at 6 months and 6 of 8 at 12 months. [8] A significant reduction of the ERs and PRs expression observed during treatment with the LNG-IUS appears to be a marker for the strong antiproliferative effect of the hormone at the cellular level. Furthermore, as the treatment is continuous, compliance is not an issue.

The most common source of endogenous unopposed estrogen is chronic anovulation which can be accompanied by either continued ovarian secretion of estradiol or conversion of circulating androstenedione and testosterone to estrone and estradiol, respectively, by aromatase in the adipocytes. Chronic anovulation is a feature of PCOS and is also a condition occurring frequently in the perimenopause. In all these women, whether they have a hyperplastic condition due to exogenous or endogenous excess estrogen, direct delivery of LNG to the target cells of the endometrium using an intrauterine device will cause substantial histologic changes. The result is usually a very uniform suppression of the endometrium, regardless of the duration of treatment, the histologic picture being independent of the distance from the delivery system. [53] Intrauterine progestin delivery, particularly LNG, is therefore probably the most effective intervention in preventing endometrial proliferation because of the uniform suppression of the endometrium throughout the whole thickness of the mucosa caused by the high tissue concentrations of the locally applied hormone. With oral progestin therapy, a higher rate of residual hyperplasia, including complex and atypical hyperplasia, has been observed. [54] It has been demonstrated that the duration of the progestin administration is more important than the daily dose for prevention of endometrial hyperplasia. Again, continuous intrauterine progestin delivery seems optimal. [55]

Over the past 5 to 10 years many reports on the management of atypical endometrial hyperplasia and early cancer of the endometrium with LNG-IUS have been published. [56-63] Remissions were frequent, but also failures occurred. Some consider that at present there is no sufficient evidence because most studies were underpowered or contained a high proportion of patients lost to follow-up. [64] A meta-analysis and systematic review of the literature concludes that the available evidence suggests that treatment with oral or intrauterine progestin are of comparable effectiveness. The risk of progression during treatment is small, but longer follow-up is required. [65] As recently highlighted by Scarselli et al., who followed patients for over 15 years, LNG-IUS represents an option to treat hyperplasia and prevent endometrial carcinoma in at least 85% of patients. [66] Consistent with that study, in order to support stable regression over long periods of time, we recommend continued preventive LNG-IUS use on a life-long basis using a suitable LNG-IUS as the uterine cavity is often very small. Annual assessment of the endometrial thickness by ultrasound is probably sufficient unless vaginal bleeding occurs.

6. Concluding remarks — The future

Endometrial cancer is the fourth most common malignancy in women. Many women die each year of this potentially preventive disease. Uterine precancerous conditions and even early endometrioid cancer of the endometrium have a reasonably studied potential to respond to

http://dx.doi.org/10.5772/59211

hormonal therapy. A growing body of evidence suggests that progestin therapy by means of local long-acting release of a potent progestin can promote early endometrial tumor regression and long-term remission.

Conservative management with LNG-IUS of precancerous changes and early well differentiated endometrial cancer seems particularly promising in women who wish to preserve their fertility. It is emerging as an alternative to oral progestins as higher regression and lower hysterectomy rates for the treatment of complex and atypical hyperplasia are achieved with the device. LNG-IUS should, therefore, be the first-line primary prevention treatment. [67-75] However, conservative treatment carries an inherent oncologic risk as no correct staging is possible and the risk of missing a concurrent ovarian cancer cannot be neglected. Pre-treatment evaluation should include assessment for genetic conditions predisposing to cancer, such as Lynch syndrome. It is apparent that the ideal candidates for conservative cancer treatment are young women with grade 1, early stage endometrioid endometrial cancer (T1) with no detectable myometrial invasion who are highly motivated to maintain their reproductive potential and understand and are willing to accept the risk associated with deviation from the established standard of care. [59, 76] Progestins rather than progesterone should be considered the ultimate tumor suppressors as they powerfully promote differentiation, cell cycle arrest and apoptosis, and reduce inflammation and the invasion associated with metastasis. [37] Patients in whom the treatment fails should be evaluated by immunochemistry on endometrial biopsies as treatment failure is often caused by loss of PR expression. Clinical research is currently underway focusing on maintaining PR levels or identifying novel therapeutic approaches that restore PR expression in tumors from which it has been lost. [38, 77] Failure could also occur simply due to the downward displacement of the hormone-releasing IUS causing less impact on areas away from the IUS. Proper distribution of the hormone to the deeper layers of the endometrium seems essential to achieve maximum impact.

As the lifetime risk of endometrial cancer in anovulating obese women is 15% or more, one could assume that many of these cancers could be prevented using LNG-IUS. We support such an approach together with others who believe that it could be successful provided that suitable LNG-releasing intrauterine delivery systems are used. The latter is important as the uterine cavities in women of any age are often small and even become smaller with the use of LNG-IUS. Side effects such as displacement, embedment and expulsion are not rare, leading to early discontinuation. [78] Leslie at al. hope that the following will be possible in the future: "As a profession, we should ask ourselves if we can not only treat, but prevent a substantial proportion of endometrial cancers with more liberal use of progestin-containing IUDs?" [79]

Apart from the emerging role of LNG-IUS for endometrial cancer prevention, as reviewed recently by Jóźwik et al. [80], the future might lead us to even more effective hormone-releasing IUDs. It was proposed that local delivery of other drugs such as mifepristone or ulipristal, with their strong antiprogestin activity and antiestrogenic effect at the endometrial level, may be more suitable than LNG to act as tumor suppressor. No studies with intrauterine delivery of these agents have been conducted so far. However, one example is worth mentioning which indicates the potential of these compounds: A 48-year old nulliparous woman was consulted by one of the authors (DW) in 2007 for bleeding problems. It was known that she suffered from multiple uterine leiomyomas which tended to increase in size significantly over the past years. A pipelle biopsy revealed atypical hyperplasia. On MRI, the uterus was increased in size with several leiomyomas, the largest being of 65 mm in diameter. A frameless mifepristone-releasing IUS was inserted on 20 January 2007. The first follow-up was done one month later. At that time, the patient mentioned some spotting and a repeat biopsy showed residual focal atypical hyperplasia. Three months after insertion, breakthrough bleeding stopped completely, the diameter of the largest myoma was reduced to 33 mm and a histological specimen showed deficient endometrium without signs of atypia. All further follow-up examinations were uneventful with no abnormal bleeding. The patient was kept on this experimental mifepristone-releasing IUS for approximately 5 years. It was replaced by a LNG-IUS at the end of 2011 and, at annual check-ups, she has remained asymptomatic.

Finally, it is worth mentioning that several large epidemiological studies pointed out the potential of metformin as an anticancer drug. Metformin is an oral antidiabetic drug and is the first-line drug for the treatment of type 2 diabetes, in particular, in overweight and obese subjects with normal kidney function. It is used for the treatment of PCOS and has been investigated for other diseases where insulin resistance seems an important factor. Metformin acts by suppressing glucose production in the liver and has a vast safety track record. Preclinical and early clinical trials suggest a role for metformin in the prevention and treatment of cancer. Its potential is still unproven, but seems extremely promising. [81] Recently, a phase 2 study was designed in Australia combining LNG-IUS with oral metformin for the treatment of complex endometrial hyperplasia with atypia and grade 1 endometrial endometrioid adenocarcinoma. [82] Hopefully, this and other careful clinical studies will path a new approach to the prevention and treatment of early endometrial cancer.

Author details

Dirk Wildemeersch[1*], Maciej Jóźwik[2] and Marcin Jóźwik[3]

*Address all correspondence to: d.wildemeersch@skynet.be

1 Gynecological Outpatient Clinic and IUD Training Center, Ghent, Belgium

2 Department of Gynecology and Gynecologic Oncology, Medical University of Białystok, Białystok, Poland

3 Department of Gynecology and Obstetrics, Faculty of Medical Sciences, University of Varmia and Masuria, Olsztyn, Poland

Maciej Jóźwik and Marcin Jóźwik declare no conflict of interest. Dirk Wildemeersch is the developer of the frameless GyneFix® IUD, the frameless FibroPlant® LNG-IUS and the framed Femilis® LNG-IUS. He has also been involved in the development and optimization of new, innovative drug delivery systems for use in the uterus. Currently he acts as a trainer

http://dx.doi.org/10.5772/59211

in the insertion procedure of GyneFix® during training sessions organized by commercial companies distributing the product. He is also advisor in devising new concepts in controlled release for contraception and gynecological treatment, and receives financial compensation for these activities.

References

[1] Siegel R, Naishadham D, Jemal A. Cancer statistics. CA Cancer J Clin 2013;63:11-30.

[2] Bray F, dos Santos Silva I, Moller H, Weiderpass E. Endometrial Cancer Trends in Europe: Underlying Determinants and Prospects for Prevention. Cancer Epidemiol Biomarkers Prev 2005;14:1132-1142.

[3] Hubbs J, Saig, RM, Abaid LN, Bae-Jump VL, Gehrig PA. Systemic and Local Hormonal Therapy for Endometrial Hyperplasia and Early Adenocarcinoma. Obstet Gynecol 2013;121:1172-1180.

[4] Nevadunsky NS, Van Arsdale A, Strickler HD, Moadel A, Kaur G, Levitt J, Girda E, Goldfinger M, Goldberg GL, Einstein MH. Obesity and age at diagnosis of endometrial cancer. Obstet Gynecol 2014;124:300-306.

[5] Chuback J, Tworoger SS, Yasui Y, Ulrich CM, Stanczyk FZ, McTiernan A. Associations between reproductive and menstrual factors and sexual hormone concentrations. Cancer Epidemiol Biomarkers Prev 2004;13:1296-1301.

[6] Hinkula M, Pakkala E, Jyyrönen P, Kauppila A. Grand multiparity and incidence of endometrial cancer: a population-based study in Finland. Int J Cancer 2001;98:912-915.

[7] The North American Menopause Society (NAMS). Role of progestin in hormone therapy for postmenopausal women: position statement of The North American Menopause Society. Menopause 2003;10:113-132.

[8] Riphagen FE. Intrauterine application of progestins in hormone replacement therapy: a review. Climacteric 2000;3:199-211.

[9] The Writing Group for the PEPI Trial. Effects of hormone replacement on endometrial histology in postmenopausal women. The Postmenoapausal Estrogen/Progestin Intervention (PEPI) Trial. JAMA 1996;275:370-380.

[10] Bain C, Kitchener HC. 1998. Post-menopausal bleeding. In: Cameron IT, Fraser IS, Smith SK, editors. Clinical disorders of the endometrium and menstrual cycle. Oxford: Oxford University Press. pp. 266-278.

[11] Kurman RJ, Kaminski PF, Norris HJ. The behavior of endometrial hyperplasia. A long-term study of 'untreated' hyperplasia in 170 patients. Cancer 1985;56:403-412.

[12] Lethaby A, Farquhar C, Sarkis A, Roberts H, Jepson R, Barlow D. Hormone replacement therapy in postmenopausal women: endometrial hyperplasia and endometrial bleeding. Cochrane Database Syst Rev 2000;2:CD00402.

[13] Writing Group for the Women's Health Initiative Investigators. Risks and benefits of estrogen plus progestin in healthy postmenopausal women. JAMA 2002;288:321-333.

[14] Li CI, Malone KE, Porter PL, Weiss NS, Tang M-TC, Cushing-Haugen KL, Daling JR. Relationship between long durations and different regimens of hormone therapy and risk of breast cancer. JAMA 2003;289:3254-3263.

[15] Chlebowski RT, Hendrix SL, Langer RD, Stefanick ML, Gass M, Lane D, Rodabough RJ, Gilligan M, Cyr MG, Thomson CA, et al. Influence of estrogen plus progestin on breast cancer and mammography in healthy postmenopausal women. JAMA 2003;289:3243-3253.

[16] Million Women Study Collaborators. Breast cancer and hormone-replacement therapy in the Million Women Study. Lancet 2003;362:419-427.

[17] Weiss LK, Burkman RT, Cushing-Haugen KL, Voigt LF, Simon MS, Daling JR, Norman SA, Bernstein L, Ursin G, Marchbanks PA, et al. Hormone replacement therapy regimens and breast cancer risk (1). Obstet Gynecol 2002;100:1148-1158.

[18] Olsson HL, Ingvar C, Bladström A. Hormone replacement therapy containing progestins and given continuously increases breast carcinoma risk in Sweden. Cancer 2003;97:1387-1392.

[19] Nilsson CG, Laähteenmaki PLA, Luukainen T, Robertson DN. Sustained intrauterine release of levonorgestrel over five years. Fertil Steril 1986;45:805-807.

[20] Andersson K, Mattsson LA, Rybo G, Stadberg E. Intrauterine release of levonorgestrel – a new way of adding progestin in hormone replacement therapy. Obstet Gynecol 1992;79:963-967.

[21] Mirena. Product Monograph. Finland: Schering AG and Leiras Oy; 2002.

[22] Wildemeersch D, Pylyser K, De Wever N, Pauwels P. Endometrial safety after 5 years of continuous combined transdermal estrogen and intrauterine levonorgestrel delivery for postmenopausal hormone substitution. Maturitas 2007;57:205-209.

[23] Jaakkola S, Lyytinen HK, Dyba T, Ylikorkla O. Pukkala E. Endometrial cancer associated with various forms of postmenopausal hormone therapy: a case control study. Int J Cancer 2010;128:1644-1651.

[24] Haoula Z, Salman M, Atiomo W. Evaluating the association between endometrial cancer and polycystic ovary syndrome. Hum Reprod 2012;27:1327-1331.

[25] The Amsterdam ESHRE/ASRM-Sonsored 3rd PCOS Consensus Working Group. Consensus on women's health aspects of polycystic ovary syndrome (PCOS). Hum Reprod 2012;27:14-24.

[26] Duska LR, Garrett A, Rueda BR, Haas J, Chang Y, Fuller AF. Endometrial cancer in women 40 years old or younger. Gynecol Oncol 2001;83:388-393.

[27] Broekmans FJ, Knauff EAH, Valkenburg O, Laven JS, Eijkemans MJ, Fauser BC. PCOS according to the Rotterdam consensus criteria: Change in prevalence among WHO-II anovulation and association with metabolic factors. BJOG 2006;113:1210-1217.

[28] Diamanti-Kandarakis E. PCOS in adolescents. Best Pract Res Clin Obstet Gynaecol 2010;24:173-183.

[29] ACOG Practical Bulletin Number 108. Polycystic ovary syndrome. Obstet Gynecol 2009;114:936-949.

[30] Schmandt RE, Iglesias DA, Co, NN, Lu KH. Understanding obesity and endometrial cancer risk: opportunities for prevention. Am J Obstet Gynecol 2011;205:518-525.

[31] Renehan AG, Tyson M, Egger M, Heller RF, Zwahlen M. Body-mass index and incidence of cancer: a systematic review and meta-analysis of prospective observational studies. Lancet 2008;371:569-578.

[32] Key TJA, Pike MC. The dose-effect relationship between 'unopposed' oestrogens and endometrial mitotic rate: its central role in explaining and predicting endometrial cancer risk. Br J Cancer 1988;57:205-212.

[33] Hampel H, de la Chapelle A. The search for unaffected individuals with Lynch Syndrome: do the ends justify the means? Cancer Prev Res 2011;4:1-5.

[34] Dunlop MG, Farrington SM, Nicholl I, Aaltonen L, Petersen G, Porteous M, Carothers A. Population carrier frequency of hMSH2 and hMLH1 mutations. Br J Cancer 2000; 83:1643-5.

[35] Early Breast Cancer Trialists' Collaborative Group. Effects of chemotherapy and hormonal therapy for early breast cancer on recurrence and 15-year survival: an overview of randomized trials. Lancet 2005;365:1687-1717.

[36] Garuti G, Grossi F, Cellani F, Centinaio G, Colonnelli M, Luerti M. Hysteroscopic assessment of menopausal breast-cancer patients taking tamoxifen; there is a bias from the mode of endometrial sampling in estimating endometrial morbidity? Breast Cancer Res Treat 2002;72:245-253.

[37] Wong AWY, Chan SSC, Yeo W, Yu MY, Tam WH. Prophylactic use of levonorgestrel-releasing intrauterine system in women with breast cancer treated with tamoxifen. Obstet Gynecol 2013;121:943-950.

[38] Yang S, Thiel KW, Leslie KK. Progesterone: the ultimate endometrial suppressor. Trends Endocrinol Metab 2011;22:145-152.

[39] Connaghan-Jones KD, Heneghan AF, Miura MT, Bain DL. Thermodynamic analysis of progesterone receptor-promoter interactions reveals a molecular model for isoform-specific function. Proc Natl Acad Sci USA 2007; 104: 2187-2192.

[40] Herkert O, Kuhl H, Sandow J, Busse R, Schini-Kerth VB. Sex steroids used in hormonal treatment increase vascular procoagulant activity by inducing thrombin receptor (PAR-1) expression: role of the glucocorticoid receptor. Circulation 2001;104:2826-2831.

[41] Stanczyk FZ. All progestins are not created equal. Steroids 2003; 68: 879-890.

[42] Nayak NR, Slayden Ov D, Mah K, Chwalisz K, Brenner RM. Antiprogestin-releasing intrauterine devices: a novel approach to endometrial contraception. Contraception 2007;75:S104-S111.

[43] Heikinheimo O., Vani S, Carpén O, Tapper A, Härkki P, Rutanen EM, Critchley H. Intrauterine release of progesterone antagonist ZK230211 is feasible and results in novel endometrial effects: a pilot study. Hum Reprod 2007;22:2515-2522.

[44] Chabbert N, Meduri G, Bouchard P, Spitz IM. Selective progesterone receptor modulators and progesterone antagonists: mechanism of action and clinical applications. Hum Reprod Update 2005;11:293-307.

[45] Wildemeersch D, Dhont M. Treatment of non-atypical and atypical endometrial hyperplasia with a levonorgestrel-releasing intrauterine system. Am J Obstet Gynecol 2003;138:1297-1298.

[46] Wildemeersch D, Janssens D, Pylyser K, De Wever N, Verbeeck G, Dhont M, Tjalma W. Management of patients with non-atypical and atypical endometrial hyperplasia with a levonorgestrel-releasing intrauterine system: Long-term follow-up. Maturitas 2007; 57: 210-213.

[47] Wildemeersch D, Anderson E, Lambein K, Pauwels P, Dhont M. Successful treatment of early endometrial carcinoma by local delivery of levonorgestrel: a case report. Obstet Gynecol Int 2010;2010:431950.

[48] Lacey Jr JV, Sherman ME, Rush BB, Ronnett BM, Ioffe OB, Duggan MA, Glass AG, Richesson DA, Chatterjee N, Langholz B. Absolute Risk of Endometrial Carcinoma During 20-Year Follow-Up Among Women With Endometrial Hyperplasia. J Clin Oncol 2010;28:788-792.

[49] Gal D, Edman CD, Vellios F, Forney JP. Long-term effect of megestrol acetate in the treatment of endometrial hyperplasia. Am J Obstet Gynecol 1983;146:316-322.

[50] Silverberg SG, Haukkamaa M, Arko H, Nilsson CG, Luukkainen T. Endometrial morphology during long-term use of levonorgestrel-releasing intrauterine devices. Int J Gynecol Pathol 1986;5:235-241.

[51] Schindler AE. Progestins, endometrial hyperplasia and endometrial cancer. Gynaecol Forum 2004;9:31-33.

[52] Montz FJ, Bristow RE, Bovicelli A, Tomacruz R, Kurman RJ. Intrauterine progesterone treatment of early endometrial cancer. Am J Obstet Gynecol 2002;186:651-657.

[53] Nilsson CG, Luukainen T, Arco H. Endometrial morphology of women using a d-norgestrel-releasing intrauterine device. Fertil Steril 1978;29:397-401.

[54] Sturdee DW, Barlow DH, Ulrich LG, Wells M, Gydesen H, Campbell M, O'Brien K, Vessey M. Is the timing of withdrawal bleeding a guide to endometrial safety during sequential oestrogen-progestin replacement therapy? Lancet 1994;344:979-982.

[55] Whitehead MI, Townsend PT, Pryse-Davies J, Ryder TA, King RJB. Effects of estrogens and progestins on the biochemistry and morphology of the postmenopausal endometrium. N Engl J Med 1981;305:1599-1605.

[56] Wang HY, Shen L, Sun Z. [Endometrial adenocarcinoma in women 40 years old or younger by treatment with progestins: report of 6 cases and review of the literatures]. Zhonghua Fu Chan Ke Za Zhi 2006;41:237-241.

[57] Yu M, Yang J-X, Wu M, Lang J-H, Huo Z, Shen K. Fertility-preserving treatment in young women with well-differentiated endometrial carcinoma and severe atypical hyperplasia of endometrium. Fertil Steril 2009;92:2122-2124.

[58] Tanmahasamut P, Wongwananuruk T. Challenging regimen for long-term conservative treatment of endometrial adenocarcinoma in young women: A case report and review of the literature. Case Rep Oncol 2010;3:380-385.

[59] Chiva L, Lapuente F, González-Cortijo L, Carballo N, García JF, Rojo A, Gonzalez-Martín A. Sparing fertility in young patients with endometrial cancer. Gynecol Oncol 2008;111(2 Suppl):S101-S104.

[60] Giannopoulos T, Butler-Manuel S, Tailor A. Levonorgestrel-releasing intrauterine system (LNG-IUS) as a therapy for endometrial carcinoma. Gynecol Oncol 2004;95:762-764.

[61] Shah MM, Wright JD. Management of Endometrial Cancer in Young Women. Clin Obstet Gynecol 2011;54:219-225.

[62] Gallos ID, Krishan P, Shehmar M, Ganesan R, Gupta JK. LNG-IUS versus oral progestin treatment for endometrial hyperplasia: a long-term comparative cohort study. Hum Reprod 2013;28:2966-2971.

[63] Chhabra S, Kutchi I. Fertility preservation in gynecological cancers. Clin Med Insights Reprod Health 2013;7:49-59.

[64] Ewies A, Alfhaily F. Use of levonorgestrel-releasing intrauterine system in the prevention and treatment of endometrial hyperplasia. Obstet Gynecol Surv 2012;67:727-733.

[65] Baker J, Obermair A, Gebski V, Janda M. Efficacy of oral or intrauterine device-delivered progestin in patients with complex endometrial hyperplasia with atypia or early endometrial adenocarcinoma: a meta-analysis and systematic review of the literature. Gynecol Oncol 2012;125:263-270.

[66] Scarselli G, Bargelli B, Taddei GL, Marchionni M, Peruzzi E, Pieralli A, Mattei A, Buccoliero AM, Fambrini, M. Levonorgestrel-releasing intrauterine system (LNG-IUS) as an effective treatment option for endometrial hyperplasia: a 15-year follow-up study. Fertil Steril 2011;95:420-422.

[67] Gallos ID, Ganesan R, Gupta JK. Prediction of regression and relapse of endometrial hyperplasia with conservative therapy. Obstet Gynecol 2013;121:1165-1171.

[68] Hubbs JL, Saig RM, Abaid LN, Bae-Jump VL, Gehrig PA. Systemic and local hormone therapy for endometrial hyperplasia and early adenocarcinoma. Obstet Gynecol 2013;121:1172-1180.

[69] Varma R, Soneja H, Bhatia K, Ganesan R, Rollason T, Clark TJ, Gupta JK. The effectiveness of a levonorgestrel-releasing intrauterine system (LNG-IUS) in the treatment of endometrial hyperplasia – a long-term follow-up study. Eur J Obstet Gynecol Reprod Biol 2008;139:169-175.

[70] Ramirez PT, Frumovitz M, Bodurka DC, Sun CC, Levenback C. Hormonal therapy for the management of grade 1 endometrial adenocarcinoma: a literature review. Gynecol Oncol 2004;95:133-138.

[71] Lee SY, Kim MK, Park H, Yoon BS, Seong SJ, Kang JH, Jun HS, Park CT. The effectiveness of levonorgestrel releasing intrauterine system in the treatment of endometrial hyperplasia in Korean women. J Gynecol Oncol 2010;21:102-105.

[72] Bahamondes L, Ribeiro-Huguet P, de Andrade KC, Leon-Martins O, Petta CA. Levonorgestrel-releasing intrauterine system (Mirena®) as a therapy for endometrial hyperplasia and carcinoma. Acta Obstet Gynecol Scand 2003;82:580-582.

[73] Ørbo A, Arnes M, Hancke C, Vereide AB, Pettersen I, Larsen K. Treatment results of endometrial hyperplasia after prospective D-score classification: a follow-up study comparing effect of LNG-IUD and oral progestins versus observation only. Gynecol Oncol 2008;111:68-73.

[74] Giannopoulos T, Butler-Manuel S, Tailor A. Levonorgestrel-releasing intrauterine system (LNG-IUS) as a therapy for endometrial carcinoma. Gynecol Oncol 2004;95:762-764.

[75] Haoula ZJ, Walker KF, Powell MC. Levonorgestrel intra-uterine system as a treatment option for complex endometrial hyperplasia. Eur J Obstet Gynecol Reprod Biol 2011;159:176-179.

[76] Cade TJ, Quinn MA, Rome RM, Neesham D. Progestogen treatment options for early endometrial cancer. BJOG 2010; 117: 879-884.

[77] Yang S, Thiel KW, De Geest K, Leslie KK. Endometrial cancer: reviving progesterone therapy in the molecular age. Discov Med 2011;12:205-212.

[78] Wildemeersch D. Intrauterine contraceptives that do not fit well contribute to early discontinuation. Eur J Contracept Reprod Health Care 2011;16:135-141.

[79] Leslie KK, Thiel KW, Yang S. Endometrial cancer: potential treatment and prevention with progestin-containing intrauterine devices. Obstet Gynecol 2012;119:419-420.

[80] Jóźwik M, Jóźwik M, Wildemeersch D. The emerging role of long-term levonorgestrel-releasing intrauterine systems for the prevention of malignancies in women: a systematic review (In preparation).

[81] Sivalingam VN, Meyers J, Nicholas S, Balen AH, Crosbie EJ. Metformin in reproductive health, pregnancy and gynaecological cancer: established and emerging indications Hum. Reprod Update 2014;20: 853-868.

[82] Queensland Centre for Gynaecological Cancer. A Phase II Randomised Clinical Trial of Mirena® ± Metformin ± Weight Loss Intervention in Patients With Early Stage Cancer of the Endometrium. ClinicalTrials.gov Identifier: NCT01686126. Accessed on 31 August 2014.

Section 5

Twins Pregnancy

Chapter 10

Monochorionic Twin Pregnancy— Potential Risks and Perinatal Outcomes

Julio Elito Júnior, Eduardo Félix Martins Santana and Gustavo Nardini Cecchino

Additional information is available at the end of the chapter

1. Introduction

Since the most ancient times, mythical stories concerning twins were described both in religion and art [1]. Examples of twin gods and heroes are numerous: from the twin sons of Zeus to Rome's founders, Romulus and Remus. Such legendary conception connected to twins may still be found in contemporary primitive societies [2]. The evolution of medicine has led to a different perception of the twinning phenomenon, with several implications for the obstetric care [3].

The frequency of multiple pregnancies has been increasing since the 1970s. Contributing factors include the wide use of fertility drugs and assisted reproductive technologies, along with a higher number of women giving birth at older ages [4]. Nevertheless, many physicians still underestimate the adversities of multiple pregnancies. [5].

2. Importance

The number of twins has doubled and the rate of twin births has risen from 18.9 to 33.2 per 1, 000 births in the United States. Recent data brief from the National Center for Health Statistics states that one in every 30 infants born in 2009 was a twin. Twin birth rates increased in all US states from 1980 to 2009, mainly among non-Hispanic white mothers and women aged 40 and over, which demonstrated the largest increase by more than 200 percent as shown in Figure 1 [6].

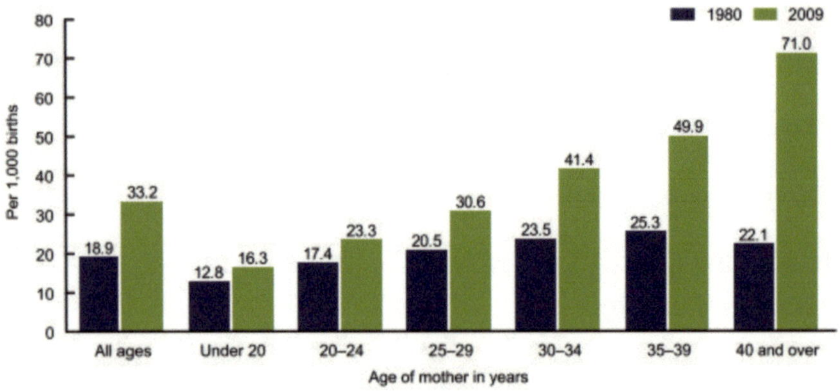

Source: CDC/NCHS, National Vital Statistics System [6]

Figure 1. Twin birth rates, by age of mother. United States, 1980 and 2009.

A consistent growth in the number of multiple births in England has also been well documented [7]. Analysis from the North of England Multiple Pregnancy Register during 1998 and 2002 showed an increasing twinning rate of 13.6 to 16.6 per 1, 000 maternities [8]. Similarly, secular changes in twinning rates were demonstrated by previous study, in which 15 out of 17 European countries listed significant increasing proportions between 1972 and 1996 [9]. Records from the Danish National Birth Cohort revealed an overall frequency of twin deliveries of 22 per 1000 [10].

Over the last 20 years in Japan, the incidence of twin births increased until 2003, when it started to decrease reaching similar rates to those registered in the 1990s [11]. The reported Chinese twinning rates range from 2.8 to 15.4 per 1000 births. This wide variation may be explained by the lack of systematic vital records [12]. Historically, the lowest twinning rates are registered in Asian countries (5-6 per 1000 maternities), and the highest rates are seen in Sub-Saharan-Africa (23 per 1000 maternities), notably Nigeria, with rates up to 40 per 1000 births [13].

The average rate of twin births in Brazil is 10 per 1000. Cândido Godói is a modest town in South Brazil universally known as "Twins' Town", considering its twinning rate of 2% and an estimated rate of 10% in the very small district of Linha São Pedro. It was hypothesized that such a high rate of twin births could be due to Nazi's experiments commanded by Joseph Mengele in the 1960s. Recent data suggest that this phenomenon is much better explained by a genetic founder effect [14].

There is a global tendency of an increased number of multiple gestations, with the exception of triplets and higher-order multiple gestations [15]. This fact was largely attributed to an elevated amount of dizygotic pregnancies, without significant variations in monozygotic births over the past few decades [4]. The dizygotic twinning rate is affected by innumerous factors such as race, parental consanguinity, maternal age and parity, lifestyle, season, use of fertility drugs and treatments, genetics and others [4, 5, 12].

Currently, it is very difficult to estimate trends in spontaneous twinning regardless of the use of fertility treatments [4]. Assisted reproductive technology has played a major role in multiple birth rates, especially after the 1980s. Evidences indicate that 30-50% of twins and at least 75% of triplets occur after infertility treatment. Therefore, several physicians and reproductive medicine societies have recommended rigorous strategies for reducing the risk of multiple pregnancies, like single-embryo transfer [16].

3. Impact of multiple gestations

Multiple pregnancies are strongly associated with greater maternal morbidity. Studies demonstrate a maternal mortality risk as much as three times higher and the numbers of intensive care unit admissions are nearly twice as those in singleton [16]. Major obstetrics complications include: miscarriage, growth retardation, pre-eclampsia, gestational diabetes, caesarean section, preterm delivery and post-partum hemorrhage [17].

Multiple children are at increased lifetime risk of developing medical complications, mainly due to the extremely high rate of preterm delivery and low birth weight among twins. Of all factors contributing to perinatal mortality, preterm newborns alone account for 70%. Likewise, infants born with less than 2500g are almost 40 times more likely to die during early infancy [18, 19]. Population-based data show greater proportions of disabilities in twins compared to singleton, with up to 3 to 7-fold increase in cerebral palsy [5, 20]. Furthermore, twinning phenomenon is associated with a higher incidence of congenital anomalies, especially among monozygotic pregnancies [16, 20].

Becoming pregnant of more than one baby imposes supplementary social implications during the antenatal and the postnatal periods. Most parents exhibit feelings of shock and isolation, which may often lead to psychological consequences such as postnatal depression. Moreover, women carrying multiples are more likely to suffer with the severity of pregnancy symptoms. Also, myths and misunderstandings regarding multiples generate many issues that the maternity care provider should be prepared to explain. Lack of sleep and personal time, chronic stress, fatigue, exhaustion and financial strains are common dilemmas experienced by parents. Delayed development, attention deficit and learning difficulties usually affect multiple children, especially due to lack of sufficient one-to-one stimulation. The prevalence of disabilities is estimated to be at least 50% higher in twins and 100% in triplets [17, 20].

In addition to all negative consequences of multiples, economic implications should also be considered. The increase in multiple births defies the current trend to lower medical costs [19]. A large study conducted in the Brigham and Women's Hospital by Callahan et al. [21] showed that multiple pregnancies contribute to a dramatic rise in hospital charges. Total family charges for a 29-year-old white mother in 1991 was estimated to be US$ 9, 845 for a singleton, compared to US$ 37, 947 for a mother of twins and US$ 109, 765 for higher-order multiple-gestation [21]. In large scale it could trigger a public health collapse.

4. Pathogenesis of twinning

4.1. Monozygotic gestation

One-egg twins result from a single fertilized oocyte. Depending on the spontaneous embryo preimplantation division at various stages of development into two genetically identical structures, three types of monozygotic pregnancies are distinguished according to Corner's embryologic theory as shown in Figure 2 [22]:

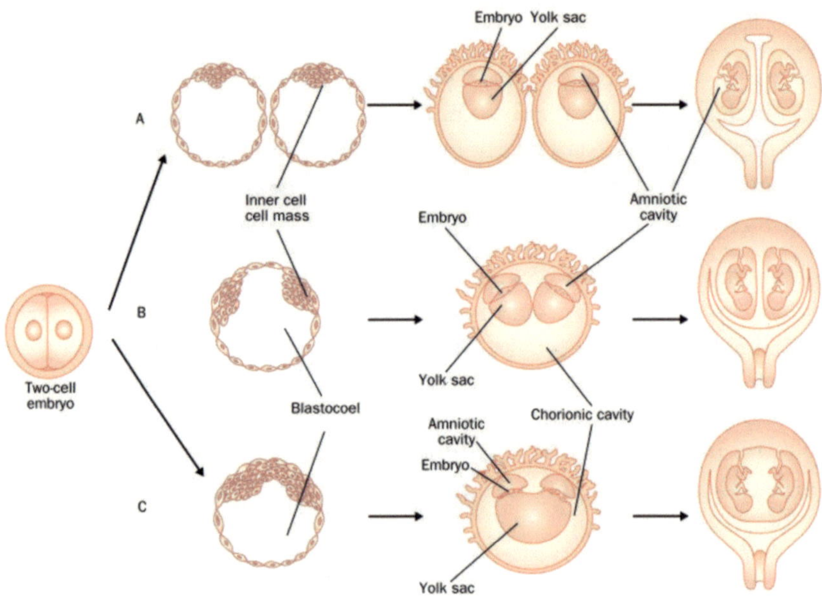

Figure 2. Three types of monozygotic placenta and membrane. A: dichorionic diamniotic. B: monochorionic diamniotic. C: monochorionic monoamniotic. From The Lancet, *JudithGHall* [23], with permission from the publisher.

- Dichorionic diamniotic if the division of the blastomerers occurs within 72 hours post-fertilization. The amnion and the chorion have not yet developed, resulting in two independent embryonic discs and diplacental monozygotic twins.
- Monochorionic diamniotic when the division of the blastocyst occurs between day 4 and day 7 post-fertilization. The chorion is already formed but not the amnion, culminating in monoplacental monozygotic twins.
- Monochorionic monoamniotic if the division of the embryoblast occurs after day 8 post-fertilization. The chorion and the amnion are fully grown, configuring monoplacental monozygotic twins as well. Even later division, usually after the 13th day, gives rise to conjoined twins, since the germ disc is completed.

The monozygotic twinning phenomenon happens in a proportion of 1:250 multiple pregnancies [5]. Usually, they share the same genetic and physical features; however, a simultaneous chromosomal error may result in heterokaryotypic monozygotes, especially in very early splits [24]. Mothers originated from a monozygotic pregnancy have exceeding rates of monozygotic twins. Despite being relatively constant and independent of factors such as ethnicity, maternal age and parity, the occurrence of monozygotic twinning is increased with in vitro fertilization and ovarian stimulation [5].

4.2. Dizygotic gestation

Two-egg twins result from simultaneous ovulation of two ova fertilized by two different spermatozoa. Thus, necessarily, two chorionic sacs are developed even in cases of fused placenta [25]. Both zygotes have different genetic constitutions, on average sharing 50% of their genes, and they can be of the same or opposite sexes [13]. Almost 75% are of the same sex, with both male twins in 45% of cases [24]. An excessive follicular recruitment occurs in 31% of mothers of dizygotic twins, who have greater basal follicle-stimulating hormone (FSH) concentration and pulse frequency, associated with elevated secretion of gonadotropin-releasing hormone (GnRH). These findings suggest that multiple ovulations are extragonadally determined [5].

Season is known to influence the dizygotic twinning process as well as the use of folic acid and oral contraceptives. Evidences suggest a slight tendency for dizygotic twins to be conceived at summer and autumn, which probably reflects the light's effect on pineal gland and the release of higher titles of FSH [5, 13]. A recent systematic review indicates a possible positive association between the use of periconceptional folic acid and increased twinning, but additional well-designed studies are needed [26]. Several researches showed raised risk for multiple pregnancies after discontinuation of oral contraceptives due to a temporary increase of FSH levels [27, 28].

Whether there is a recessive or dominant inheritance pattern for dizygotic twinning is still controversial. The fact is that a substantially greater female genetic contribution was observed, in contrast with limited evidence for a paternal effect [29, 30]. Genetic mutations could not yet be definitively associated as a cause of hereditary dizygotic twinning, but genetic mapping studies support a mechanism of inheritance connected to chromosomes 2, 7 and 18. Further investigations are needed [13].

4.3. Other forms of multiple gestation

Superfecundation is the fertilization of two or more ova from the same ovulation cycle by sperm released at intercourse on different occasions, not necessarily from the same partner (heteropaternal superfecundation). Cases of twins with different fathers have been reported since 1940 by red cell antigen typing, and these findings were later endorsed by human leukocyte antigen (HLA) typing [31, 32]. Genetic disease studies and circumstances of disputed paternities allowed more accurate diagnosis [33]. Recently, a case of heteropaternal superfecundation was reported in a pair of Danish twins [34].

Superfetation is the fertilization of 2 ova released in different menstrual cycles, resulting in the onset of a subsequent pregnancy during an ongoing pregnancy. The occurrence is more rare than superfecundation and only few human cases have been described [35]. Confirmation requires ultrasound scanning during the first trimester, but neurosonography with detailed ophthalmic examination may support the diagnosis. Superfetation has innumerous antenatal implications although it is very difficult to retrospectively confirm the diagnosis postnatally [36]. Considering the absence of substantial evidence, we believe the superfetation mechanism could only be possible in theory.

5. Diagnosis of chorionicity

Chorionicity, different from zygosity, refers to the type of placentation and it directly impacts obstetric management (Figure 3) [37]. Distinguishing the placental chorionicity plays a critical role in clinical practice since perinatal mortality rates are 2-5 times higher in cases of monochorionicity, which is present in 20% of all twin pregnancies [37, 38]. Monochorionic placentas may present vascular communications that can induce several syndromes. These vascular anastomoses also explain the existence of chimerism and mosaicism upon monozygotic twins [23].

Correct antenatal assignment of chorionicity is very important not only for risk stratification and prenatal monitoring, but also for genetic counseling, invasive procedures, diagnosis of twin-twin transfusion syndrome (TTTS) and growth abnormalities, as well as for the management of conditions affecting only one twin [39, 40]. Thus, the ascertainment of chorionicity has enabled the prevention of undesired repercussions.

Currently, early sonographic study is the gold standard for the antenatal twin chorionicity prediction. When assessed before 14 weeks' gestation it is extremely precise, with reported accuracy rates ranging from 77 to 100% [40, 41]. Such large variation can be mainly explained by the use of different ultrasound markers and by the time of scanning. Combining first-trimester sonographic parameters makes it possible to reach accuracy close to 100% [41, 42].

The identification of two clearly separate placentas or gestational sacs during the earliest first-trimester ultrasound scanning indicates dichorionic twinning, with more than 97% sensibility and 100% specificity. In cases of single or even fused placenta, the chorionicity can be assessed either by the presence of lambda sign or T-sign (Figure 4). Measurement of the inter-twin membrane thickness and counting of the layers of the inter-twin membrane are less useful indicators [37, 42].

In 1981, Bessis and Papiernik [43] first described the lambda sign as a reference for the triangular projection of placental tissue observed at the base of the inter-twin membrane in cases of dichorionic placentation. It has been mutually used with the twin peak sign, described later in 1992 by Finberg [44]. The lambda-sign is better perceived in the late first and early second trimester ultrasound scanning, and may disappear by week 20 in 7% of dichorionic pregnancies with fused placenta [41, 42]. The absence of twin peak sign neither excludes dichorionic pregnancy nor implies monochorionicity [37].

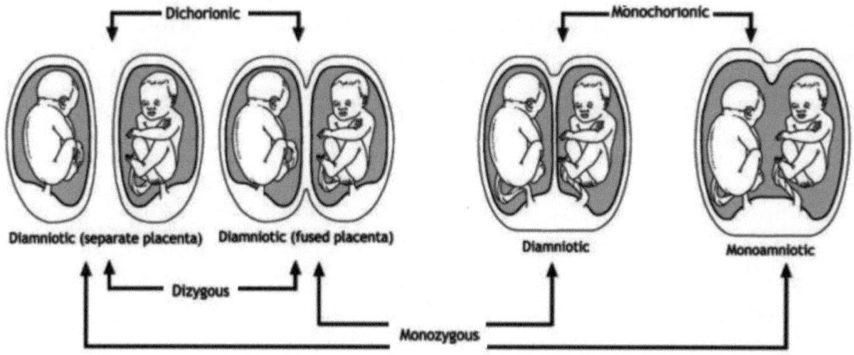

Figure 3. Different patterns of placentation for twins. Adapted from Prenatal Diagnosis, *Shetty&Smith* [37], with permission from the publisher.

The T-sign has been traditionally used to describe the point where the two opposing amnions at the base of the separating membrane approach the placenta at almost a 90^0 angle, characterizing a monochorionic placentation [37, 42]. In 2002, Carroll et al [38] performed the very first robust study evaluating sonographic signs between 10-14 weeks of gestation. In their series of 150 cases, the prenatal chorionicity diagnosis was confirmed postnatally by placental histology. They identified a sensitivity and specificity of the T-sign in predicting monochorionicity of 100% and 98.2%, respectively. The combination of the lambda sign or two separate placentas showed a sensitivity of 97.4% and specificity of 100% to predict dichorionicity. Innumerous studies were subsequently carried out and similar sensitivity and specificity percentages were reported [41].

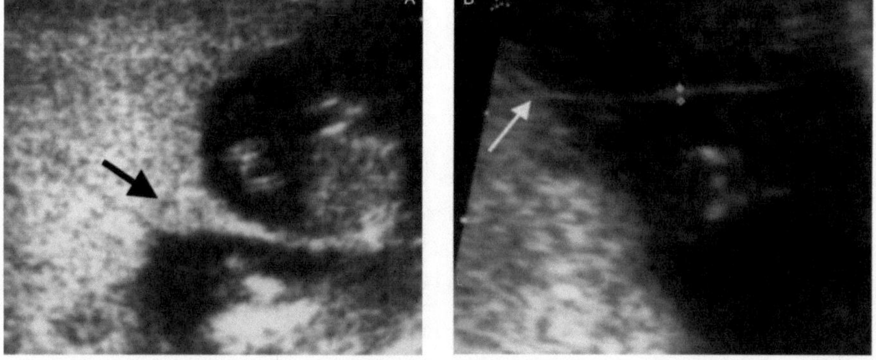

Figure 4. First trimester ultrasound image of a fused dichorionic placenta with lambda sign (A) and first trimester ultrasound image of a monochorionic placenta with T sign (B). Adapted from BJOG, *Carrolletal.* [38], with permission from the publisher.

The antenatal chorionicity determination is remarkably precise. Yet, eventual mistakes have a major impact on patient counseling, pregnancy monitoring and perinatal outcome. Some researchers are going for 3-D ultrasound but its contribution for chorionicity determinations is still unclear. Further studies should be encouraged [39, 40].

Recognition of zygosity is more difficult to be predicted and can be either performed by ultrasound or noninvasive molecular genetic tests. Only 55-65% of twin pregnancies zygosity can be determined by correlating chorion type with the sex of twins [45, 46]. Invasive approaches combined with microsatellite DNA markers could also detect zygosity, but they have the inconvenience of a miscarriage risk of 0.5-1%. Recently, Zheng et al [47] developed a noninvasive method based on maternal plasma target region sequencing through a bioinformatics' model with promising results.

6. Placental characteristics in monochorionic twins

Monochorionic placentation is associated with higher perinatal morbidity and mortality as a result of placental morphologic characteristics and vascular problems (Figure 5) [48]. Overall, almost 1% of all monozygotic twin gestations are monoamniotic, which consist of both single amniotic cavity and placenta, sharing two umbilical cord insertions. This may lead to a complication specific to monoamniotic twins: cords entanglement and knotting [49]. For decades it was believed that cord entanglement was responsible for most fetal deaths, but recent studies, including a systematic review, showed no contribution of cord entanglement to prenatal morbidity and mortality [50, 51].

Superficial vascular anastomoses are present in all monoamniotic placentas, with the majority being of arterioarterial and arteriovenous type. Also, a small distance between cords' insertion are observed in most cases, as well as a low incidence of velamentous cord insertion (4%). No significant association among various morphologic or histophatologic characteristics of monochorionic monoamniotic placentas and perinatal mortality were reported. Furthermore, no relation between severe birth weight discordance (≥20%) and unequally shared placenta or velamentous cord insertion were described. Twin-twin transfusion syndrome is a rare condition in monochorionic monoamniotic placentas due to the protector effect of the arterio-arterial anastomoses [49, 52].

Likewise, monochorionic diamniotic placentas did not demonstrate a clear relation between placental angioarchitecture, intercord distance and shared placental territories with greater perinatal mortality. Twins with unequally shared placentas and velamentous cord insertion significantly lower mean birth weight. Perinatal mortality was found to be substantially higher in the presence of velamentous cord insertion [48].

Additionally, in cases of TTTS, vascular anastomoses are more likely to be of deep other than superficial type. Most anastomoses are arteriovenous, and vascular communications are fewer in number without compensating superficial arterioarterial flow [53]. Moreover, evidences suggest that unequally shared placentas and velamentous cord insertion are not mandatory for the occurrence of TTTS [54].

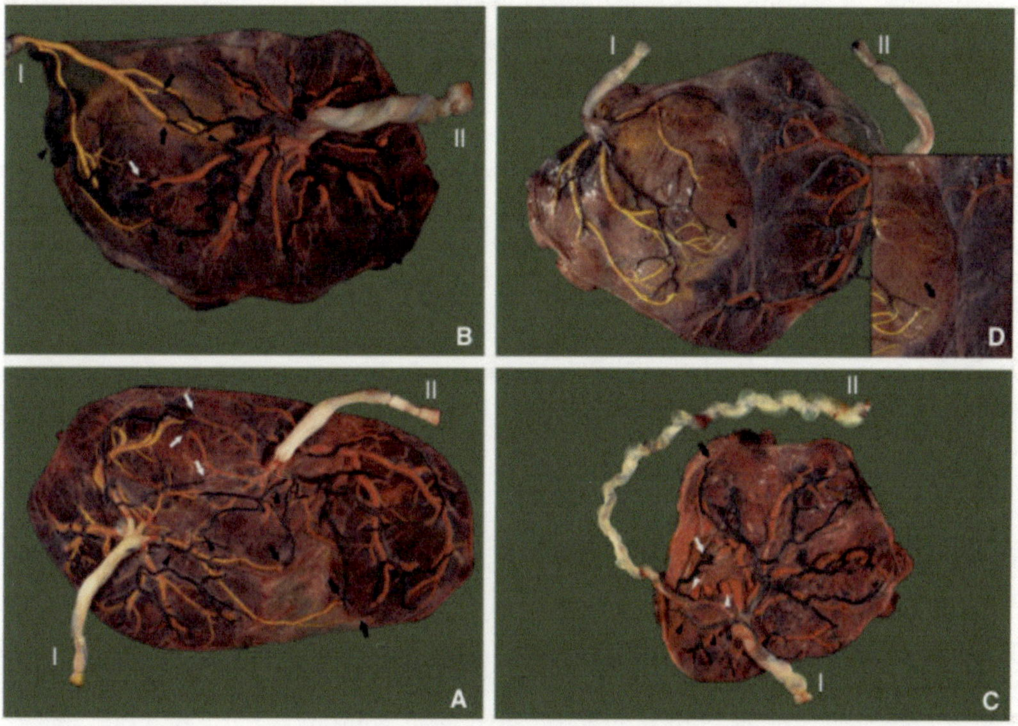

Figure 5. Monochorionic placentas after injection with coloured dye. The veins are coloured yellow or orange and the arteries are black or blue. The white arrows indicate arteriovenous anastomoses from twin I towards twin II; the black arrows indicate arteriovenous anastomoses from twin II towards twin I. The white arrowheads indicate venovenous anastomoses and the black arrowheads indicate arterioarterial anastomoses. **(A)** Placenta of monochorionic twin without TTTS, delivered at 36^{+6} weeks of gestation. Similar placental territory for both twins. **(B)** Placenta of monochorionic twin with selective intrauterine growth restriction. Caesarean section at 32 weeks of gestation after determination of lung maturity. The growth-restricted twin I has a velamentous cord insertion and placental territory of 28%. **(C)** Placenta of monochorionic twin with mild TTTS. Caesarean section at 32 weeks of gestation due to TTTS. The ex-recipient twin I has a placental territory of 82%. **(D)** Placenta of monochorionic twin with TTTS, conservative management. Caesarean section at 31^{+5} weeks for signs of anemia in the donor twin. Adapted from Placenta, *Hack et al.* [48], with permission from the publisher.

7. Antenatal care in monochorionic pregancies

Multiple pregnancies impose a higher risk of complications for both mother and baby; therefore, adverse outcomes take place more often [55]. Intensive antenatal care should be provided along with a multidisciplinary team. Furthermore, an effective interpersonal communication between healthcare professionals and women is fundamental [56].

The very first step for quality assistance is an early detection of multiple pregnancies along with appropriate amnionicity and chorionicity determination as soon as possible. Whenever the diagnosis of chorionicity is uncertain, the woman should be referred to a specialist or a senior ultrasonographer before 14 weeks. If still indeterminate, even after referral, the pregnancy should be managed as monochorionic until proven otherwise [55-57]. Parents should be thoroughly informed about the implications of a monochorionic pregnancy [58].

Nuchal translucency should be offered as a screening for fetal aneuploidies. The detection accuracy is better when combining maternal age, nuchal fold, crown-rump length, and serum markers [42, 55]. Some professionals do not recommend the routine use of serum markers neither in the first trimester nor during the second trimester [59], while others do recommend for both situations [56].

The prevalence of congenital anomalies is almost twice when comparing monochorionic twins with dichorionic, although in both cases only one fetus is affected in 90% of the time. In case of a suspicious screening exam, a fetal echocardiographic assessment should be considered. The same applies for in vitro fertilization conceived twins and cases of severe TTTS [42]. First trimester surveillance for TTTS is not advised [55, 56, 58]. When applicable, chorionic villus sampling is preferred over amniocentesis and the transabdominal route is the best choice [59].

Placental evaluation and cervical length assessment are also important. Placenta previa is 40% more common in twins, and so is vasa previa. The placental cord insertion should be determined once velamentous cord insertion is associated with greater risk of TTTS, unequal placental sharing and perinatal mortality. Cervical length smaller than 20-25 mm raises the likelihood of preterm delivery in 3-5 times [42].

Serial sonographic monitoring for intrauterine growth restriction (IUGR) or discordance is warranted rather than abdominal palpation, symphysis-fundal height measurement or umbilical artery Doppler [42, 55, 56]. Only an estimated fetal weight discordance greater than 25% is clinically important [55, 56]. Both IUGR and twin discordance are associated with increased risk for fetal and perinatal death [42]. A recent prospective cohort study showed that twin birth weight discordance might be predicted with an abdominal circumference ratio cutoff of 0.93, with a sensitivity and specificity of 61% and 84%, respectively [60].

Additionally, it is also mandatory to monitor for maternal complications, especially for hypertensive disorders that present an increased likelihood of 2 to 3-fold. Concerning gestational diabetes, whether its occurrence is increased or not is still controversial. The management of all maternal complications shall not be different from singleton pregnancies [55].

Table 1 shows an overview of ultrasound applications for twin pregnancies [42]. Monthly prenatal consultations are strongly recommended for all monochorionic pregnancies, as well as ultrasound scanning every 4 weeks for uncomplicated dichorionic pregnancy and every 2 weeks for uncomplicated monochorionic twins [42, 59].

Indication	Timing	Comment
Pregnancy dating	First trimester	Optimal at 7–10 weeks using CRL
Determination of chorionicity	First trimester	Close to 100% accuracy if done prior to second trimester
Nuchal translucency assessment	10–13 weeks	Increased with aneuploidy, malformations, TTTS
Anatomical survey	Second trimester	Optimal at 18–22 weeks; fetal echocardiography for IVF twins and/or monochorionic twins
Placental evaluation	Second trimester	Transvaginal imaging to exclude previa and vasa previa; color imaging for PCI
Baseline cervical length	Second trimester	Transvaginal imaging optimal
Twin growth studies	Second and third trimester	Every 4 weeks for uncomplicated twins
Serial surveillance	Second and third trimester	Every 2 weeks for uncomplicated monochorionic twins; daily testing at viability for monoamniotic twins; frequency and type of testing of twins depends on chorionicity, risk, and complications

CRL = crown-rump length; TTTS = twin-twin transfusion syndrome; IVF = in vitro fertilization; PCI = placental cord insertion.

From Seminars in Perinatology, *Lynn Simpson* [42], with permission from the publisher.

Table 1. Ultrasound in twins

8. Antenatal complications

Certainly, preterm birth is the most relevant complication related to multiple pregnancies. Current available data in the literature are insufficient to determine effective preventive strategies, limiting the applicability of routine screening methods to predict preterm delivery [55].

Two recent systematic reviews and meta-analysis concerning the use of transvaginal sonographic cervical length to predict spontaneous preterm birth in twin pregnancies concluded that women with a short cervix are at increased risk [61, 62]. Testing for fetal fibronectin should not be used as a single approach to suppose a greater risk of preterm delivery in twins. If combined with cervical length measurement it might be valuable [55, 56]. Also, women with a history of previous preterm singleton delivery are at increased risk of preterm birth in a subsequent twin pregnancy [63].

All studied interventions to prevent spontaneous preterm labour in twin pregnancies up to date failed, including hospitalization and bed rest, progesterone treatment, prophylactic cervical cerclage or pessary and the use of betamimetics [64-69]. This is the rationale for worldwide guidelines to discourage any of the above-mentioned strategies [56, 59, 70]. Further well-designed, properly powered, prospective randomized trials are warranted prior to widespread implementation in clinical practice.

It is well known that both antenatal corticosteroids and magnesium sulphate reduce neonatal complications in preterm babies related to lung maturity and neurological development respectively, regardless of fetal number [71, 72]. Although, there is no evidence to support neither the routine use of untargeted course of steroids nor magnesium sulphate therapy, except when preterm labour or birth is imminent [55, 56, 70].

Other antenatal complications, including those specific to monochorionic twins, were exhaustively discussed along the chapter.

9. Monochorionic twin pregnancies specific complications

9.1. Twin-Twin Transfusion Syndrome (TTTS)

Chronic twin-to-twin transfusion syndrome is a specific complication of monochorionic pregnancies, almost exclusively to monochorionic diamniotic placentation. It results from an unbalanced unidirectional blood flow through placental arteriovenous anastomoses, and the proportion is up to 15% of all monochorionic pregnancies [73]. Additional factors such as vasoactive hormones are also believed to influence the development of TTTS [74].

Commonly diagnosed during routine second-trimester ultrasound scanning, its predicted peak in incidence is around 20-21 weeks of gestation [75]. The presentation is highly variable and the recipient twin may present circulatory overload and polycythemia, possibly leading to congestive heart failure and hydrops. Contrarily, the donor twin shows oliguria and oligohydramnios, as well as anemia and growth restriction. Acute unbalancement can also occur at any time before birth, threatening the prognosis [76].

Data shows that 17% of the overall twin's perinatal mortality and 50% of all perinatal deaths in monochorionic diamniotic twins are attributed for TTTS [77].

9.2. Diagnostic criteria

TTTS is properly diagnosed after confirmation of monochorionic twin pregnancy in early sonography demonstrating T-sign. In late diagnosed cases, chorionicity is supposed when single placental mass and a thin intertwin membrane are seen [78]. Besides the confirmation of a monochorionic diamniotic gestation, the presence of oligohydramnios (maximal vertical pocket <2 cm) within the donor sac, instead of polyhydramnios (maximal vertical pocket >8 cm) in the recipient sac are also essential [74, 77]. Differential diagnoses include selective intrauterine growth restriction and other causes of amniotic fluid abnormalities [77].

Additional sonographic findings usually coexist with TTTS such as significant growth discordance, absent or reversed a-wave in the ductus venous and velamentous cord insertion [74]. TTTS frequently occurs acutely and a meticulous follow-up in a specialized center is strongly recommended. The initial ultrasound assessment should include detailed anatomy scan and Doppler study, along with cervical length measurement. Fetal echocardiography is a valuable option for cardiac function evaluation [75].

9.3. Severity staging

In cases of sudden TTTS aggravation, acute polyhydramnios develops between 16 and 24 weeks. Mortality rates are high, reaching 80 to 100% in untreated disorders. There is also high occurrence of miscarriage, premature rupture of membranes, preterm delivery and spontaneous death of one or both siblings [79].

Quintero's et al. [80] major classification considers cumulative evolving stages (Table 2). Initial stages only differ in the amount of amniotic fluid in both cavities, followed by signs of anuria in the donor twin (anidramnios or absence of bladder content). An abnormality in the dopplervelocimetry of the donor twin precedes anasarca in the recipient twin. Final stages come with death of one or both fetuses.

I	*Maximum vertical pocket <2 cm in donor and >8 cm in recipient sac*
II	*I + Donor anuria (anidramnios / absence of bladder)*
III	*I + II + Doppler anomalies in donor*
IV	*I + II + III + Fetal hydrops*
V	*I + II + III + IV + Fetal demise*

Adapted from Quintero et al, 1999 [80].

Table 2. Quintero's staging of twin-twin transfusion syndrome

This system has some prognostic significance, but the stages not always correlate perfectly with perinatal outcomes. Over 75% of stage I TTTS cases remain stable or regress with conservative management. If treated with suboptimal approaches in non-specialized centers, the consequences can be fatal [75, 77].

9.4. Management

In order to improve the prognosis of TTTS, many options were proposed throughout the years, including specific strategies (selective fetoscopic laser coagulation of placental anastomoses) and non-specific strategies such as expectant management, amnioreduction, septostomy and selective reduction [75, 77]. An algorithm proposed by the Society for Maternal-Fetal Medicine for management of TTTS is shown in Figure 6 [77].

Selectivefetoscopiclaserphotocoagulation: first-line treatment for early-onset severe TTTS, requiring highly qualified professionals and specific equipment [75]. Advances in endoscopic surgery allowed proper identification of arteriovenous anastomoses and its coagulation. The rate of survival of at least one fetus is close to 75% and almost 40% of both twins. The overall frequency of neurological impairment is around 4% [81]. This procedure is only performed in severe stages and requires specialized tertiary center, trained staff, and adequate equipment. Maternal morbidity is minimal and complications include miscarriage, preterm premature rupture of membranes, placental abruption, and stillbirth. The Eurofetus trial showed significantly higher survival rate of at least one fetus when comparing laser photocoagulation with amnioreduction (76% vs. 56%) as well as lesser neurological abnormalities (31% vs. 52%) [82].

Amnioreduction: progressive polyhydramnios in TTTS increases the risk of preterm premature rupture of membranes and preterm birth, often causing maternal distress. The rationale is to temporary relieve intrauterine pressure. Serial amnioreduction is usually required, with an average of three procedures until the pregnancy reaches an acceptable gestational age [83]. Complications are similar to fetoscopy, although less frequent and with decreased maternal morbidity. Mean survival rate is 40-50% of at least one fetus and 20% for both. Reported neurological sequels are just about 20 to 30% [84]. The main advantage is that amnioreduction is inexpensive, easy to perform and widely available [74].

Septostomy: performed to balance the amniotic fluid amount in both sacs by needle-opening the intertwin membrane. It relieves cameras pressure and may be performed during amnioreduction, with 40 to 83 % survival rate. Septostomy increases the risk of severe complications like cord entanglement and eventual disruption of the membrane. [85]. This procedure has generally been abandoned [75, 77].

Selectivereduction: therapeutic option through cord coagulation in order to improve the outcome of the surviving twin whenever there is an imminent risk of spontaneous intrauterine death of one fetus. It can be performed either by ultrasound guided vascular embolization or cord clamping through fetoscopy. A maximum of 50% survival is reached and most services have not supported this technique [86].

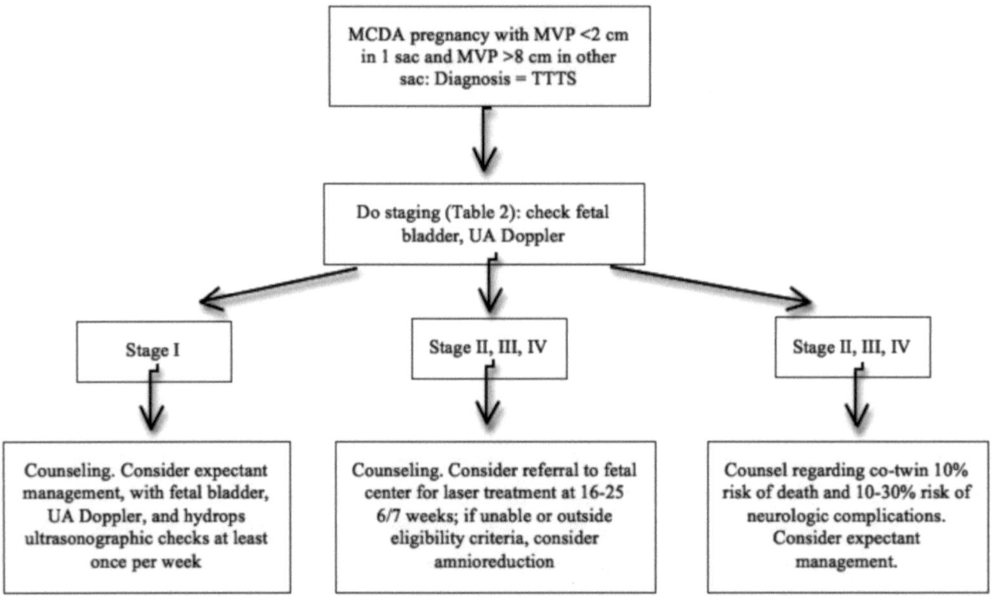

MCDA: monochorionic diamniotic; MVP: maximum vertical pocket; UA: umbilical artery

Figure 6. Algorithm for management of TTTS. Adapted from American Journal of Obstetrics and Gynecology, *LynnSimpson* [77], with permission from the publisher.

9.5. Twin Anemia Polycythemia Sequence (TAPS)

Twin anemia polycythemia sequence (TAPS) occurs spontaneously in up to 5% of all monochorionic pregnancies or even after fetoscopic laser photocoagulation, with an estimated prevalence of 13%. This syndrome is characterized by a substantial difference in hemoglobin levels among twins, in absence of discordance in the amniotic fluid. It could be mainly explained by the presence of few persistent arteriovenous anastomoses besides the reduced placental territory where the circulating blood is transferred from donor to the receiver twin, in a unidirectional flow [87].

Prenatal diagnosis may be assessed through the determination of the peak systolic velocity in the middle cerebral artery (PSV-MCA) by dopplervelocimetry. The anemic twin will have a PSV-MCA >1, 5MoM in contrast to a decreased PSV-MCA <0, 8MoM in the polycythemic co-twin [88]. In the postnatal period, diagnostic criteria are based on different levels of hemoglobin between fetuses over 8g/dL, reticulocytes amount over 1.7% or small anastomoses <1mm [89].

Treatment includes expectant management, labor induction, intrauterine blood transfusion (intravenous or intraperitoneal), selective feticide and fetoscopic laser coagulation. Survival rates up to 80% are achieved when identified in early stages, although there are no studies of long-term neurological outcome [87].

10. Selective Intrauterine Growth Restriction (sIUGR)

10.1. Causes

Selective intrauterine growth restriction (sIUGR) happens in 10% of monochorionic gestations, similar to dichorionic twins. It is diagnosed when the fetal weight of one twin is under the 10th percentile, and frequently there is 25% of discordance. In most cases the origin is in the placental territory discrepancy. Vascular anastomoses between both fetuses intrinsically justify IUGR, and one twin receives better-oxygenated blood [90].

10.2. Classification

Although a wide spectrum of vascular anastomoses variations establish different standards for fetal growth, three known patterns of umbilical artery dopplervelocimetry are inclined to develop sIUGR. Type I shows normal diastolic flow in this artery. Constantly absent or reverse flow characterizes type II. Finally, in type III, absent or reverse flow appears intermittently [91].

Prognosis is quite better in type I, contrasting with types II and III, which have been associated to an increased risk of neurological disorders, preterm births and stillbirths. In type III, massive blood transfusion through arterioarterial anastomoses is usually identified [91].

10.3. Differential diagnosis between TTTS and early sIUGR

In spite of the available evidence, causes of severe weight discordance in monochorionic pregnancies are still challenging for proper identification. Differential diagnosis demands early sonographic scanning, along with the exclusion of fetal abnormalities. The development of TTTS is probable once detected any abnormality in the amniotic volume with the larger compartment over 8 cm in one fetus cavity and bellow 2 cm in the other's.. If there is no disturb of the amniotic fluid and either the estimated weight of one twin is below the 10th percentile, or the weight discordance is over 25%, sIUGR may be presumed. Additionally, the evaluation of peak systolic velocity in the middle cerebral artery can be helpful. Finally, if not fitting any of the above criteria, a thorough follow up is recommended [91].

10.4. Management

Type I sIUGR has better prognosis and expectant management is reasonable until 34-35 weeks. Types II and III are associated with worse prognosis, and the therapeutic choice largely depends on the gestational age and severity staging. In these cases, laser therapy and cord occlusion may be practicable alternatives [91].

A fetal medicine specialist must follow monochorionic twins with routine sonographic assessment starting from 16 weeks. Finding any discordance in amniotic fluid or fetal weight, weekly interval is strongly recommended. Except for these cases, monochorionic gestations are expected to undergo an elective resolution around 37 weeks [91].

In our department, types II and III of sIUGR are closely monitored until 26 weeks of gestation, when the patient should be admitted at the hospital for daily Doppler ultrasound scanning, biophysical profile and cardiotocographic exam.

10.5. Twin reversed arterial perfusion sequence (trap sequence)

Twin reversed arterial perfusion sequence is a rare malformation in monochorionic pregnancies. The reported incidence is of 1:35000 deliveries and 1:100 monochorionic gestations. Usually, there are multiple structural abnormalities in one of the fetus, varying from a rudimentary heart to its complete absence, and an undeveloped head, associated or not to upper limbs alterations [92].

Generally an edema of the fetal trunk is observed or seen as an amorphous mass. A specific angioarchitecture characterized by an arterioarterial and a venovenous anastomosis supports the development of the acardiac twin. The normal twin acts like an infusion pump, with an increased mortality rate of 50 to 70%. Furthermore, this fetus is threatened by a raised risk of congestive cardiac failure, preterm labor, preterm premature rupture of membranes, premature delivery, polyhydramnios and intrauterine fetal death [75, 93].

Therapeutic options include expectant management, which showed good results when associated to thorough vitality surveillance [94]. There are also invasive procedures to interrupt blood flow to the acardiac twin. Innumerous surgical approaches have been described such as endoscopic cord ligation or compression, bipolar or laser coagulation of the umbilical cord, radiofrequency ablation or even embolization of the vessels inside the abdomen of the acardiac fetus. Despite the success of various techniques, intrafetal ablation is recommended as the best choice concerning its simplicity, safety and effectiveness when compared to others [95].

10.6. Conjoined twins and abnormal variations

The union of twins happens once in 50, 000 gestations, and it is related to imperfect segmentation of a single zygote after the 13th day of fecundation [96]. A marked female predominance of 72% is registered [97]. Diagnosis is held through early sonography in the first trimester [96]. Attachment may be rostral: omphalopagus, thoracopagus and cephalopagus; caudal: ischiopagus; lateral: parapagus, or dorsal: craniopagus, rachipagus and pygopagus (Figure 7) [98].

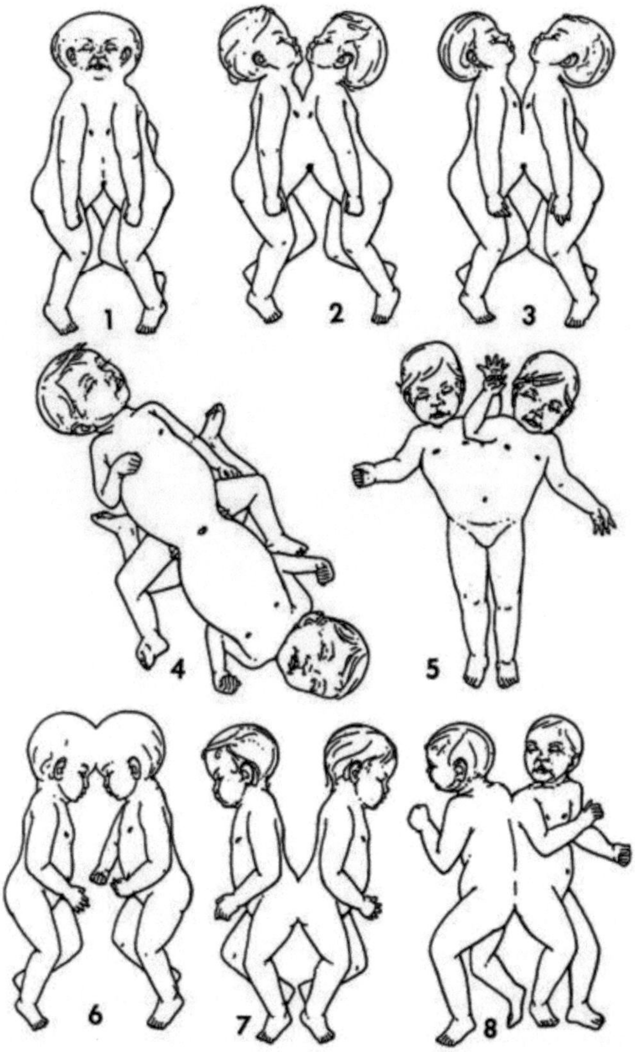

Figure 7. The eight types of conjoined twins: **(1)** cephalopagus, **(2)** thoracopagus, **(3)** omphalopagus, **(4)** ischiopagus, **(5)** parapagus, **(6)** craniopagus, **(7)** pygopagus, **(8)** rachipagus. From Journal of Pediatric Surgery, *Rowena Spencer* [98], with permission from the publisher.

Prognosis is determined according to the site of attachment, organs involved, presence and extension of associated malformations. About 10% of conjoined twins are unequally distributed and 50% have structural anomalies of major organs. Thus, planning for the best correction strategy requires knowledge of cardiac abnormalities, which are frequent in these cases. When a poor outcome is foreseen, vaginal delivery is preferable, although it depends on gestational week and fetuses' dimension [23, 96].

10.7. Externally attached parasitic twin

Externally attached parasitic twin is also an infrequent finding in 1:1, 000, 000 births. They are asymmetric conjoined twins in whom a fetus with defect, or a fetal part, is externally attached in a relatively normal twin. Also known as heteropagus twins, it is believed that this type of union results from atrophic ischemia of monozygotic conjoined twins and the parasite twin depends on the cardiovascular system of the other. In most cases the parasite fetus does not have a functional heart or brain [96].

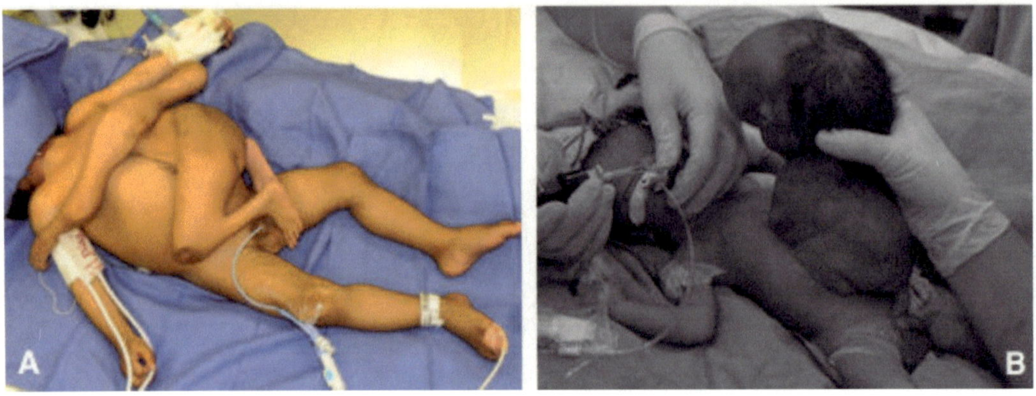

Figure 8. Epigastric heteropagus twins. **(A)** Adapted from Journal of Pediatric Surgery, *Sharma et al.* [97], with permission from the publisher. **(B)** Adapted from Journal of Pediatric Surgery, *Ribeiro et al.* [99], with permission from the publisher.

10.8. Fetus In Fetu (FIF)

Fetus in fetu is a seldom finding in monochorionic twins, with incidence of 1:500, 000 deliveries. It has been also detected in adults. Even though already reported elsewhere, the most frequent localization is in the abdominal cavity. It is defined as a fetiform mass incorporated inside a host twin coming from abnormal embryogenesis [100].

FIF happens whenever there is an unequal division of totipotent cells of a blastocyst, resulting in the inclusion of a small cellular mass into a more mature embryo. The main sites of presentation by frequency order are vertebral column, limbs, central nervous system, digestive tract, vessels and genitourinary tract [101]. Karyotype is usually normal and surgery is encouraged to remove the included fetus, not only to relive its mass effect, but also considering its potential of malignization [100].

10.9. Internal teratoma

Internal teratomas are rare congenital tumors, usually benign and of multifactorial etiology. They are constituted by a complex combination of microscopically identifiable tissues inside the fetus, which derivate from mesoderm, endoderm and ectoderm. In its interior, structures like teeth, intestine and hair are covered by connective tissue receiving vascularization from small vessels. It has independent potential of growth and also of malignization [96].

Although prenatal diagnosis can be held by a simple sonographic study within 15-16 weeks, tridimensional evaluation and the use of magnetic resonance may improve diagnostic precision, allowing the establishment of its precise localization, extension, and dissemination.

11. Monochorionic twins discordant for fetal defects

The rate of congenital anomalies in twins is 2 times higher than in singletons [102, 103]. In monozygotic twins it is around 5-fold greater. However, in dizygotic twins this rate is similar to singletons. One of the main causes of congenital anomalies in monochorionic twins is related to vascular disruption. The past concept that all monozygotic twins are always identical has changed. The rate of concordant congenital anomalies is 9-18%, even in monozygotic twins [104]. Actually, monozygotic twins are rarely identical once genetic differences exist [105].

There are specific anomalies related to multiple pregnancies, explained by the twinning process and aspects of placentation. The abnormalities of monozygotic twinning include: conjoined twins, TRAP sequence, parasitic twins, and fetus-in-fetu [106]. Monochorionic twin pregnancies have placental vascular anastomoses that could result in TTTS in 15% of cases [107]. Congenital heart defects is 3-fold increased in monochorionic pregnancies with TTTS predominantly affecting the recipient twin, such as ventricular septal defects, pulmonary stenosis and atrial septal defects [108, 109]. The rate of fetal anomaly in monoamniotic pregnancies is around 25%, even if conjoined twins are excluded [106].

A discordant fetal defect in a dizygotic twin pregnancy is easy to explain, since the genetic material is distinct. However, in monozygotic pregnancies, discordant congenital anomalies are related to several mechanisms: missegregation of cytoplasmic material (resulting in different characteristics due to post-zygotic mitotic crossing over or non-disjunction), inactivation or expression of selected genes, imprinting and telomere size differences, X-inactivation and discordant cytoplasmic segregation [110, 111]

Whenever there is a post zygotic non-disjunction in one of the twins, there might be an eventual chromosomal aneuploidy discordance related to chromosomal mosaicism in various degrees. Thus, monozygotic 46, XY and 46, XX twins may be a product of a 46, XXY zygote. Single gene mutation discordances involving either nuclear or mitochondrial DNA as well as X-inactivation and imprinting discordances have occurred. Environmental factors play a major role in epigenetic differences, considering its greatest impact lays on monozygotic twins who were apart the longest [105].

In monochorionic placentas the risk of vascular anastomoses could result in disruption that compromises the fetus. These hemodynamic abnormalities are more prevalent after the death of one co-twin; however, it can happen even in surviving infants. This process of hypoxia and ischemia could affect several organs such as the brain (microcephaly, hydrocephalus or hydranencephaly), the gastrointestinal system (intestinal atresia), the kidney, and the skin (aplasia cutis) [112].

Malformations in twins affect the abdominal wall, skull, and chest, as well as the cardiac, musculoskeletal, urogenital and central nervous systems. They are related to embryonic midline fates (neural tube and cardiac defects), hemodynamic instability of the placenta (brain lesions, limb reduction, cardiac defects, renal agenesis, aplasia cutis and intestinal atresia), and anomalies associated with prematurity (patent ductus arteriosus and retinopathy) [113].

The management of discordant anomalies in monochorionic twins is a great challenge when parents decide to keep the pregnancy. The normal fetus is at increased risk of prematurity and its consequences. The major problem occurs after the death of the discordant fetus for congenital anomalies, which increases the risk of death of the normal co-twin around 10-25%. The risk of brain lesions in the surviving infant is approximately 25% [114]. Also, the rate of perinatal death in twins associated with congenital malformations is approximately 15% [115, 116]. Therefore, it is very important to maintain a strict surveillance during the prenatal in order to diminish the risks for the normal co-twin.

12. Fetal death

In general, it is known that multiple pregnancies increase the risk for fetal death. Whenever there is death of one fetus, there is also increased rates of prematurity, neurological sequel and death of the other twin. Chorionicity is determinant in these cases, with more unfavorable prognosis in monochorionic pairs [117].

The vanishing twin syndrome occurs after the sonographic diagnosis of a twin pregnancy, in which a subsequent ultrasound study fails to identify both fetuses. The dead embryo may be completely reabsorbed or even become incorporate into placental membranes, resulting in fetus papyraceous [23, 118].

Later single twin demise in monochorionic twins could also happen due to multiple reasons such as infection, chromosomal or structural anomaly, placental factors or even maternal problems (hypertensive disorder, thrombophilia) [118]. In this scenario, the chance of death of the other fetus and the risk of neurological sequel is around 25% [119]. This can be explained by hemodynamic fluctuations and ischemia, where the blood volume of the living fetus is diverted to the vascular space of the dead fetus, thereby causing multicystic encephalomalacia. Serial ultrasonographic monitoring for brain damage is mandatory and it can be complemented by magnetic resonance imaging. Although the results were inconsistent, some physicians have reported fetal blood sampling and intrauterine transfusion in the surviving twin [118, 120]. Others highlighted the use of ultrasonographic evaluation of the peak systolic velocity in the middle cerebral artery for detection of fetal anemia [121].

It is important to remember the risk of maternal coagulopathy, which although infrequent, is hard to reverse. Even after single fetal demise, the mode of delivery may be vaginal. The exact time of pregnancy's termination depends on a balance between the need to break the unfavorable gradual evolution of the remaining fetus and the establishment of iatrogenic prematurity [118].

13. Time and mode of delivery in monochorionic pregnancies

There are many suitable recommendations for twin gestation term in the literature. It is known that the risk of fetal death becomes gradually increased from 38 weeks of pregnancy and it is greater in case of monochorionic pairs [122]. Thus, in many universities' protocols, resolution is recommended for dichorionic pregnancies around 38 weeks, at 37 weeks for monochorionic (devoid of complications) and at 32 to 34 weeks in cases of single amniotic chamber [123].

The main risk associated with vaginal delivery is connected to the possibility of anoxia of the second twin. Thus, studies have shown that elective cesarean delivery at term pregnancy can reduce to 75% the risk of perinatal death [124]. However, a Cochrane systematic review showed that cesarean delivery performed by non-cephalic presentation of the second twin is associated with increased maternal morbidity without improved neonatal outcome [125].

The most important factors in the decision of the delivery mode include the presentation of the fetus, gestational age, and weight or the weight difference between the fetuses. In term births, if only the first twin is in cephalic presentation without detected adversities, vaginal delivery may proceed. If the first twin is neither cephalic, nor presents weight difference for the second fetus, being equal or less than to 500g, caesarean section seems to be a good indication. In preterm pregnancies without other complications or fetal weight lower than 1.500g, a cesarean remains as the best option [126].

Results from the biggest randomized trial conducted by the Twin Birth Study Collaborative Group established major key points [127]. Caesarean section is indicated for all monoamniotic twins, conjoined twins, non-vertex first twin and other classic indications similar to singleton pregnancies. During labour and delivery of a twin pregnancy, neuroaxial anesthesia is preferable. Whenever there is a non-vertex second twin, vaginal delivery is indicated as long as the estimated weight is between 1500-4000g and the obstetrician feels comfortable and skilled [127, 128].

14. Conclusion

The frequency of multiple pregnancies has been increasing in the last decades. Currently, it seems to have stabilized mainly due to a more strict regulation of assisted reproductive techniques. Advances in medicine allowed for earlier diagnosis not only of twin pregnancy but also chorionicity and amnionicity characteristics, which are directly implied in adverse outcomes and prognosis. Despite the various abnormalities related to monochorionic pregnancies, efforts have been made to overcome medical and parenting challenges. Even though twin pregnancies have many peculiarities and must be followed regularly by well-trained professionals, there is no evidence that planned cesarean delivery may diminish fetal morbidity and death.

Author details

Julio Elito Júnior, Eduardo Félix Martins Santana and Gustavo Nardini Cecchino

Department of Obstetrics, Universidade Federal de São Paulo (UNIFESP), Hospital São Paulo, São Paulo, Brazil

References

[1] Fava JL, Guerzet EA, Mattar R, Souza E, Camano L. Twins in the mythology and religion. Femina 2002;30(2):137-140.

[2] De Rachewiltz B, Parisi P, Castellani V. [Twins in myth (author's transl)]. Acta Geneticae Medicae et Gemellologiae (Roma) 1976;25:17–9.

[3] Camano L, Elito Junior J. Gestação múltipla. In: Moron AF, Camano L, Kulay Júnior L. Obstetrícia. Såo Paulo: Manole; 2011. p1221-1271.

[4] Bortolus R, Parazzini F, Chatenoud L, Benzi G, Biachi MM, Marini A. The epidemiology of multiple births. Human Reproduction Update 1999;5(2):179-87.

[5] The ESHRE Capri Workshop Group. Multiple gestation pregnancy. Human Reproduction 2000;15(8):1856-64.

[6] Martin JA, Hamilton BE, Osterman MJK. Three decades of twin births in the United States, 1980-2009. NCHS data brief, no 80. Hyattsville, MD: National Center for Health Statistics. 2012.

[7] Macfarlane A, Mugford M, Henderson J, Furtado A, Stevens J, Dunn A. Birth counts: Statistics of pregnancy and childbirth. London: The Stationery Office; 2000.

[8] Ward Platt MP, Glinianaia SV, Rankin J, Wright C, Renwick M. The North of England Multiple Pregnancy Register: a five-year results of data collection. Twin Research and Human Genetics: the official journal of the International Society for Twin Studies 2006;9(6):913-8.

[9] Imaizumi Y. A comparative study of twinning and triplet rates in 17 countries, 1972-1996. Acta Geneticae Medicae et Gemellologiae (Roma) 1998;47(2):101-14.

[10] Zhu JL, Basso O, Obel C, Christensen K, Olsen J. Infertility, infertility treatment and twinning: the Danish National Birth Cohort. Human Reproduction 2007;22(4): 1086-90.

[11] Kurosawa K, Masuno M, Kuroki Y. Trends in occurrence of twin births in Japan. American Journal of Medical Genetics Part A 2012;158A(1):75-7.

[12] Gan JP, Wu ZH, Tu ZM, Zheng J. The comparison of twinning rates between urban and rural areas in China. Twin Research and Human Genetics: the official journal of the International Society for Twin Studies 2007;10(4):633-7.

[13] Hoekstra C, Zhao ZZ, Lambalk CB, Willemsen G, Martin NG, Boomsma DI, Montgomery GW. Dizygotic twinning. Human Reproduction Update 2008;14(1):37-47.

[14] Tagliani-Ribeiro A, Oliveira M, Sassi AK, Rodrigues MR, Zagonel-Oliveira M, Steinman G, Matte U, Fagundes NJ, Schuler-Faccini L. Twin Town in South Brazil: a Nazi's experiment or a genetic founder effect? PLoS One 2011;6(6):e20328.

[15] Collins J. Global epidemiology of multiple birth. Reproductive Biomedicine Online 2007;15(3):45-52.

[16] Blondel B, Kaminski M. Trends in the occurrence, determinants, and consequences of multiple births. Seminars in Perinatology 2002;26(4):239-49.

[17] Fauser BC, Devroey P, Macklon NS. Multiple birth resulting from ovarian stimulation for subfertility treatment. The Lancet 2005;365(9473):1807-16.

[18] Blondel B, Kogan MD, Alexander GR, Dattani N, Kramer MS, Macfarlane A, Wen SW. The impact of the increasing number of multiple births on the rates of preterm birth and low birthweight: an international study. American Journal of Public Health 2002;92(8):1323-30.

[19] Elster N. Less is more: the risks of multiple births. The Institute for Science, Law, and Technology Working Group on Reproductive Technology. Fertility and Sterility 2000;74(4):617-23.

[20] Campbell D, van Teijlingen ER, Yip L. Economic and social implications of multiple birth. Best Practice & Research: Clinical Obstetrics & Gynaecology 2004;18(4):657-68.

[21] Callahan TL, Hall JE, Ettner SL, Christiansen CL, Greene MF, Crowley WF Jr. The economic impact of multiple-gestation pregnancies and the contribution of assisted-reproduction techniques to their incidence. The New England Journal of Medicine 1994;331(4):244-9.

[22] Corner GW. The morphological theory of monochorionic twins as illustrated by a series of supposed early twin embryos of the pig. Johns Hopkins Hospital Bulletin 1922;33:389-92.

[23] Hall JG. Twinning. The Lancet 2003;362(9385):735-43.

[24] Bush MC, Pernoll ML. Multiple pregnancy. In: DeCherney AH, Nathan L, Goodwin TM, Laufer N. Current Diagnosis & Treatment Obstetrics & Gynecology. 10th ed. New York: Lange Medical Books/McGraw-Hill; 2006.p301-310.

[25] Cameron AH. The Birmingham twin survey. Proceedings of the Royal Society of Medicine 1968;61(3):229-34.

[26] Muggli EE, Halliday JL. Folic acid and risk of twinning: a systematic review of the recent literature, July 1994 to July 2006. The Medical Journal of Australia 2007;186(5): 243-8.

[27] Murphy MF, Campbell MJ, Bone M. Is there an increased risk of twinning after discontinuation of the oral contraceptive pill? Journal of Epidemiology and Community Health 1989;43(3):275-9.

[28] Jernstrom H, Knutsson M, Olsson H. Temporary increase of FSH levels in healthy, nulliparous, young women after cessation of low-dose oral contraceptive use. Contraception 1995;52(1):51-6.

[29] White C, Wyshak G. Inheritance in human dizygotic twinning. The New England Journal of Medicine 1964;271:1003-5.

[30] Meulemans WJ, Lewis CM, Boomsma DI, Derom CA, Van den Berghe H, Orlebeke JF, Vlietinck RF, Derom RM. Genetic modeling of dizygotic twinning in pedigrees of spontaneous dizygotic twins. American Journal of Medical Genetics 1996;61(3): 258-63.

[31] Terasaki PI, Gjertson D, Bernoco D, Perdue S, Mickey MR, Bond J. Twins with two different fathers identified by HLA. The New England Journal of Medicine 1978;299(11):590-2.

[32] Verma RS, Luke S, Dhawan P. Twins with different fathers. The Lancet 1992;339:63-4.

[33] Girela E, Lorente JA, Alvarez JC, Rodrigo MD, Lorente M, Villanueva E. Indisputable double paternity in dizygous twins. Fertility and Sterility 1997;67(6):1159-61.

[34] Hansen HE, Simonsen BT. A case of heteropaternal superfecundation in a pair of Danish twins. Forensic Science International: Genetics Supplement Series 2008;1(1): 514-5.

[35] Tuppen GD, Fairs C, de Chazal RC, Konje JC. Spontaneous superfetation diagnosed in the first trimester with successful outcome. Ultrasound in Obstetrics & Gynecology: the official journal of The International Society of Ultrasound in Obstetrics and Gynecology 1999;14(3):219-21.

[36] Harrison A, Valenzuela A, Gardiner J, Sargent M, Chessex P. Superfetation as a cause of growth discordance in a multiple pregnancy. The Journal of Pediatrics 2005;147(2): 254-5.

[37] Shetty A, Smith AP. The sonographic diagnosis of chorionicity. Prenatal Diagnosis 2005;25(9):735-9.

[38] Carroll SG, Soothill PW, Abdel-Fattah SA, Porter H, Montague I, Kyle PM. Prediction of chorionicity in twin pregnancies at 10-14 weeks of gestation. BJOG: An International Journal of Obstetrics and Gynaecology 2002;109(2):182-6.

[39] Stenhouse E, Hardwick C, Maharaj S, Webb J, Kelly T, Mackenzie FM. Chorionicity determination in twin pregnancies: how accurate are we? Ultrasound in Obstetrics & Gynecology: the official journal of The International Society of Ultrasound in Obstetrics and Gynecology 2002;19(4):350-2.

[40] Lee YM, Cleary-Goldman J, Thaker HM, Simpson LL. Antenatal sonographic prediction of twin chorionicity. American Journal of Obstetrics and Gynecology 2006;195(3):863-7.

[41] Dias T, Arcangeli T, Bhide A, Napolitano R, Mahsud-Dornan S, Thilaganathan B. First-trimester ultrasound determination of chorionicity in twin pregnancy. Ultrasound in Obstetrics & Gynecology: the official journal of The International Society of Ultrasound in Obstetrics and Gynecology 2011;38(5):530-2.

[42] Simpson LL. Ultrasound in twins: dichorionic and monochorionic. Seminars in Perinatology 2013;37(5):348-58.

[43] Bessis R, Papiernik E. Ecographic imagery of amniotic membranes in twin pregnancies. Progress in Clinical and Biological Research 1981;69A:183-7.

[44] Finberg HJ. The "twin peak" sign: reliable evidence of dichorionic twinning. Journal of Ultrasound in Medicine: official journal of the American Institute of Ultrasound in Medicine 1992;11(11):571-7.

[45] Tong S, Vollenhoven B, Meagher S. Determining zygosity in early pregnancy by ultrasound. Ultrasound in Obstetrics & Gynecology: the official journal of The International Society of Ultrasound in Obstetrics and Gynecology 2004;23(1):36-7.

[46] Yang MJ, Tzeng CH, Tseng JY, Huang CY. Determination of twin zygosity using a commercially available STR analysis of 15 unlinked loci and gender-determining marker amelogenin – a preliminary report. Human Reproduction 2006;21(8):2175-9.

[47] Zheng J, Xu C, Guo J, Wei Y, Ge H, Li X, Zhang C, Jiang H, Pan L, Tang W, Xie W, Zhang H, Zhao Y, Jiang F, Chen S, Wang W, Xu X, Chen F, Huang H, Jiang H. Effective noninvasive zygosity determination by maternal plasma target region sequencing. PLoS One 2013;8(6):e65050.

[48] Hack KE, Nikkels PG, Koopman-Esseboom C, Derks JB, Elias SG, van Gemert MJ, Visser GH. Placental characteristics of monochorionic diamniotic twin pregnancies in relation to perinatal outcome. Placenta 2008;29(11):976-81.

[49] Hack KE, van Gemert MJ, Lopriore E, Schaap AH, Eggink AJ, Elias SG, van den Wijngaard JP, Vandenbussche FP, Derks JB, Visser GH, Nikkels PG. Placental charac-

teristics of monoamniotic twin pregnancies in relation to perinatal outcome. Placenta 2009;30(1):62-5.

[50] Dias T, Mahsud-Dornan S, Bhide A, Papageorghiou AT, Thilaganathan B. Cord entanglement and perinatal outcome in monoamniotic twin pregnancies. Ultrasound in Obstetrics & Gynecology: the official journal of The International Society of Ultrasound in Obstetrics and Gynecology 2010;35(2):201-4.

[51] Rossi AC, Prefumo F. Impact of cord entanglement on perinatal outcome of monoamniotic twins: a systematic review of the literature. Ultrasound in Obstetrics & Gynecology: the official journal of The International Society of Ultrasound in Obstetrics and Gynecology 2013;41(2):131-5.

[52] Umur A, van Gemert MJ, Nikkels PG. Monoamniotic-versus diamniotic-monochorionic twin placentas: anastomoses and twin-twin transfusion syndrome. American Journal of Obstetrics and Gynecology 2003;189(5):1325-9.

[53] Bajoria R, Wigglesworth J, Fisk NM. Angioarchitecture of monochorionic placentas in relation to the twin-twin transfusion syndrome. American Journal of Obstetrics and Gynecology 1995;172(3):856-63.

[54] Lopriore E, Sueters M, Middeldorp JM, Oepkes D, Walther FJ, Vandenbussche FP. Velamentous cord insertion and unequal placental territories in monochorionic twins with and without twin-to-twin-transfusion syndrome. American Journal of Obstetrics and Gynecology 2007;196(2):159.e1-5.

[55] Bricker L. Optimal antenatal care for twin and triplet pregnancy: the evidence base. Best Practice & Research. Clinical Obstetrics & Gynaecology 2014;28(2):305-17.

[56] National Collaborating Centre for Women's and Children's Health. Multiple pregnancy: the management of twin and triplet pregnancies in the antenatal period. London: RCOG Press; 2011.

[57] RCOG. Management of monochorionic twin pregnancy. Green-top Guideline, number 51; 2008.

[58] Royal Australian and New Zealand College of Obstetricians and Gynaecologists. Management of monochorionic twin pregnancy (C-Obs 42); 2014.

[59] Vayssière C, Benoist G, Blondel B, Deruelle P, Favre R, Gallot D et al. Twin pregnancies: guidelines for clinical practice from the French College of Gynaecologists and Obstetricians (CNGOF). European Journal of Obstetrics, Gynecology and Reproductive Biology 2011;156(1):12-7.

[60] Klam SL, Rinfret D, Leduc L. Prediction of growth discordance in twins with the use of abdominal circumference ratios. American Journal of Obstetrics and Gynecology 2005;192(1):247-51.

[61] Conde-Agudelo A, Romero R, Hassan SS, Yeo L. Transvaginal sonographic cervical length for the prediction of spontaneous preterm birth in twin pregnancies: a system-

atic review and metaanalysis. American Journal of Obstetrics and Gynecology 2010;203(2):128.e1-12.

[62] Lim AC, Hegeman MA, Huis In 'T Veld MA, Opmeer BC, Bruinse HW, Mol BW. Cervical length measurement for the prediction of preterm birth in multiple pregnancies: a systematic review and bivariate meta-analysis. Ultrasound in Obstetrics & Gynecology: the official journal of The International Society of Ultrasound in Obstetrics and Gynecology 2011;38(1):10-7.

[63] Facco FL, Nash K, Grobman WA. Are women who have had a preterm singleton delivery at increased risk of preterm birth in a subsequent twin pregnancy. American Journal of Perinatology 2008;25(10):657-9.

[64] Crowther CA, Han S. Hospitalisation and bed rest for multiple pregnancy. The Cochrane Database of Systematic Reviews 2010;(7):CD000110.

[65] Rouse DJ, Caritis SN, Peaceman AM, Sciscione A, Thom EA, Spong CY et al. A trial of 17 alpha-hydroxyprogesterone caproate to prevent prematurity in twins. The New England Journal of Medicine 2007;357(5):454-61.

[66] Norman JE, Mackenzie F, Owen P, Mactier H, Hanretty K, Cooper S et al. Progesterone for the prevention of preterm birth in twin pregnancy (STOPPIT): a randomised, double-blind, placebo-controlled study and meta-analysis. The Lancet 2009;373(9680):2034-40.

[67] Newman RB, Krombach RS, Myers MC, McGee DL. Effect of cerclage on obstetrical outcome in twin gestations with a shortened cervical length. American Journal of Obstetrics and Gynecology 2002;186(4):634-40.

[68] Liem S, Schuit E, Hegeman M, Bais J, de Boer K, Bloemenkamp K et al. Cervical pessaries for the prevention of preterm birth in women with a multiple pregnancy (ProTWIN): a multicentre, open-label randomised controlled trial. The Lancet 2013;382(9901):1341-9.

[69] Yamasmit W, Chaithongwongwatthana S, Tolosa JE, Limpongsanurak S, Pereira L, Lumbiganon P. Prophylactic oral betamimetics for reducing preterm birth in women with a twin pregnancy. The Cochrane Database of Systematic Reviews 2012;9:CD004733.

[70] ACOG Practice Bulletin, number 56. Multiple gestation: complicated twin, triplet and high-order multifetal pregnancy. Obstetrics and Gynecology 2004;104(4):869-83.

[71] Roberts D, Dalziel S. Antenatal corticosteroids for accelerating fetal lung maturation for women at risk of preterm birth. The Cochrane Database of Systematic Reviews 2006;(3):CD004454.

[72] Doyle LW, Crowther CA, Middleton P, Marret S, Rouse D. Magnesium sulphate for women at risk of preterm birth for neuroprotection of the fetus. The Cochrane Database of Systematic Reviews 2009;(1):CD004661.

[73] Sebire NJ, Snijders RJ, Hughes K, Sepulveda W, Nicolaides KH. The hidden mortality of monochorionic twin pregnancies. British Journal of Obstetrics and Gynaecology 1997;104(10):1203-7.

[74] Mosquera C, Miller RS, Simpson LL. Twin-twin transfusion syndrome. Seminars in Perinatology 2012;36(3):182-9.

[75] Chalouhi GE, Stirnemann JJ, Salomon LJ, Essaoui M, Quibel T, Ville Y. Specific complications of monochorionic twin pregnancies: twin-twin transfusion syndrome and twin reversed arterial perfusion sequence. Seminars in Fetal & Neonatal Medicine 2010;15(6):349-56.

[76] Rausen AR, Seki M, Strauss L. Twin transfusion syndrome. A review of 19 cases studied at one institution. The Journal of Pediatrics 1965;66:613-28.

[77] Society for Maternal-Fetal Medicine, Simpson LL. Twin-twin transfusion syndrome. American Journal of Obstetrics and Gynecology 2013;208(1):3-18.

[78] D'Antonio F, Bhide A. Early pregnancy assessment in multiple pregnancies. Best Practice & Research. Clinical Obstetrics & Gynaecology 2014;28(2):201-14.

[79] Antsaklis A, Daskalakis G, Souka AP, Kavalakis Y, Michalas S. Fetal blood sampling in twin pregnancies. Ultrasound in Obstetrics & Gynecology: the official journal of The International Society of Ultrasound in Obstetrics and Gynecology 2003;22(4): 377-9.

[80] Quintero RA, Morales WJ, Allen MH, Bornick PW, Johnson PK, Kruger M. Staging of twin-twin transfusion syndrome. Journal of Perinatology: official journal of the California Perinatal Association 1999;19(8 Pt 1):550-5.

[81] De Lia JE, Cruikshank DP, Keye WR Jr. Fetoscopic neodymium: YAG laser occlusion of placental vessels in severe twin-twin transfusion syndrome. Obstetrics and Gynecology 1990;75(6):1046-53.

[82] Senat MV, Deprest J, Boulvain M, Paupe A, Winer N, Ville Y. Endoscopic laser surgery versus serial amnioreduction for severe twin-twin transfusion syndrome. The New England Journal of Medicine 2004;351(2):136-44.

[83] Montan S, Jörgensen C, Sjöberg NO. Amniocentesis in treatment of acute polyhydramniosis in twin pregnancies. Acta Obstetricia et Gynecologica Scandinavica 1985;64(6):537-9.

[84] Saunders NJ, Snijders RJ, Nicolaides KH. Therapeutic amniocentesis in twin-twin transfusion syndrome appearing in the second trimestrer of pregnancy. American Journal of Obstetrics and Gynecology 1992;166(3):820-4.

[85] Saade GR, Belfort MA, Berry DL, Bui TH, Montgomery LD, Johnson A, O'Day M, Olson GL, Lindholm H, Garoff L, Moise KJ Jr. Amniotic septostomy for the treatment of

twin oligohydramnios-polyhydramnios sequence. Fetal Diagnosis and Therapy 1998;13(2):86-93.

[86] Lopriore E, Slaghekke F, Middeldorp JM, Klumper FJ, Oepkes D, Vandenbussche FP. Residual anastomoses in twin-to-twin transfusion syndrome treated with selective fetoscopic laser surgery: localization, size, and consequences. American Journal of Obstetrics and Gynecology 2009;201(1):66.e1-4.

[87] Slaghekke F, Kist WJ, Oepkes D, Pasman SA, Middeldorp JM, Klumper FJ, Walther FJ, Vandenbussche FP, Lopriore E. Twin anemia-polycythemia sequence: diagnosis criteria, classification, perinatal management and outcome. Fetal Diagnosis and Therapy 2010;27(4):181-90.

[88] Robyr R, Lewi L, Salomon LJ, Yamamoto M, Bernard JP, Deprest J, Ville Y. Prevalence and management of late fetal complications following successful selective laser coagulation of chorionic plate anastomoses in twin-to-twin transfusion syndrome. American Journal of Obstetrics and Gynecology 2006;194(3):796-803.

[89] Lopriore E, Slaghekke F, Oepkes D, Middeldorp JM, Vandenbussche FP, Walther FJ. Hematological characteristics in neonates with twin anemia-polycythemia sequence (TAPS). Prenatal Diagnosis 2010;30(3):251-5.

[90] Lewi L, Cannie M, Blickstein I, Jani J, Huber A, Hecher K, Dymarkowski S, Gratacós E, Lewi P, Deprest J. Placental sharing, birthweight discordance, and vascular anastomoses in monochorionic diamniotic twin placentas. American Journal of Obstetrics and Gynecology 2007;197(6):587.e1–8.

[91] Gratacós E, Ortiz JU, Martinez JM. A systematic approach to the differential diagnosis and management of the complications of monochorionic twin pregnancies. Fetal Diagnosis and Therapy 2012;32(3):145–55.

[92] James WH. A note on the epidemiology of acardiac monsters. Teratology 1977;16(2): 211–6.

[93] Moore TR, Gale S, Benirschke K. Perinatal outcome of forty-nine pregnancies complicated by acardiac twinning. American Journal of Obstetrics and Gynecology 1990;163(3):907–12.

[94] Sullivan AE, Varner MW, Ball RH, Jackson M, Silver RM. The management of acardiac twins: a conservative approach. American Journal of Obstetrics and Gynecology 2003;189(5):1310-3.

[95] Tan TY, Sepulveda W. Acardiac twin: a systematic review of minimally invasive treatment modalities. Ultrasound in Obstetrics & Gynecology: the official journal of The International Society of Ultrasound in Obstetrics and Gynecology 2003;22(4): 409–19.

[96] Spencer R. Parasitic conjoined twins: external, internal (fetuses in fetu and teratomas), and detached (acardiacs). Clinical Anatomy 2001;14(6):428–44.

[97] Sharma G, Mobin SS, Lypka M, Urata M. Heteropagus (parasitic) twins: a review. Journal of Pediatric Surgery 2010;45(12):2454-63.

[98] Spencer R. Anatomic description of conjoined twins: a plea for standardized terminology. Journal of Pediatric Surgery 1996;31(7):941-4.

[99] Ribeiro RC, Maranhão RF, Moron AF, Leite MT, Cordioli E, Hisaba W, Martins JL. Unusual case of epigastric heteropagus twinning. Journal of Pediatric Surgery 2005;40(3):E39-41.

[100] Hoeffel CC, Nguyen KQ, Phan HT, Truong NH, Nguyen TS, Tran TT, Fornes P. Fetus in fetu: a case report and literature review. Pediatrics 2000;105(6):1335–44.

[101] Pourang H, Sarmadi S, Mireskandari SM, Soleimani M, Mollaeian M, Alizadeh H, Alehosein SM. Twin fetus in fetu with immature teratoma: a case report and review of the literature. Archives of Iranian Medicine 2009;12(5):507–10.

[102] Kohl SG, Casey G. Twin gestation. The Mount Sinai Journal of Medicine 1975;42(6): 523-39.

[103] Sebire NJ. Anomalous development in twins including monozygotic duplication. In: Kilby M, Baker P, Critchley H, Field D. Multiple pregnancy. London: RCOG Press; 2006. p59-88.

[104] Little J, Bryan E. Congenital anomalies in twins. Seminars in Perinatology 1986;10(1): 50-64.

[105] Machin G. Non-identical monozygotic twins, intermediate twin types, zygosity testing, and the non-random nature of monozygotic twinning: a review. American Journal of Medical Genetics. Part C, Seminars in Medical Genetics 2009;151C(2):110-27.

[106] Baldwin VJ. Pathology of multiple pregnancy. New York: Springer-Verlag; 1994.

[107] Fisk NM, Duncombe GJ, Sullivan MH. The basic and clinical science of twin-twin transfusion syndrome. Placenta 2009;30(5):379-90.

[108] Karatza AA, Wolfenden JL, Taylor MJ, Wee L, Fisk NM, Gardiner HM. Influence of twin-twin transfusion syndrome on fetal cardiovascular structure and function: prospective case-control study of 136 monochorionic twin pregnancies. Heart 2002;88(3): 271-7.

[109] Bahtiyar MO, Dulay AT, Weeks BP, Friedman AH, Copel JA. Prevalence of congenital heart defects in monochorionic/diamniotic twin gestations: a systematic literature review. Journal of Ultrasound in Medicine: official journal of the American Institute of Ultrasound in Medicine 2007;26(11):1491-8.

[110] Hall JG. Genomic imprinting: review and relevance to human diseases. American Journal of Human Genetics 1990;46(5):857-73.

[111] Côté GB, Gyftodimou J. Twinning and mitotic crossing over: some possibilities and their implications. American Journal of Human Genetics 1991;49(1):120-30.

[112] Jung JH, Graham JM Jr, Schultz N, Smith DW. Congenital hydranencephaly/porencephaly due to vascular disruption in monozygotic twins. Pediatrics 1984;73(4):467-9.

[113] Harper LM, Odibo AO, Roehl KA, Longman RE, Macones GA, Cahill AG. Risk of preterm delivery and growth restriction in twins discordant for structural anomalies. American Journal of Obstetrics and Gynecology 2012;206(1):70.e1-5.

[114] Powers WF, Kiely JL. The risks confronting twins: a national perspective. American Journal of Obstetrics and Gynecology 1994;170(2):456-61.

[115] Liapis AE, Hassiakos DK, Panagopoulos PP. Perinatal morbidity and mortality rates in twin pregnancies e a 15-year review study from Athens. Acta Geneticae Medicae et Gemellologiae (Roma) 1997;46(4):185-91.

[116] Glinianaia SV, Pharoah P, Sturgiss SN. Comparative trends in cause-specific fetal and neonatal mortality in twin and singleton births in the North of England, 1982-1994. BJOG: an international journal of obstetrics and gynaecology 2000;107(4): 452-60.

[117] Carlson NJ, Towers CV. Multiple gestation complicated by the death of one fetus. Obstetrics and Gynecology 1989;73(5 Pt 1):685-9.

[118] Hillman SC, Morris RK, Kilby MD. Single twin demise: consequence for survivors. Seminars in Fetal & Neonatal Medicine 2010;15(6):319-26.

[119] Pharoah PO, Adi Y. Consequences of in-utero death in a twin pregnancy. The Lancet 2000;355(9215):1597-602.

[120] Tanawattanacharoen S, Taylor MJ, Letsky EA, Cox PM, Cowan FM, Fisk NM. Intrauterine rescue transfusion in monochorionic multiple pregnancies with recent single intrauterine death. Prenatal Diagnosis 2001;21(4):274-8.

[121] Senat MV, Loizeau S, Couderc S, Bernard JP, Ville Y. The value of middle cerebral artery peak systolic velocity in the diagnosis of fetal anemia after intrauterine death of one monochorionic twin. American Journal of Obstetrics and Gynecology 2003;189(5):1320-4.

[122] Soucie JE, Yang Q, Wen SW, Fung Kee Fung K, Walker M. Neonatal mortality and morbidity rates in term twins with advancing gestational age. American Journal of Obstetrics and Gynecology 2006;195(1):172-7.

[123] Winer N, Caroit Y, Le Vaillant C, Philippe HJ. Monoamniotic twins: diagnosis and management. Journal de Gynécologie, Obstétrique et Biologie de la Reproduction (Paris) 2009;38(8 Suppl):S85-9.

[124] Smith GC, Shah I, White IR, Pell JP, Dobbie R. Mode of delivery and the risk of delivery-related perinatal death among twins at term: a retrospective cohort study of 8073

births. BJOG: an international journal of obstetrics and gynaecology 2005;112(8): 1139-44.

[125] Crowther CA. Caesarean delivery for the second twin. The Cochrane Database of Systematic Reviews 2000;(2):CD000047.

[126] Lee YM. Delivery of twins. Seminars in Perinatology 2012;36(3):195-200.

[127] Barrett JF, Hannah ME, Hutton EK, Willan AR, Allen AC, Armson BA et al. A randomized trial of planned cesarean or vaginal delivery for twin pregnancy. The New England Journal of Medicine 2013;369(14):1295-305.

[128] Barrett JF. Twin delivery: method, timing and conduct. Best Practice & Research: Clinical Obstetrics & Gynaecology 2014;28(2):327-38.